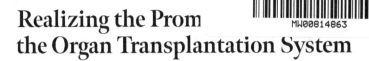

# Realizing the Prom
# the Organ Transplantation System

Kenneth W. Kizer, Rebecca A. English, Meredith Hackmann, *Editors*

Committee on A Fairer and More Equitable, Cost-Effective, and Transparent System
of Donor Organ Procurement, Allocation, and Distribution

Board on Health Sciences Policy

Board on Health Care Services

Health and Medicine Division

A Consensus Study Report of

*The National Academies of*
SCIENCES · ENGINEERING · MEDICINE

THE NATIONAL ACADEMIES PRESS
*Washington, DC*
**www.nap.edu**

**THE NATIONAL ACADEMIES PRESS**     **500 Fifth Street, NW**     **Washington, DC 20001**

This activity was supported by Contract No. HHSN263201800029I/75N98020F00011 between the National Academy of Sciences and The National Institutes of Health. Any opinions, findings, conclusions, or recommendations expressed in this publication do not necessarily reflect the views of any organization or agency that provided support for the project.

International Standard Book Number-13: 978-0-309-27072-4
International Standard Book Number-10: 0-309-27072-3
Digital Object Identifier: https://doi.org/10.17226/26364

Additional copies of this publication are available from the National Academies Press, 500 Fifth Street, NW, Keck 360, Washington, DC 20001; (800) 624-6242 or (202) 334-3313; http://www.nap.edu.

Suggested citation: National Academies of Sciences, Engineering, and Medicine. 2022. *Realizing the promise of equity in the organ transplantation system.* Washington, DC: The National Academies Press. https://doi.org/10.17226/26364.

*The National Academies of*
# SCIENCES · ENGINEERING · MEDICINE

The **National Academy of Sciences** was established in 1863 by an Act of Congress, signed by President Lincoln, as a private, nongovernmental institution to advise the nation on issues related to science and technology. Members are elected by their peers for outstanding contributions to research. Dr. Marcia McNutt is president.

The **National Academy of Engineering** was established in 1964 under the charter of the National Academy of Sciences to bring the practices of engineering to advising the nation. Members are elected by their peers for extraordinary contributions to engineering. Dr. John L. Anderson is president.

The **National Academy of Medicine** (formerly the Institute of Medicine) was established in 1970 under the charter of the National Academy of Sciences to advise the nation on medical and health issues. Members are elected by their peers for distinguished contributions to medicine and health. Dr. Victor J. Dzau is president.

The three Academies work together as the **National Academies of Sciences, Engineering, and Medicine** to provide independent, objective analysis and advice to the nation and conduct other activities to solve complex problems and inform public policy decisions. The National Academies also encourage education and research, recognize outstanding contributions to knowledge, and increase public understanding in matters of science, engineering, and medicine.

Learn more about the National Academies of Sciences, Engineering, and Medicine at **www.nationalacademies.org**.

*The National Academies of*
# SCIENCES · ENGINEERING · MEDICINE

**Consensus Study Reports** published by the National Academies of Sciences, Engineering, and Medicine document the evidence-based consensus on the study's statement of task by an authoring committee of experts. Reports typically include findings, conclusions, and recommendations based on information gathered by the committee and the committee's deliberations. Each report has been subjected to a rigorous and independent peer-review process and it represents the position of the National Academies on the statement of task.

**Proceedings** published by the National Academies of Sciences, Engineering, and Medicine chronicle the presentations and discussions at a workshop, symposium, or other event convened by the National Academies. The statements and opinions contained in proceedings are those of the participants and are not endorsed by other participants, the planning committee, or the National Academies.

For information about other products and activities of the National Academies, please visit www.nationalacademies.org/about/whatwedo.

## COMMITTEE ON A FAIRER AND MORE EQUITABLE, COST-EFFECTIVE, AND TRANSPARENT SYSTEM OF DONOR ORGAN PROCUREMENT, ALLOCATION, AND DISTRIBUTION

**KENNETH W. KIZER** (*Chair*), Chief Healthcare Transformation Officer and Senior Executive Vice President, Atlas Research
**ITAI ASHLAGI,** Associate Professor, Stanford University
**CHARLES BEARDEN,** Senior Organ Transplant Coordinator, Clinical Consulting Associates
**YOLANDA T. BECKER,** Professor of Surgery, University of Chicago (*until September 2021*)
**ALEXANDER CAPRON,** University Professor, Scott H. Bice Chair in Healthcare Law, Policy, and Ethics, and Professor of Medicine and Law, University of Southern California
**BERNICE COLEMAN,** Director, Nursing Research Department and Assistant Professor, Biomedical Sciences, Cedars-Sinai
**LEIGH ANNE DAGEFORDE,** Transplant Surgeon and Assistant Professor, Massachusetts General Hospital, Harvard Medical School
**SUE DUNN,** Chief Executive Officer (Retired), Donor Alliance (Former)
**ROBERT GIBBONS,** Blum-Riese Professor of Biostatistics, The University of Chicago
**ELISA J. GORDON,** Professor, Department of Surgery, Center for Health Services and Outcomes Research, Center for Bioethics and Medical Humanities, Northwestern University Feinberg School of Medicine
**RENÉE M. LANDERS,** Professor and Director, Health Law, Faculty Director, Law Life Sciences, Suffolk University
**MARIO MACIS,** Professor, Carey Business School, Johns Hopkins University
**JEWEL MULLEN,** Associate Dean for Health Equity, University of Texas at Austin, Dell Medical School
**NEIL R. POWE,** Chief of Medicine, Zuckerberg San Francisco General Hospital, and Professor of Medicine, University of California, San Francisco
**DORRY SEGEV,** Marjory K. and Thomas Pozefsky, Professor of Surgery and Epidemiology, Johns Hopkins University[1]
**DENNIS WAGNER,** Principal and Managing Director, Yes And Leadership, LLC
**JAMES YOUNG,** Executive Director of Academic Affairs, Cleveland Clinic; Professor of Medicine and Vice-Dean for Academic Affairs, Cleveland Clinic Lerner College of Medicine of Case Western Reserve University George & Linda Kaufman Chair, Heart & Vascular Institute

*Study Staff*

**REBECCA A. ENGLISH,** Study Director
**AMANDA WAGNER GEE,** Program Officer (*until November 2021*)
**SIOBHAN ADDIE,** Program Officer (*until August 2021*)
**MEREDITH HACKMANN,** Associate Program Officer
**ELIZABETH TOWNSEND,** Associate Program Officer (*until October 2021*)
**EMMA FINE,** Associate Program Officer
**DEANNA GIRALDI,** Associate Program Officer (*from October 2021*)
**RUTH COOPER,** Associate Program Officer (*from June 2021*)

---

[1] As of February 1, 2022, Dr. Segev is Professor of Surgery and Population Health and Vice Chair for Research in the Department of Surgery, New York University.

# Reviewers

This Consensus Study Report was reviewed in draft form by individuals chosen for their diverse perspectives and technical expertise. The purpose of this independent review is to provide candid and critical comments that will assist the National Academies of Sciences, Engineering, and Medicine in making each published report as sound as possible and to ensure that it meets the institutional standards for quality, objectivity, evidence, and responsiveness to the study charge. The review comments and draft manuscript remain confidential to protect the integrity of the deliberative process.

We thank the following individuals for their review of this report:

**DIANE BROCKMEIER,** Mid-America Transplant Center
**JAMES F. CHILDRESS,** University of Virginia
**GABRIEL M. DANOVITCH,** University of California, Los Angeles
**DAVID C. MULLIGAN,** Yale University
**GLENDA V. ROBERTS,** University of Washington
**JOHN ROSENDALE,** Senior Performance Analyst (retired)
**LAINIE FRIEDMAN ROSS,** University of Chicago
**MARTY SELLERS,** Tennessee Donor Services
**MARION SHUCK,** Gift of Hope
**MARYAM VALAPOUR,** Cleveland Clinic
**BRUCE C. VLADECK,** Greater New York Hospital Association
**BETSY WALSH,** Novant Health
**WINFRED W. WILLIAMS,** Harvard University

Although the reviewers listed above provided many constructive comments and suggestions, they were not asked to endorse the conclusions or recommendations of this report nor did they see the final draft before its release. The review of this report was overseen by **BOBBIE BERKOWITZ,** University of Washington, and **SARA ROSENBAUM,** George Washington University. They were responsible for making certain that an independent examination of this report was carried out in accordance with the standards of the National Academies and that all review comments were carefully considered. Responsibility for the final content rests entirely with the authoring committee and the National Academies.

# Acknowledgments

The study committee and project staff would like to thank the study sponsor, the National Institutes of Health, for their leadership in the development of this study. The committee wishes to express its particular gratitude to the patients and family members who shared their stories and advice with the committee. The committee also wishes to thank the many individuals who participated in public workshops and shared their expertise throughout the course of the study.

The committee thanks the authors whose commissioned papers provided valuable information and analysis for the committee including Abigail Alyesh, Yolanda Becker, Robert Gibbons, Kathleen Giblin, Allie Herr, Kim Ibarra, Samantha Klitenic, Elaine Ku, Jennifer Lai, Carolee Lantigua, Macey Levan, Sumit Mohan, Josh Mooney, William Parker, Chris Queram, Jesse Schold, and Sri Lekha Tummalapalli. The committee also acknowledges the Health Resources and Services Administration and the Centers for Medicare & Medicaid Services (CMS) for verifying for accuracy relevant technical content pertaining to the Organ Procurement and Transplantation Network and to CMS programs related to transplantation. The committee is grateful for the many staff within the Health and Medicine Division who provided support for the project. Special thanks are extended to Rebecca Morgan, senior librarian, who compiled literature searches and provided fact checking assistance; Christie Bell, the financial business partner; and Mark Goodin, for his editorial assistance provided in preparing the final report.

# Preface

Since the first successful kidney transplant was performed in 1954, organ transplantation has become a lifesaving treatment for a growing number of conditions. Each year, the individuals and organizations in the U.S. organ donation, procurement, allocation, and distribution system work together to provide lifesaving transplants to many thousands of persons, but thousands more will die before getting a transplant because of the ongoing shortage of deceased donor organs. The combination of deceased donor organs as a scarce resource and the high value of transplantation—both for individual patients and their families and for society broadly—creates a setting for high-stakes health care decision making.

While the U.S. deceased donor organ transplantation system benefits tens of thousands of individuals each year, the system is demonstrably inequitable. Too many persons, especially in minority and underserved populations, are disadvantaged in accessing the services that lead to transplantation, and experience worse outcomes than others. Across the country, donor hospitals and organ procurement organizations have dramatically different performance in identifying potential donors and procuring organs. Transplant centers differ significantly in the rates of accepting or declining organs on behalf of patients on their waiting list and struggle to make individual transplant center- and patient-level decisions that reflect the best use of organs on a national scale. Overall, the transplantation system—donor hospitals, organ procurement organizations, transplant centers, regulators, payers—has much work to do to improve fairness and equity in who receives an organ transplant.

Akin to the changes implemented to improve patient safety and health care quality over the past 25 years, we know that improving the performance of the health care system for patient benefit is possible. The transplantation system is composed of many dedicated and committed professionals trying to do their best, but the overall organ transplantation system is not producing the synergistic results that we should expect from it. As a nation, we must do better.

This study—focused on increasing fairness, equity, cost-effectiveness, and transparency in the deceased donor organ procurement, allocation, and distribution system—occurs at a time when the transplantation system is under intense scrutiny, and thus, at an opportune time for making significant change. In this report we discuss multiple changes that would create a more equitable organ transplantation system, beginning with reconceptualizing the system as beginning well before an individual is added to an organ transplant waiting list. Because many individuals from minority and underserved populations, as well as women, are never added to the waiting list, bringing these individuals into the system, combined with improved fairness in the allocation policies that govern how patients are prioritized on the waiting list, would help create a more equitable system.

During the committee's deliberations, some members were startled by the statistics showing the large number of donated organs that are never transplanted—and especially by the lack of transparency that accompanies organ offer acceptance or decline decisions. Most individuals on the waiting list are never made aware of the organ offers that are declined on their behalf. Of course, there are appropriate reasons based on sound medical judgment for a transplant team to decline an organ offered to a particular patient, but there also are many instances when the process would benefit from bringing the patient into the decision-making process. The benefits of shared decision making with patients have been proven and incorporating more shared decision making into organ offer processes would provide an opportunity for the transplantation system to be more transparent and accountable.

In responding to the study's broad task—which includes looking into policy-making processes, allocation modeling, and quality improvement processes and performance metrics—this report provides an overview of the current organ transplantation system and advances multiple near- and longer-term actionable recommendations to improve fairness, equity, transparency, and cost-effectiveness.

The committee's work was informed by and materially benefited from the compelling insights shared by individuals waiting for a donor organ, transplant recipients, families of individuals who had donated organs, individuals and organizations advocating on behalf of minority or marginalized individuals, the disabled, women, and rural populations needing transplants, and organizations and associations working in transplantation every day. We carefully reflected on the comments received and the possibilities for improving access to transplantation, especially for those who have historically experienced difficulties in gaining access to the system.

The committee greatly appreciated the information provided by workshop speakers and the many others who shared information with the committee. The feedback from the report reviewers was invaluable. And, we especially thank the study sponsor, the National Institutes of Health, for its work in organ transplantation and for its support of this study.

It was my great privilege to work with such dedicated committee members, each of whom thoroughly engaged in the study, generously shared their expertise, and contributed substantial time and effort to the endeavor. This was a complex task, and the committee members stepped up to meet the challenge. Their reasoned and thoughtful discussions made this report possible. The committee was very fortunate to work with a diligent and outstanding team of National Academies of Sciences, Engineering, and Medicine staff, and we deeply thank Rebecca English, Meredith Hackmann, Deanna Giraldi, Elizabeth Townsend, Amanda Wagner Gee, Emma Fine, Ruth Cooper, Siobhan Addie, and Kendall Logan, led by Andrew Pope and Sharyl Nass, board directors in the Health and Medicine Division. We also thank Anna Nicholson and Jon Weinisch for writing and editing work as well as the National Academies' library staff for assistance in conducting detailed literature searches for the committee and staff.

The committee considered a large body of evidence on the components of the organ transplantation system and worked to develop this report in an objective manner. The committee was cognizant of the large amount of data reported on organ transplantation but was surprised at the gaps in knowledge in some areas. For instance, why do so many individuals who ostensibly would be candidates for organ transplantation not gain access to the waiting list? Disaggregated data by race and ethnicity, gender/sex, age, and language are needed to better understand current inequities so that appropriate interventions can demonstrably improve the system and make it more equitable.

As requested in the study charge, the committee also considered the Organ Procurement and Transplantation Network (OPTN) policy-making process and opportunities for improving it. While the steps in the general policy-making process are well documented, the dynamics of the OPTN committee interactions and the true impact on final policies was not always clear. The OPTN is not alone in its efforts to work with a broad range of stakeholders to craft policies to complicated and contentious issues in health care and the policy-making process for organ procurement, allocation, and distribution should be informed by the expertise and experience of other entities.

Overall, we are confident system improvement is possible and are hopeful for the future.

Kenneth W. Kizer, *Chair*
Committee on A Fairer and More Equitable, Cost-Effective,
and Transparent System of Donor Organ Procurement,
Allocation, and Distribution

# Contents

## APPENDIXES

# Boxes, Figures, and Tables

## BOXES

# FIGURES

## TABLES

# Acronyms and Abbreviations

| | |
|---|---|
| CMS | Centers for Medicare & Medicaid Services |
| CPRA | calculated panel reactive antibody |
| | |
| DCDD | donation after circulatory determination of death |
| DCU | donor care unit |
| DDKT | deceased donor kidney transplant |
| DNDD | donation after neurological determination of death |
| DSA | donor service area |
| | |
| eGFR | estimated glomerular filtration rate |
| EPTS | estimated posttransplant survival |
| ESKD | end-stage kidney disease |
| | |
| HCV | hepatitis C virus |
| HHS | U.S. Department of Health and Human Services |
| HLA | human leukocyte antigen |
| HRSA | Health Resources and Services Administration |
| | |
| IOM | Institute of Medicine |
| | |
| KAS | kidney allocation system |
| KDPI | Kidney Donor Profile Index |
| | |
| LAS | lung allocation score |
| LDKT | living donor kidney transplantation |
| LOS | length of stay |
| | |
| MELD | Model for End-Stage Liver Disease |

NHBD    non–heart-beating donor
NOTA    National Organ Transplant Act
NQF     National Quality Forum

OPO     organ procurement organization
OPTN    Organ Procurement and Transplantation Network

PELD    Pediatric End-Stage Liver Disease
QALY    quality-adjusted life year

SAM     simulated allocation model
SDOH    social determinants of health
SES     socioeconomic status
SRTR    Scientific Registry of Transplant Recipients

UNOS    United Network for Organ Sharing
USRDS   United States Renal Data System

VAD     ventricular assist device
VCA     vascularized composite allotransplantation

# Summary

## ABSTRACT

*Despite the many individual successes of transplantation in the United States, key components of the transplantation system—donor hospitals, organ procurement organizations (OPOs), transplant centers, and the Organ Procurement and Transplantation Network—suffer from significant variations in performance, which often creates an inefficient and inequitable system. An individual's chance of referral for transplant evaluation, being added to the waiting list, and receiving a transplant varies greatly based on race and ethnicity, gender, geographic location, socioeconomic status, disability status, and immigration status. Given these issues, the U.S. Congress requested that the National Institutes of Health sponsor a National Academies of Sciences, Engineering, and Medicine study to review the fairness, equity, transparency, and cost-effectiveness in the system of procuring, allocating, and distributing deceased donor organs. The resulting analysis emphasizes that a combination of immediate or near-term (1–2 years) corrections and longer-term actions (3–5 years) are needed. Immediate or near-term actions include establishing national performance goals, requiring each OPO to establish a donor care unit, increasing the use of procured organs, modernizing information technology infrastructure and data collection requirements, increasing shared decision making with waiting patients, improving the policy development process, sustaining and expanding quality improvement efforts, removing predialysis waiting time "points" from the kidney allocation system, resolving the use of race in the Kidney Donor Profile Index and other clinical equations, and aligning financial incentives with the goal of equity. Longer-term solutions that should begin immediately include extending regulatory oversight of the organ transplantation system to encompass patients needing transplant but not yet on the waiting list.*

While the U.S. deceased donor organ transplantation system has seen significant growth in the number of transplants performed, the number of individuals waiting for a transplant continues to outpace the number of transplants performed. Organ transplantation—the surgical removal of a healthy organ from one deceased or living individual and its placement into another person—has been a lifesaving treatment since its introduction in the mid-twentieth century. In 2021, there were 41,354 transplants performed—an increase of 5.9 percent over 2020, despite the complications of the COVID-19 pandemic (OPTN, 2022).

Receiving an organ transplant can provide significant health benefits for a variety of conditions that result in organ failure. Individuals with kidney, liver, or uterus failure can receive transplants from living donors, but for individuals with heart, lung, pancreas, or intestinal failure, or the failure of an extremity or tissue system, an organ from a deceased donor is usually the only possibility.[1] Although living donation is an option, most individuals seeking a kidney, liver, or uterus transplant ultimately receive an organ from a deceased donor. There is a shortage of all types of deceased donor organs. Individuals waiting for a kidney make up approximately 84.7 percent of the total number of candidates on the waiting list for any organ.[2] Far fewer individuals are on a waiting list for liver, heart, lung, pancreas, and intestine donor organs. Dialysis is an alternative form of renal replacement therapy for individuals with end-stage kidney disease or kidney failure. Other types of organ failure sometimes have no alternative lifesaving treatments.

Despite the many successes of organ procurement and transplantation in the United States, the components of the system suffer from significant variations in performance, creating an inefficient and inequitable system. An individual's chance of being referred for a transplant evaluation, being added to the waiting list, and receiving a transplant varies greatly based on race and ethnicity, gender, geographic location, socioeconomic status, disability status, and immigration status (Ahearn et al., 2021; Axelrod et al., 2010; Darden et al., 2021; Harding et al., 2021; Lee and Terrault, 2020; Patzer et al., 2012; Richards et al., 2009). Disparities and inequities in the organ transplantation system are not new and have been a topic of debate and frequent efforts at reform since the United States formalized the national Organ Procurement and Transplantation Network (OPTN) in 1986.

The U.S. Congress requested that the National Institutes of Health sponsor this study to examine the fairness, equity, transparency, and cost-effectiveness of the deceased donor organ procurement, allocation, and distribution system. See Box S-1 for the Statement of Task.[3] To accomplish the task, the National Academies of Sciences, Engineering, and Medicine (the National Academies) empaneled a committee of 17 members with expertise in the areas of bioethics, health equity, biostatistics, economics, law and regulation, transplant surgery, nephrology, epidemiology, organ procurement, management science, and quality improvement (see Appendix C for biographical sketches of the committee members and staff).

---

[1] Although uncommon, in some cases it may be possible to receive a portion of a lung, pancreas, or intestine from a living donor. See https://www.organdonor.gov/learn/process/living-donation (accessed January 31, 2022).

[2] As of February 3, 2022, there were 90,315 candidates waiting for a kidney transplant out of a total of 106,616 candidates waiting for any type of organ transplant. 90,135/106,616 = 84.7 percent. See https://optn.transplant.hrsa.gov/data/view-data-reports/national-data (accessed February 3, 2022).

[3] The study task did not include a focus on living donors and living donation, nor issues around tissue procurement and transplantation. The committee's work includes heart, lung, liver, kidney, kidney–pancreas, intestinal, vascular composite allotransplantations, dual organ, and multiorgan transplants. However, many of the committee's conclusions and recommendations focus on issues related to kidney transplant access given the large size of the kidney waiting list and the significant opportunity and promise for lives saved. Many of the committee's recommendations apply to all organs or, if kidneys are mentioned as a primary area for action, other organs are not excluded.

## BOX S-1    STATEMENT OF TASK

An ad hoc committee of the National Academies of Sciences, Engineering, and Medicine will conduct a consensus study to examine the economic (costs), ethical, policy, regulatory, and operational issues relevant to organ allocation policy decisions involving deceased donor organs (e.g., heart, lung, liver, kidney, kidney–pancreas, intestinal, vascular composite allografts, dual and/or multi-organ organ transplants). The committee will examine the gaps, barriers, and opportunities for improving deceased donor organ procurement, allocation, and organ distribution to waiting recipients at transplant centers with a keen eye towards optimizing the quality and quantity of donated organs available for transplantation—in a cost-effective and efficient, fair and equitable manner consistent with the National Organ Transplant Act and the Final Rule.

Specifically, the final consensus report will delineate the issues pertinent to organ allocation policy, modeling and simulation of anticipated policy changes for intended and unintended consequences, and the process for efficiently executing allocation policy changes in an open, transparent, fair, and equitable manner. The report will make recommendations to maximize public and professional trust in the organ donation, procurement, allocation, and distribution process. The report will also make recommendations to better align the performance metrics or incentives of various stakeholders within the Organ Procurement and Transplantation Network [specifically donor service areas (DSAs), organ procurement organizations (OPOs), and transplant centers] to maximize donor referrals, evaluations, procurement and organ placement/allocation while minimizing organ discard rates.

The committee will consider the following in its discussions and deliberations to address the Statement of Task:

- If deceased donor organs should be allocated to specific individuals based on need (i.e., national, continuous framework) rather than groups of individuals defined by locale, zip code, or donor service area (i.e., the donor service area, geographic framework) and if measures can be taken to reduce inequities in organ allocation affecting socioeconomically disadvantaged populations;
- Relevant factors that determine transplant recipient waitlist priority (i.e., "need") for an organ;
- Best model/method(s) to ensure fairness, equity, cost-effectiveness and efficiency, and reduce the reported socioeconomic and racial/ethnic disparities in the current organ allocation system;
- Challenges with current organ allocation policy development and policy change procedures and processes, including opportunities to update OPTN policies and processes to ensure organ allocation decisions consider the viewpoints of expert OPTN committees;
- Challenges involved in modeling proposed organ allocation policy changes and opportunities to improve modeling, including how costs should be factored into the modeling of organ allocation policy changes;
- Appropriate parameters, factors, and variables that should make up various transplant scoring systems (e.g., CPRA, EPTS, KDPI, LAS, MELD, etc.)* that determine organ allocation and patient prioritization to assure fair and equitable practices and reduce inequalities affecting socioeconomically disadvantaged patient populations;
- How to more effectively acquire needed data points to enhance transplant scoring systems (e.g., through better sharing of donor and recipient data between various federal agency databases);
- Self-reported donation metrics (e.g., "eligible deaths") and the impact on estimates of the true donor supply. Consider the development of a new, standardized, objective, and verifiable donation metric to permit the transplant community to evaluate DSAs and OPOs and establish best practices;

*continued*

> **BOX S-1**    **CONTINUED**
>
> - Data sharing and optimization opportunities, revealed by the COVID-19 pandemic, via collaboration across Department of Health and Human Services administrative databases regarding vital statistics on transplant recipients and potential donors to better inform policy makers, the OPTN, OPOs, transplant centers, transplant health care workers, patients, and the public; and relevant comparisons to international allocation policies and models.
>
> ---
>
> CPRA = calculated panel reactive antibody; EPTS = estimated posttransplant survival; KDPI = Kidney Donor Profile Index; LAS = lung allocation score; MELD = Model for End-Stage Liver Disease.

## CHALLENGES AND OPPORTUNITIES

To address its broad charge, the committee focused on three key issues and areas of opportunity for improvement in deceased donor organ procurement, allocation, and distribution—challenges of inequity in access, variation and inefficiency in system performance, and underuse of donated organs.

### Challenges of Inequity in Access

Getting onto the waiting list—being listed—is metaphorically the gateway that must open for one to have access to receiving a transplant of a deceased donor organ. The point at which an individual joins the waiting list is also the time that federal oversight traditionally has begun for the policies and processes that govern prioritization of waiting list patients, allocation of organs, and posttransplant outcomes. For many persons who would benefit from organ transplantation—and particularly racial and ethnic minorities, individuals of lower socioeconomic status, those who live in rural areas, or undocumented immigrants or individuals with an intellectual disability—this gate may be especially hard to open.

It is well established that inequities arise in access to referrals, evaluation, and the waiting list for organ transplant, yet little is known where along the trajectory in that process disparities are most likely to arise, especially for vulnerable populations. The purview of the OPTN begins when an individual patient is added to the waiting list for a deceased donor organ. The committee finds that this gap in oversight presents a significant challenge to ensuring fairness and equity in the organ transplantation system and that federal oversight should expand to begin when an individual is diagnosed with end-stage organ failure and include the steps involved in identifying patients as needing a transplant before patients are added to the waiting list.

Certain groups of patients (e.g., patients of color, lower socioeconomic status, female gender) receive organ transplants at a disproportionately lower rate and after longer waiting times than other patients with comparable medical need (Ahearn et al., 2021; Darden et al., 2021; Patzer et al., 2012). Illustrative of some disparities, black persons are three times more likely to develop kidney failure than whites in the United States but are significantly less likely to receive lifesaving kidney transplants (Saran et al., 2017). Black candidates enter the kidney transplant waiting list with double the length of dialysis time than white candidates and consequently have increased medical urgency as evidenced by their increased risk of mortality without transplantation. Under the current kidney allocation system, which prioritizes how long an individual has been on the waiting list, putting many individuals at a disadvantage, the disparity will persist.

The committee concludes that the current organ transplantation system is demonstrably inequitable. Based on available information, the committee does not find justifiable reasons for the demonstrable disparities between organ transplant rates for persons who would benefit from organ transplants and the burden of disease in many populations. These inequities undermine the trust necessary for the organ transplantation system to function optimally.

## Justice, Fairness, Equity, and Transparency— Foundations for a Trustworthy System

Even when policies are premised on all people being treated alike, measurable—in fact, often very large—disparities exist that are not explained by medical differences but rather arise from historical patterns of discrimination. Historical patterns of discrimination are embedded in social institutions (including in health care) and are perpetuated by conscious prejudices as well as unexamined practices.

Justice demands that access to health care be equitable, meaning that persons in equivalent medical circumstances actually receive equivalent medical care, free from irrelevant considerations such as their sex, race, ethnicity, religion, socioeconomic condition, physical and mental capabilities, geographic residence, and other personal attributes. Disparities in the ways that certain historically disadvantaged groups are treated or in the outcomes that the transplantation system produces for them are signals that an injustice exists. To the extent that such disparities are avoidable, an equitable system will take the steps necessary to eliminate them.

Transparency is an instrumental value in shaping public beliefs and attitudes about the trustworthiness of the organ transplantation system. Individual and societal trust in the organ transplantation system depends on health care professionals fulfilling their ethical duties to do good and not to harm, to respect the patients' autonomy, and to strive for justice and usefulness in organ allocation decisions. Additionally, such trust is contingent on other institutions—the OPOs, the OPTN, and agencies of the federal government—upholding these same values.

## Variation and Inefficiency in System Performance

Marked variations in performance exist across the organ transplantation system. In particular, the committee identified five-fold variation among OPOs[4] in their procurement of organs from donation after circulatory determination of death (DCDD) organ donors.[5] Across transplant centers, the committee found significant variation in the rate at which a center accepts the deceased donor organs offered to individual patients on the waiting list. In both cases, accountability currently does not exist for OPO performance in procuring DCDD organs and transplant center willingness to accept organs suitable for a patient. Each source of significant variation decreases the reliability and functionality of the system and directly

---

[4] OPOs are not-for-profit organizations responsible for identifying potential organ donors, working directly with a decedent's family about potential donation, receiving authorization for organ donation, obtaining organs from donors, and properly preserving these organs for quick delivery to a suitable recipient waiting for a transplant.

[5] DCDD organs are one type of medically complex organ.

affects equity in patient care. If an individual happens to join the waiting list at a transplant center with poor organ offer acceptance rates, or in an area where the OPO does not procure as many donated organs as they could, that individual is less likely to receive a transplant.

While the behaviors of OPOs and transplant centers can vary significantly across the United States, the policy development process governing how deceased donor organs are allocated to individuals on the waiting list is the purview of the OPTN. The OPTN policy-making process for organ allocation includes extensive committee reviews that aim to involve all stakeholders, but the nature of the reviews contributes to variability in the policy development processes and a general slowness in policy development and implementation.

## Underuse of Procured Organs

The committee also identified the significant issue of organ nonuse—that is, organs procured for transplantation but not transplanted. While the waiting list remains long and individuals waiting for an organ transplant die every day, too many donated organs are being procured and not used. The proportion of kidneys from deceased donors that were recovered for transplant but ultimately not transplanted in 2019 was approximately 20 percent (Israni et al., 2021), with a projected 2021 kidney nonuse rate of 23 percent (see Figure 6-4 in Chapter 6). The rate at which kidneys go unused in the United States is much higher than other developed countries (Mohan et al., 2018; Stewart et al., 2017). For example, the U.S. rate of nonuse for procured organs is nearly double the rate in France (Aubert et al., 2019). Approximately 62 percent of kidneys not used in the United States would likely have been successfully transplanted in France (Aubert et al., 2019).

## RECOMMENDATIONS

The committee developed each recommendation in this report with the interests of patients in mind and through the lens of equity (see Box S-2 for the list of recommendations). Based on the committee's review of the evidence and reflection on the experience of individual committee members, there is an opportunity to refocus the organ transplantation system around the patient experience of needing and seeking an organ transplant. The committee concluded that even at its best, the organ transplantation system is not accountable to all patients who need an organ transplant. A shift is needed toward policies that engender accountability to all patients in need of a transplant, whether they are on the waiting list yet or not, as well as organ donors and their families who donate the gift of life.

In crafting the recommendations in this report the committee often calls on the U.S. Department of Health and Human Services (HHS) to update the OPTN contract to require or hold the OPTN accountable for taking specific actions. The committee realizes that the OPTN contract will come up for bid again in 2023 and that some elements of the committee's recommendations might be best incorporated in the HHS request for proposals in 2023, while others can be immediately embedded into the priorities for the OPTN.

## Achieving Equity

While all of the committee's recommendations include a focus on increasing equity, including many related to system-level improvements, the following five recommendations stand out as being squarely focused on equity:

---

| BOX S-2 | COMMITTEE'S RECOMMENDATIONS FOR CREATING A MORE EQUITABLE, TRANSPARENT, AND EFFICIENT SYSTEM FOR DECEASED DONOR ORGANS |
|---|---|

The committee recommends the following actions—some near term (in the next 1–2 years) and others longer term (in the next 3–5 years)—to realize a more equitable, transparent, cost-effective, and efficient system for deceased donor organs:

- Develop national performance goals for the U.S. organ transplantation system (Recommendation 1).
- Improve the OPTN policy-making process (Recommendation 2).
- Achieve equity in the U.S. transplantation system in the next 5 years (Recommendation 3).
- Accelerate finalizing continuous distribution allocation frameworks for all organs (Recommendation 4).
- Eliminate predialysis waiting time points from the kidney allocation system (Recommendation 5).
- Study opportunities to improve equity and use of organs in allocation systems (Recommendation 6).
- Increase equity in organ allocation algorithms (Recommendation 7).
- Modernize the information technology infrastructure and data collection for deceased donor organ procurement, allocation, and distribution (Recommendation 8).
- Make it easier for transplant centers to say "yes" to organ offers (Recommendation 9).
- Increase transparency and accountability for organ offer declines, and prioritize patient engagement in decisions regarding organ offers (Recommendation 10).
- Require the establishment and use of a donor care unit for each organ procurement organization (Recommendation 11).
- Create a dashboard of standardized metrics to track performance and evaluate results in the U.S. organ transplantation system (Recommendation 12).
- Embed continuous quality improvement efforts across the fabric of the U.S. organ transplantation system (Recommendation 13).
- Align reimbursement and programs with desired behaviors and outcomes (Recommendation 14).

---

**Recommendation 3:[6] Achieve equity in the U.S. organ transplantation system in the next 5 years.**

Under the direction and oversight of Congress, HHS should be held accountable for achieving equity in the transplantation system in the next 5 years. Within 1 to 2 years, HHS should identify and publish a strategy with specific proposed requirements, regulations, payment structures, and other changes for elimination of disparities. Elements of the strategy should include expanding oversight and data collection, aligning providers with the goal of equity, shared decision making with patients and public education, and elevating voices of those facing disparities.

*Expanding Oversight and Data Collection*
- HHS should extend its regulatory oversight of the organ transplantation system beginning, at least, at the time a patient reaches end-stage organ failure and extending beyond 1 year posttransplant.

---

[6] Recommendations are numbered according to their appearance in the full report.

- HHS should update the OPTN contract to require the collection of disaggregated data by race and ethnicity, gender/sex, age, as well as language and the creation of new measures of inequity in the transplantation system.

### Aligning Providers with the Goal of Equity

- The Centers for Medicare & Medicaid Services (CMS) should adopt payment policies that incentivize all providers—from primary and specialty care of patients with organ failure to referral for transplant, from care while awaiting a transplant to long-term posttransplant care—to improve equity in access to care and outcomes for patients.

### Shared Decision Making with Patients and Public Education

- HHS should develop, implement, and evaluate rigorous approaches for transplant teams to communicate routinely with (1) potential transplant recipients about their status and remaining steps in the process of transplant evaluation; (2) wait-listed candidates about organs offered to them, including information about the benefits, risks, and alternatives to accepting different types of organs to facilitate shared decision making about whether to accept the organ; and (3) wait-listed candidates about the number of organs offered and declined.
- HHS should develop, implement, and evaluate rigorous approaches for routinely educating the public about the benefits, risks, and alternatives to organ transplantation as a treatment option for end-stage organ disease or for those needing transplantation of tissue or a functional unit.
- HHS should conduct ongoing culturally targeted public education campaigns to convey the need for organ donation to save lives, to eliminate misconceptions about organ donation and transplantation, and to increase the trustworthiness of the transplantation system.

### Elevating Voices of Those Facing Disparities

- The OPTN should be required to ensure that all populations facing disparities, including persons with disabilities, are represented in the transplant policy development process.
- HHS should require and support work with OPOs to increase the diversity of their workforce to better meet the needs of donor families.

**Recommendation 4: Accelerate finalizing continuous distribution allocation frameworks for all organs.**

The OPTN should accelerate the development of the continuous distribution framework for all organ types with full implementation by December 31, 2024. The OPTN should set organ-specific upper bounds on the weight of "distance to the donor hospital" in the continuous distribution equation. The weights should be proportional to the effect of increased organ travel on posttransplant survival. The OPTN should regularly reevaluate the weight assigned to this factor as advances in normothermic preservation permit travel time to be extended without impairing outcomes. The OPTN should annually evaluate the effects of the continuous distribution policy and adjust the equations for organs that are not moving toward the goals set by HHS for improved equity, organ use, and patient outcomes, as well as steady or reduced costs.

**Recommendation 5: Eliminate predialysis waiting time points from the kidney allocation system.**

To reduce racial and ethnic disparities in the application of kidney transplant allocation policies, the OPTN should discontinue the use of predialysis waiting time credit, or points, in the current kidney allocation system, leaving only the date that the patient began regularly administered dialysis as an end-stage kidney disease patient as the basis for an individual to accumulate points based on waiting time. While this committee is *not* recommending that access to the deceased donor kidney waiting list be limited to only those who have started dialysis, the committee is recommending that predialysis waiting time should be discontinued as a basis for accumulating waiting time points. This change would ultimately save more lives in a fairer and more equitable manner by eliminating the current preferential access to deceased donor kidneys for individuals able to gain timely access to referral for transplant and the transplant waiting list. Considerations may be necessary for pediatric transplant candidates, multiorgan transplant candidates, prior transplant recipients, and those currently listed with predialysis waiting time. The OPTN should closely monitor any unintended consequences of removing predialysis waiting time points. To avoid manipulating the system by earlier dialysis initiation, OPTN policy should include penalties for providers who engage in the premature initiation of dialysis.

**Recommendation 6: Study opportunities to improve equity and use of organs in allocation systems.**
HHS should require the OPTN to study the effect of changing the kidney allocation system to include a measure of survival benefit and dialysis waiting time as a method of improving access to transplant for all patients without unintended consequences for patients with disabilities, socioeconomically disadvantaged populations, and racially diverse patients. Additional endpoints for study should include patient-centered and patient-identified metrics as well as waiting list mortality, organ nonuse rates, and overall survival from the time of entry onto the waiting list.

**Recommendation 7: Increase equity in organ allocation algorithms.**
HHS should quickly resolve areas of inequity in current organ allocation algorithms. The committee identified numerous aspects of the current organ allocation algorithms that require revision, further study, or immediate implementation. The committee recommends that HHS do the following:

- Require the OPTN to update its prediction models (e.g., KDPI, EPTS, and MELD) using the most recent data no less frequently than every 5 years. During this time, the models themselves should be reconsidered by adding or removing predictors that will either improve predictive accuracy or increase equity (e.g., adding serum sodium to the MELD score, replacing race with scientifically valid biologic predictors in the KDPI). Statistical aspects of the prediction models themselves should also be reviewed to ensure that the best performance possible is achieved and that they are properly validated using data not used to derive the prediction models.
- Modify the MELD scoring system for liver allocation and prioritization or establish an alternative overall prioritization scheme to include a modifier based on body size or muscle mass to overcome the demonstrated disparities observed for patients of smaller size.
- Immediately implement the recommendations of the National Kidney Foundation and American Society of Nephrology joint task force to use the revised equation, which eliminates race, in calculating estimated glomerular filtration rate for all individuals and to use the revised equation for high-risk individuals that incorporates a blood test for cystatin C along with serum creatinine.

- Require the OPTN to ensure that all laboratories in the transplantation system become capable of conducting validated cystatin C tests within 12 months.
- Resolve the use of race in KDPI and other clinical equations. Within 12 months HHS should make a decision on the continued use of race in KDPI and how best to eliminate race from KDPI and other clinical equations used in organ allocation and access.
- Continue to gather data on factors that may result in disparities in access to, and outcomes of, organ transplantation (e.g., socioeconomic status, place of residence, access to health care, race and ethnicity, presence in patient or family of stressors caused by racism) and use such data to determine whether faster progression to end-stage kidney disease is experienced by patients with any particular factor or combination of factors, and if so whether this evidence should be used to establish a new threshold for listing on the transplant list and for allocation of an organ for transplantation.

## Improving System Performance to Increase Reliability, Predictability, and Trustworthiness

The current organ transplantation system is unduly fragmented and inefficient. The system's component parts—physicians caring for patients with organ failure, donor hospitals, OPOs, the OPTN, transplant centers, the Scientific Registry of Transplant Recipients, CMS, and other payers, among others—do not operate as a fully integrated system. Likewise, the entities with oversight responsibilities each oversee particular components, but none monitors the performance of the system as a whole in producing predictable, consistent, and equitable results. The organ transplantation system could save additional lives and be more equitable if its component parts functioned in a more cohesive fashion and were overseen by a single entity, or by several entities operating in a coordinated fashion with common goals and unified policies and processes. Such alignment of all components and oversight responsibilities would allow the public and Congress to ascertain whether the system is fairly and efficiently maximizing the benefits provided by organ donation and transplantation. The committee offered six recommendations focused on system-level improvements.

Recommendation 1: Develop national performance goals for the U.S. organ transplantation system.

HHS should identify and substantially reduce or eliminate the existing variations among donor hospitals, OPOs, and transplant centers in the rates of organ donation, DCDD procurement and transplantation, acceptance of offered organs, and nonuse of donated organs, to improve the quality of, and foster greater equity in, organ donation and transplantation. HHS should also use the proven capabilities of the highest performing donor hospitals, OPOs, and transplant centers to establish bold goals to drive national progress toward greater equity, higher rates of organ donation, procurement and transplantation of organs from DCDD donors, and acceptance of offered organs, along with lower rates of nonuse of donated organs, to increase the total number of organs procured and transplants performed.

These goals can inform the development and use of various levers of influence including organized programs of quality improvement, payment policies, regulations, technical assistance, and public education campaigns. The goals should be continuously reviewed (at least annually) and updated as results are obtained, and as new, higher levels of organizational performance are achieved. HHS should

- Build on the initial CMS goals established in the kidney transplant collaborative, and establish a national goal for all transplant centers to reduce donated kidney nonuse rates to 5 percent or less.
- Establish new national goals to do the following:
  - Improve donation among minority populations and disadvantaged populations, and increase transplantation rates among minority and disadvantaged populations, based on the proven practices of donor hospitals, OPOs, and transplant centers which have the highest rates in these areas.
  - Increase the number of organs procured from medically complex donors. In particular, increase DCDD donors to at least 45 percent of all deceased donors, with no reductions in the numbers of organs procured from donors from neurological determination of death.
  - Improve offer acceptance levels for each organ type to those achieved by the 5 to 10 percent highest-performing transplant centers for that organ type nationally.
  - Increase the number of transplants to at least 50,000 by 2026.

**Recommendation 2: Improve the Organ Procurement and Transplantation Network (OPTN) policy-making process.**

**HHS should hold the OPTN and Health Resources and Services Administration (HRSA) accountable for developing a more expedient, and responsive policy-making process including increasing racial, ethnic, professional, and gender diversity on the boards and committees responsible for developing OPTN policies. HHS should use the agreed on policy priorities established by the OPTN Policy Oversight Committee to establish contractual deadlines for completion of these policy-making priorities. HHS should consider requiring the OPTN to work with and receive support from an external organization, such as the National Quality Forum (NQF) or the National Academy of Public Administration, with expertise in guiding federal programs through unique challenges in leadership and stakeholder collaboration. HHS should require the OPTN to consider the following elements of the policy-making process:**

- Proven approaches by others, such as the NQF Measure Applications Partnership, for meeting aggressive timelines with intensive, consensus-based, multistakeholder policy development processes;
- Optimal board size and stakeholder balance;
- Continuous and concurrent versus sequential policy-making processes;
- Managing strategic priorities and ensuring priority items have sufficient momentum, institutional memory, and timelines;
- Alternative governance models; and
- Appropriate tools and processes for evaluating the effectiveness of the policy-making process.

**Recommendation 8: Modernize the information technology (IT) infrastructure and data collection for deceased donor organ procurement, allocation, distribution, and transplantation.**

**HHS should ensure that the OPTN uses a state-of-the-art information technology infrastructure that optimizes the use of new and evolving technologies to support the needs and future directions of the organ transplantation system. Toward this end, HHS should do the following:**

- Within the next 1 to 2 years, evaluate how well the current IT system meets the needs of the transplantation system by collecting and analyzing data from IT end users (e.g., OPOs and transplant teams) and other stakeholders.
- Using the user needs assessment and input from external IT experts, identify needed improvements in the current IT system used by the OPTN that would make it more efficient, equitable, and user friendly.
- Assess the pros and cons of various contracting approaches to mitigate and prevent the risks of system failures if substantial changes in IT contracting are pursued.

**Based on the evaluation of the current IT system, HHS should consider pursuing one of the following three noted courses of action:**

- Immediately separate the IT infrastructure components from the remainder of the OPTN contract and institute a new competitive process for an IT services contractor. or
- Incorporate the identified improvements in the next OPTN contract bidding process in 2023. This could include smart approaches to mitigate potential system failure risks, separating the IT infrastructure components from the OPTN contract to address necessary improvements, and keeping the contract intact but with updated expectations for the winning contractor. or
- Pursue an alternative approach that would achieve the same desired outcome.

**If HHS determines that separating the IT infrastructure from the current OPTN contract requires a change in the National Organ Transplant Act (NOTA), then HHS should work with Congress to revise NOTA accordingly.**

**Recommendation 11: Require the establishment and use of a donor care unit for each organ procurement organization.**
To better serve donors and families, increase cost-effectiveness, and foster innovation in organ rehabilitation and donor intervention research, HHS should require each of the 57 OPOs to create, establish, and manage a donor care unit (DCU). Ensuring the success of donor care units at a national level will also require CMS to revise payment incentives for transplant centers such that the transplant center is neither financially punished nor excessively rewarded for performing deceased donor organ management and recovery. Specific actions include the following:

- For DSA in the United States, HHS should require the OPO and transplant center(s) to collaborate on the development of a DCU that would be designed, established, and managed by the OPO, if one does not already exist, to serve that geographic area. Because multiple models of DCUs are in practice today, the committee recommends that HHS require the following attributes for each donor care unit:
  - Dedicated beds for deceased donors in a dedicated space;
  - Dedicated operating room with trained staff, reserved specifically for organ procurement surgery;
  - Dedicated space for donor families;
  - ICU-level care;

- o Oversight by a critical care physician;
- o Ability to conduct some in-house imaging and diagnostics of donors;
- o Ability to conduct organ rehabilitation and therapy;
- o Ability to conduct donor intervention research; and
- o Reasonable distance to an airport.
- CMS should adjust current reimbursement structures that create disincentives that dampen the willingness of some transplant centers to transfer donors to an OPO DCU. Transplant centers should not be disadvantaged financially by allowing a donor to be transferred to a DCU for donor management and organ recovery. Similarly, transplant centers should not excessively gain from transferring and managing already deceased donors from another hospital for the sole purpose of organ procurement.
- HHS should require hospitals to smooth surgical scheduling so that organ donation surgical procedures for DCDD donors and donors who cannot be transferred to a DCU can take place in a timely manner all seven days of the week.

**Recommendation 12: Create a dashboard of standardized metrics to track performance and evaluate results in the U.S. organ transplantation system.**

HHS should use a combination of currently collected data and new data elements specifically related to access to transplant to create a publicly available dashboard of standardized metrics to measure the performance of the organ transplantation system. The metrics in the dashboard should be developed to be meaningful to donor families, individuals with chronic disease or organ failure, transplant candidates, and individuals on the waiting list and their families, and to ensure accountability and partnership across the components of the system. The metrics should be used for quality improvement, and once they are deemed valid and reliable, they should be used for regulatory purposes. Specific actions HHS should take include the following:

- Establish standardized data collection requirements, with an emphasis on timeliness of reporting, for donor hospitals, OPOs, and transplant centers. All data points collected should reflect demographics—that is, the most updated way of capturing race, ethnicity, and language, as well as socioeconomic factors, disability status, a social deprivation index based on geography, and other factors to better document, understand, reduce, and eventually eliminate disparities.
- Require collaboration among the federal agencies with oversight of the transplantation system on data collection to ensure relevant, accurate, and timely data are available about the transplantation system.
- Collaborate with an organization like the National Quality Forum to develop consensus measures and measure specifications to evaluate and improve the performance of the organ transplantation system in a standardized way. Recommended data points needed from donor hospitals, OPOs, referring organizations, and transplant centers are detailed in Figure 7-1.
- Create a publicly available dashboard of standardized metrics to provide a complete human-centered picture of the patient experience—from patient referral for transplant evaluation, to time on the waiting list, to posttransplant quality of life—managed by the Scientific Registry of Transplant Recipients (SRTR) or a similar entity.

**Recommendation 13: Embed continuous quality improvement efforts across the fabric of the U.S. organ transplantation system.**

HHS should take actions to reduce variations in the performance of donor hospitals, OPOs, and transplant centers and increase the reliability, predictability, and trustworthiness of the U.S. organ transplantation system through implementing and sustaining continuous quality improvement efforts across the system. HHS should hold the component parts of the organ transplantation system accountable for achieving demonstrable performance improvement. With government leadership, quality improvement efforts should create greater systemness and accountability for the highest possible performance among all donor hospitals, OPOs, and transplant centers. Special attention and focus should be given to spreading best practices in organ procurement and transplantation that reduce and eliminate inequities and disparities. The following are specific actions HHS should take in this regard:

- Sustain continuous quality improvement work on a national scale over time as a long-term investment in lifesaving transplants.
- Align quality improvement efforts with the performance goals for the U.S. organ transplantation system (see Recommendation 1). Quality improvement efforts should improve the prework that includes identifying who would possibly benefit from a transplant and also the postwork of caring for people who receive a transplant.
- Deploy quality improvement techniques that focus on behavior change tools, implementation science, nudging, and education theory to realize uptake of best practices for organ procurement, use, and transplantation across donor hospitals, OPOs, and transplant centers.
- Promote the development, systematic sharing, adaptation, and use of best practices in areas such as rapid referral and early response by donor hospitals and OPOs, increasing donation authorization rates among diverse populations, pursuit of all possible organ donors, how to have culturally sensitive conversations with all families about organ donation, intensive waiting list management, successful use of medically complex organs, and how best to communicate with patients about organ offers.
- Urge hospitals to smooth surgical scheduling to both enable organ donation surgical procedures, and to ensure the hospital's capability to accept and use organ offers, regardless of which day of the week the gift of donation occurs.
- Explore additional tools and approaches for promoting innovation in the organ transplantation system, including the following:
  - Launch a nationwide learning process improvement collaborative to address deceased organ donors, waiting list management, the acceptance of offered organs, transplant rate, and automated organ referrals.
  - Encourage preapproved controlled experiments by OPOs and transplant centers to allow experimentation with innovation and the development of evidence to support widespread adoption of best practices.
  - Incentivize transplant centers, donor hospitals, and OPOs to actively participate in the kidney transplantation collaborative sponsored by CMS and HRSA.
  - Require the OPTN to implement an organized system of proactive communication or nudges in the form of special messages or brief reports aimed at calling attention to outlier performance by OPOs and transplant centers, based on SRTR

data. Nudges should be sent to both high and low performers. For example, OPOs with a low percentage of DCDD donors in their deceased donor organ pool could receive a special message or brief report calling attention to their current performance in comparison to other OPOs.

## Underuse of Procured Organs

While waiting lists remain long and every day many listed individuals die while awaiting an organ, too many donated organs that are procured and offered to patients at transplant centers are not accepted—leaving thousands of potentially lifesaving donated organs unused every year. Approximately 20 percent of kidneys procured from deceased donors are not used (i.e., the organs are procured for transplantation but not transplanted into individuals on the waiting list) (Israni et al., 2021). The committee agreed that this issue of unused organs represents a critical need for system improvement. Evidence indicates that many, if not a large majority, of unused organs could be successfully transplanted and benefit patients. Two facets of the organ transplantation system are in tension. On the one hand, priority for individuals on each organ waiting list is based on formal, publicly announced policies, and organs are allocated by match-run algorithms. On the other hand, a patient's access to an organ offered depends on how the transplant professionals in the program caring for the patient exercise the discretion that the system gives them regarding when to accept or reject an organ for transplantation. This divergence—which is not transparent either to the general public or even to all patients on the waiting list—has implications for equitable treatment of all patients, for adherence to the ethical principles of autonomy and beneficence, and for trust in the system. The committee offered three recommendations focused on increasing use of organs procured from deceased donors:

> **Recommendation 9: Make it easier for transplant centers to say "yes" to organ offers.**
> The OPTN should enhance organ allocation and distribution policies and processes to reduce nonuse of deceased donor organs and make it easier for transplant centers to say "yes" to organ offers. To improve the organ offer process, the OPTN should do the following:
> - Require the use of more refined filters for transplant centers to indicate their preferences for which kidneys will be accepted, if offered. The filters should especially focus on determining transplant center willingness to accept medically complex kidneys, akin to what is done in the UK's Kidney Fast Track Scheme.
> - Implement expedited placement policies, at first offer, for offered and procured kidneys at high risk of nonuse to effectively direct difficult-to-place kidneys to transplant centers with a demonstrated history of using them.
> - Since donations occur seven days a week, the OPTN should require hospitals with transplant centers to smooth surgical scheduling using proven procedures in order to ensure the capability of organ procurement operations and organ transplants all seven days of the week.
> - Adapt the process of offering an organ to gradually increase the number of simultaneous offers of a given organ to save cold ischemic time and minimize herding effects.
> - Review and standardize current requirements for organ quality assessments conducted by OPOs with the primary goal of helping transplant centers accept more organ offers by focusing on the following specific actions:

- o Develop evidence-based standards for organ quality assessment to be used by all OPOs prior to organ allocation. The standardized requirements for organ quality assessments should carefully consider the value of biopsies as it has been repeatedly shown that biopsy results deter organ acceptance, often inappropriately.
- o Develop clear guidelines for transplant centers to request any additional organ quality testing beyond the standardized requirements.

**Recommendation 10: Increase transparency and accountability for organ offer declines and prioritize patient engagement in decisions regarding organ offers.**

HHS should update the OPTN contract to require increased *transparency* around organ offer declines. The updated OPTN contract should do the following:

- Require transplant centers to share with a patient and their family the number and context of organ offer declines for that individual on the waiting list during a defined period (e.g., every 3 to 6 months).
- Require the collection of more reliable, specific, and patient-centered data on reasons organ offers were declined through improvements in refusal codes. For example, require transplant centers to provide additional justification for declining an offered kidney when survival benefit of the transplant is greater than staying on dialysis.
- Require investigation of approaches for shared decision making between patients and transplant teams in the organ offer process and implementation of models proven to be most useful and desirable.

HHS should update the OPTN contract to require transplant center *accountability* for patient engagement and partnership between transplant center professionals and patients in deciding whether to accept or reject an offered organ. The updated OPTN contract should require

- Close monitoring of any new transplant center performance metrics to ensure the desired outcomes are achieved and unintended consequences are avoided;
- Nudges in the form of reports showing a transplant center's decisions regarding offered organs, as well as comparisons to other transplant centers, to be proactively developed from SRTR data and shared with individual transplant centers on a monthly basis; and
- Transplant programs to document shared decision making that includes a discussion of survival benefit, relative to staying on the waiting list or dialysis, before deciding to accept or reject an offered deceased donor organ.

**Recommendation 14: Align reimbursement and programs with desired behaviors and outcomes.**

CMS should align payment and other policies to meet the national performance goals for the organ transplantation system (see Recommendation 1). Within 2 years, CMS should

- Continue and expand funding, as needed, for the current quality improvement initiative aimed at reducing the kidney nonuse rate, and pursuing simultaneous expansion of kidney donation by spreading the best practices of transplant centers and OPOs.

- Sustain and expand current work in the End-Stage Renal Disease (ESRD) program to
  - refer more eligible patients for transplant,
  - help referred patients to get both evaluated and listed by transplant centers,
  - assist patients in fully understanding and engaging with transplant centers when organs that are offered are declined on their behalf, and
  - work with Congress to update and increase the existing and outdated dialysis withholding payment to fund ESRD quality improvement activities.
- Sustain and expand model tests and other payment policies to increase reimbursement for nephrologists and dialysis centers to educate and refer patients for transplant evaluation.
- Increase reimbursement for referral for transplant evaluation for all organ types, and in the case of kidney transplant, even before dialysis begins.
- Update the CMS Interpretive Guidelines to reflect current practices and promote a collaborative relationship between the donor hospital and OPO, and institute measurable reporting mechanisms for donor hospital data. Address this systematically as part of both CMS hospital surveys and surveys by deemed organizations such as The Joint Commission.
- Explore financial incentives and make changes to Interpretive Guidelines to make hospitals accountable for smoothing surgical scheduling to ensure the capacity to recover and transplant donated organs seven days a week.

**HHS, CMS, and other payers should consider new opportunities to increase the use of organs. HHS, CMS, and other payers should take the following steps:**

- Increase payment for improving the procurement and transplantation of all types of organs, as CMS did in the 2021 Inpatient Prospective Payment System Final Rule when it created new Diagnosis Related Groups with higher payments for kidney transplants that required a higher level of medical care.
- Incentivize OPOs and transplant centers to learn from the organizations and centers that already make extensive use of medically complex organs, and actively work to spread the practices for obtaining and transplanting these organs that have proven to be most successful and cost effective.
- Within the next 2 years, the CMS Innovation Center should design and implement one or more model tests to assess the effects of additional increased payments to address the added costs of rehabilitating and using more organs that are medically complex and increasing equitable access to a broader pool of patients. These model tests should also measure the potential improvement in health care quality and financial savings of providing transplants more quickly to patients who would otherwise require continued extensive medical support, such as an artificial organ or hospitalization.

# REFERENCES

Ahearn, P., K. L. Johansen, J. C. Tan, C. E. McCulloch, B. A. Grimes, and E. Ku. 2021. Sex disparity in deceased-donor kidney transplant access by cause of kidney disease. *Clinical Journal of the American Society of Nephrology* 16(2):241-250.

Aubert, O., P. P. Reese, B. Audry, Y. Bouatou, M. Raynaud, D. Viglietti, C. Legendre, D. Glotz, J. P. Empana, X. Jouven, C. Lefaucheur, C. Jacquelinet, and A. Loupy. 2019. Disparities in acceptance of deceased donor kidneys between the United States and France and estimated effects of increased US acceptance. *JAMA Internal Medicine* 179(10):1365-1374.

Axelrod, D. A., N. Dzebisashvili, M. A. Schnitzler, P. R. Salvalaggio, D. L. Segev, S. E. Gentry, J. Tuttle-Newhall, and K. L. Lentine. 2010. The interplay of socioeconomic status, distance to center, and interdonor service area travel on kidney transplant access and outcomes. *Clinical Journal of the American Society of Nephrology* 5(12):2276-2288.

Darden, M., G. Parker, E. Anderson, and J. F. Buell. 2021. Persistent sex disparity in liver transplantation rates. *Surgery* 169(3):694-699.

Harding, J. L., A. Perez, and R. E. Patzer. 2021. Nonmedical barriers to early steps in kidney transplantation among underrepresented groups in the United States. *Current Opinion in Organ Transplantation* 26(5):501-507.

Israni, A. K., D. Zaun, J. D. Rosendale, C. Schaffhausen, W. McKinney, and J. J. Snyder. 2021. OPTN/SRTR 2019 annual data report: Deceased organ donors. *American Journal of Transplantation* 21(S2):567-604.

Lee, B. P., and N. A. Terrault. 2020. Liver transplantation in unauthorized immigrants in the United States. *Hepatology* 71(5):1802-1812.

Mohan, S., M. C. Chiles, R. E. Patzer, S. O. Pastan, S. A. Husain, D. J. Carpenter, G. K. Dube, R. J. Crew, L. E. Ratner, and D. J. Cohen. 2018. Factors leading to the discard of deceased donor kidneys in the United States. *Kidney International* 94(1):187-198.

OPTN (Organ Procurement and Transplantation Network). 2022. *All-time records again set in 2021 for organ transplants, organ donation from deceased donors.* https://optn.transplant.hrsa.gov/news/all-time-records-again-set-in-2021-for-organ-transplants-organ-donation-from-deceased-donors (accessed January 20, 2022).

Patzer, R. E., J. P. Perryman, J. D. Schrager, S. Pastan, S. Amaral, J. A. Gazmararian, M. Klein, N. Kutner, and W. M. McClellan. 2012. The role of race and poverty on steps to kidney transplantation in the southeastern United States. *American Journal of Transplantation* 12(2):358-368.

Richards, C. T., L. M. Crawley, and D. Magnus. 2009. Use of neurodevelopmental delay in pediatric solid organ transplant listing decisions: Inconsistencies in standards across major pediatric transplant centers. *Pediatric Transplantation* 13(7):843-850.

Saran, R., B. Robinson, K. C. Abbott, L. Y. Agodoa, P. Albertus, J. Ayanian, R. Balkrishnan, J. Bragg-Gresham, J. Cao, J. L. Chen, E. Cope, S. Dharmarajan, X. Dietrich, A. Eckard, P. W. Eggers, C. Gaber, D. Gipson, H. Gu, S. M. Hailpern, Y. N. Hall, Y. Han, K. He, H. Hebert, M. Helmuth, W. Herman, M. Heung, D. Hutton, S. J. Jacobsen, N. Ji, Y. Jin, K. Kalantar-Zadeh, A. Kapke, R. Katz, C. P. Kovesdy, V. Kurtz, D. Lavalee, Y. Li, Y. Lu, K. McCullough, M. Z. Molnar, M. Montez-Rath, H. Morgenstern, Q. Mu, P. Mukhopadhyay, B. Nallamothu, D. V. Nguyen, K. C. Norris, A. M. O'Hare, Y. Obi, J. Pearson, R. Pisoni, B. Plattner, F. K. Port, P. Potukuchi, P. Rao, K. Ratkowiak, V. Ravel, D. Ray, C. M. Rhee, D. E. Schaubel, D. T. Selewski, S. Shaw, J. Shi, M. Shieu, J. J. Sim, P. Song, M. Soohoo, D. Steffick, E. Streja, M. K. Tamura, F. Tentori, A. Tilea, L. Tong, M. Turf, D. Wang, M. Wang, K. Woodside, A. Wyncott, X. Xin, W. Zang, L. Zepel, S. Zhang, H. Zho, R. A. Hirth, and V. Shahinian. 2017. US Renal Data System 2016 annual data report: Epidemiology of kidney disease in the United States. *American Journal of Kidney Diseases* 69(3 Suppl 1):A7-A8.

Stewart, D. E., V. C. Garcia, J. D. Rosendale, D. K. Klassen, and B. J. Carrico. 2017. Diagnosing the decades-long rise in the deceased donor kidney discard rate in the United States. *Transplantation* 101(3):575-587.

# 1

# Introduction and Study Context

From its beginnings on December 23, 1954—when a surgical team in Boston removed a healthy kidney from one 23-year-old and implanted it in his identical twin whose own kidneys had failed—the modern era of transplantation has engendered both admiration and disapproval. Over the next 13 years, surgeons performed successful transplantation of livers, lungs, and hearts, using organs obtained from recently deceased patients, and soon most kidney transplants were also relying mostly on such "cadaver donors." In the 1980s, the introduction of more effective immune rejection drugs, beginning with cyclosporine, made "matching" organs to recipients easier. Over the past seven decades, more than 875,000 patients with organ failure have been able to live better and longer lives with transplanted organs,[1] about 700,000 of which came from deceased donors while the rest—almost all kidneys—were provided by living donors, a category that rose rapidly in the 1990s (from 2,123 in 1990, to 5,939 in 2000).[2] At the request of the sponsor, this study and report focus on organ transplants from deceased donors.

## MOVEMENT TOWARD A NATIONAL SYSTEM

In the early years, hospitals that created transplant programs established relationships with other hospitals in their locality from which they could obtain deceased patients'

---

[1] The term "organ transplantation" encompasses a range of procedures, including transplantation of solid organs from living donors; transplantation of donated organs from persons after neurological or circulatory determination of death; multiorgan transplantation (e.g., kidney and pancreas for diabetics with renal failure); and vascularized composite allotransplantations (such as face, hand, penis, uterus). Kidney, liver, pancreas, heart, and lung transplants are the most common forms of organ transplantation; indeed, by the end of 2021, kidneys alone had accounted for 58.9% of all U.S. transplants and 95.1% of those involving a living donor, versus 49.7% of all transplants from deceased donors. See https://optn.transplant.hrsa.gov/data/view-data-reports/national-data (accessed January 20, 2022).

[2] The number of living donors annually, which had increased to 7,397 by 2019, fell by more than 1,600 donors in 2020 on account of the COVID-19 pandemic; half that loss was reversed in 2021, when 6,541 living donors were recorded. The annual number of deceased donors (from each of whom multiple organs can usually be obtained) has been rising fairly steadily for decades and reached 34,813 in 2021, more than double the number in 2000. *Id.*

organs. The groups handling this function—now known as organ procurement organizations (OPOs)—developed expertise in the psychosocial as well as the medical aspects of facilitating organ donations. While some of these organizations remained based in a transplant program, the scope of others broadened to serve transplant teams at several hospitals in their area. The Uniform Anatomical Gift Act (UAGA), promulgated in 1968 and rapidly adopted by all states, facilitated the task of obtaining organs by allowing people to fill out a simple, wallet-sized card donating their organs upon death and by empowering the next of kin to donate if the deceased had not filled out a donor card. The UAGA also established that the persons doing the procurement and transplantation were the custodians rather than the owners of the donated organs.

Nonetheless, from the beginning, the gap between the number of patients with organ failure and the number of transplants increased each year. This was especially true for kidneys; not only were more patients added to the waiting list than were transplanted but an even larger number received dialysis for chronic kidney disease than were listed for a transplant. At a 1983 congressional hearing on improving organ procurement, H. Barry Jacobs, a Virginia physician who established the "International Kidney Exchange, Ltd." after losing his medical license, described his plan to serve as a broker between U.S. patients needing a kidney transplant and people from poor countries who would be willing to sell one of theirs. Opposition to—actually, disgust at—his proposal helped to push the bill that emerged from the House committee to rapid, bipartisan passage. The National Organ Transplant Act of 1984 (NOTA) not only forbids the giving or receiving of "valuable consideration" for an organ for transplantation but also established a unified, standardized system to oversee and support the procuring and distribution of deceased donor organs for transplantation, to coordinate other aspects of the transplant process, and to gather and analyze data about outcomes. NOTA began the still-ongoing process of creating a national system out of the patchwork of transplant centers and OPOs, which had grown organically in response to local circumstances, along with other professionals involved in patient care, with responsibility to ensure equitable and efficient use of donated organs as a "national resource."[3]

## COMPLEXITY, SCARCITY, AND PUBLIC CONCERNS

Organ transplants depend on the generosity of organ donors and their families as well as the successful completion of a highly complex array of specialized tasks performed by numerous individuals and organizations, referred to in this report as the "organ transplantation system" or "transplantation system." The term "system" is somewhat metaphorical since many of the activities involved in obtaining, allocating, and transplanting organs are carried out independently by health care professionals and organizations rather than under the direction or review of a single controlling authority. As concerns deceased donation (the topic of this report), the specific activities and tasks include

- identifying persons who may be candidates for receiving organs and referring them for transplant evaluation;

---

[3] NOTA instructed the Department of Health and Human Services to appoint a Task Force on Organ Transplantation to develop the basis for regulating the system established by the Act. In its 1986 report, the Task Force recommended "that each donated organ be considered a national resource to be used for the public good; the public must participate in the decisions of how this resource can be used to best serve the public interest." *Organ Transplantation: Issues and Recommendations: Report of the Task Force on Organ Transplantation,* Jan 1986. U.S. Department of Health and Human Services, Public Health Service, Health Resources and Services Administration, Office of Organ Transplantation, at p. xxi, 9 (Jan. 1986).

- medically evaluating these candidates for their suitability to receive an organ;
- treating and, when appropriate, diagnosing death in potential donors;
- procuring organs from potential donors;
- allocating donated organs to individuals who have been medically screened and placed on an organ transplant waiting list;
- matching donated organs with waiting list candidates;
- transporting organs to hospitals where the matched recipients will receive a transplant;
- surgically transplanting the donated organs;
- caring for the organ recipients after transplantation, both immediately after surgery and often for many years or decades afterwards; and
- compiling, analyzing, and reporting data on transplants and patient outcomes.

Importantly, the organ transplantation journey for most patients actually begins well before they are placed on the waiting list for an organ transplant when the person is diagnosed and treated for a condition that has significant likelihood of ending in organ failure, has already gotten to that point, or has significant tissue damage that is unresponsive to reconstructive surgery. Figure 1-1 shows the points encountered along the path of a typical recipient of an organ transplant. Yet many factors—such as patients' gender, economic resources, or ethnicity—affect how they experience the journey and, indeed, whether they survive it and receive a transplant.

The gap between patients on waiting lists and the number of transplants performed is largest for kidneys. In 2020, 91,099 kidneys were needed by individuals on the waiting list, but only 22,817 (25 percent) were transplanted (HRSA, 2021b). While data sources vary, it is estimated that 17 people die waiting for an organ transplant each day and one person is added to the transplant waiting list every 9 minutes (HRSA, 2021a). Yet deaths on the waiting list provide an imperfect picture of the number of patients who need, but do not receive, a transplant. The Organ Procurement and Transplantation Network (OPTN) reports that 5,758 patients were removed from the waiting list in 2021 because they died and another 5,371 because they became "too sick to transplant." This means that 11,129 patients—about 30 a day—who had been listed for an organ transplant died without receiving one that year. Additionally, and as expounded upon elsewhere in this report, many patients whose lives could be saved by an organ transplant never even reach the waiting list.

Additionally, many patients whose lives could be saved or improved by an organ transplant never even reach the waiting list. For example, the pool of possible kidney transplant candidates in 2020 was even larger than the 91,099 on the waiting list, since more than 558,000 patients with end-stage kidney disease (ESKD) received dialysis in 2020. As explicated later in this report, notable disparities exist between patients who could benefit and those who are placed on a transplant waiting list based on race, ethnicity, gender, age, socioeconomic status, geographic place of residence and location of the transplant center visited, intellectual ability, and immigration status. For instance, black patients are significantly less likely than white patients to be referred for transplant evaluation and then wait longer for a transplant once listed. Disparities and inequities in transplantation are discussed throughout the report and in detail in Chapter 4.

Whenever a system is created to allocate a scarce resource that cannot be left to market distribution, favoritism and discrimination among the decision makers can produce inequities. In the case of the shortage of organs donated for transplantation, the resulting concerns seem to be exacerbated by deficiencies in public understanding of organ donation, allocation, and transplantation, which is not surprising given the complexity of the transplanta-

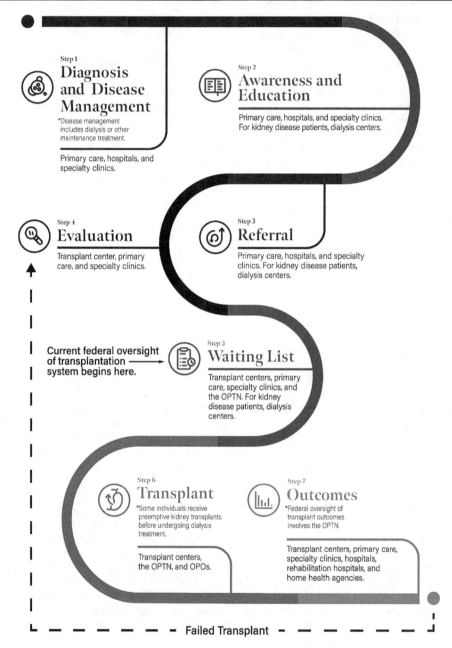

**Step 1**
## Diagnosis and Disease Management

*Disease management includes dialysis or other maintenance treatment.

Primary care, hospitals, and specialty clinics.

**Step 2**
## Awareness and Education

Primary care, hospitals, and specialty clinics. For kidney disease patients, dialysis centers.

**Step 4**
## Evaluation

Transplant center, primary care, and specialty clinics.

**Step 3**
## Referral

Primary care, hospitals, and specialty clinics. For kidney disease patients, dialysis centers.

**Current federal oversight of transplantation system begins here.** →

**Step 5**
## Waiting List

Transplant centers, primary care, specialty clinics, and the OPTN. For kidney disease patients, dialysis centers.

**Step 6**
## Transplant

*Some individuals receive preemptive kidney transplants before undergoing dialysis treatment.

Transplant centers, the OPTN, and OPOs.

**Step 7**
## Outcomes

*Federal oversight of transplant outcomes involves the OPTN.

Transplant centers, primary care, specialty clinics, hospitals, rehabilitation hospitals, and home health agencies.

**Failed Transplant**

**FIGURE 1-1** Transplant patient journey showing each step in the journey as well as the institutions responsible for creating the resources, setting the policies, or providing patients with the services that are relevant to that step.
NOTE: OPTN = Organ Procurement and Transplantation Network; OPO = organ procurement organization.

tion system and the sources on which members of the public mostly rely for information. Respondents in the 2019 National Survey of Organ Donation Attitudes and Practices[4] reported learning about organ donation primarily through news coverage (51.5 percent), their Department of Motor Vehicles[5] (46.5 percent), discussion with family (43.3 percent), discussion with a friend (42.0 percent), movie or TV show (42.0 percent), social media (40.9 percent), and advertisement on TV (40.1 percent). Medical professionals accounted for 29.5 percent and donation organizations accounted for 25.7 percent of the public's source of information (HHS, 2019). The survey also revealed that only 46.6 percent of respondents had heard, read, or seen information about organ donation or transplantation in the past year (HHS, 2019). The proportion of the public exposed to such information has dropped over time, by nearly 10 percent from 2012 (56.0 percent), and by nearly 18 percent from 2005 (63.3 percent). Since public support for organ donation is essential for the transplantation system to work, the survey's conclusion that roughly half the respondents believe that wealth and race affect access to a transplant (as reported in Box 1-1) indicate that steps need to be taken to increase the system's transparency and trustworthiness, a topic to which this report turns in Chapter 3.

---

[4] For more information about the 2019 National Survey of Organ Donation Attitudes and Practices, see https://www.organdonor.gov/professionals/grants-research/research-reports (accessed August 24, 2021).

[5] The organ donation statute in most states provides that people should be offered the opportunity, when obtaining or renewing their driver's license, to express their willingness to be a deceased organ donor, to be indicated by a statement or sticker on their license.

---

**BOX 1-1  ATTITUDES AND BELIEFS ABOUT ORGAN DONATION AND ALLOCATION**

The 2019 National Survey of Organ Donation Attitudes and Practices presents the percentage of people who agree with various descriptions of the organ transplant system, including the following that are particularly relevant to the present report.

- **86.3%:** "All people who need an organ transplant should be able to receive a transplant." (Significant differences in beliefs emerged along racial, ethnic, education, and age categories.)
- **66.6%:** "The U.S. transplant system uses a fair approach to distribute organs to patients."
- **52.5%:** "Given equal need, a poor person has as good a chance as a rich person of getting an organ transplant."
- **47.9%:** "Minority patients are less likely to receive organ transplants."
- **53.7%:** "Organs should be distributed so that the expected life of the organ is similar to the expected life of the recipient. For example, older people should generally get older organs and younger people should get younger organs."
- **84.1%:** "Doctors do everything they can to save a person's life before organ donation is even considered."
- **31.9%:** "If you indicate you intend to be a donor, doctors will be less likely to save your life."
- **42.1%:** "It is possible for a brain-dead person to recover from his or her injuries."
- **33.1%:** "It is important for a person's body to have all of its parts when it is buried."

SOURCE: HHS, 2019.

## STUDY CHARGE

This study was mandated by the U.S. Congress in the Consolidated Appropriations Act of 2020.[6] Specifically, the National Academies of Sciences, Engineering, and Medicine (the National Academies) was asked to examine and recommend improvements to research, policies, and activities related to deceased donor organ procurement, allocation, and distribution. The congressional language requested that the report include

(1) identification of the current challenges involved in modeling proposed organ allocation policy changes and recommendations to improve modeling; (2) recommendations about how costs should be factored into the modeling of organ allocation policy changes; (3) a review of the scoring systems (e.g., CPRA, EPTS, KDPI, LAS, MELD)[7] or other factors that determine organ allocation and patient prioritization and recommendations to assure fair and equitable practices are established, including reducing inequities affecting socioeconomically disadvantaged patient populations; (4) recommendations to update the Organ Procurement and Transplantation Network's (OPTN's) policies and processes to ensure that organ allocation decisions take into account the viewpoints of expert OPTN committees; and (5) such other issues as may be identified.[8]

At the direction of Congress, the National Institutes of Health (NIH) via the National Institute of Allergy and Infectious Diseases sponsored and funded this study. The Statement of Task from NIH, found in Box 1-2, directs the committee to examine the economic (costs), ethical, policy, regulatory, and operational issues related to organ allocation policy decisions involving a range of deceased donor organs. This study follows a history of work conducted by the Institute of Medicine (IOM) and the National Academies, which began some 3 decades

---

[6] The complete congressional language requesting this consensus study can be found in Division A of the Joint Explanatory Statement that accompanied H.R. 1865, the Further Consolidated Appropriations Act, 2020 (P.L. 116-94) on PDF page 82 here: https://www.appropriations.senate.gov/imo/media/doc/HR%201865%20-%20SOM%20FY20.pdf (accessed February 22, 2022).

[7] CPRA = calculated panel reactive antibody; EPTS = estimated posttransplant survival; KDPI = Kidney Donor Profile Index; LAS = lung allocation score; MELD = Model for End-Stage Liver Disease.

[8] H.R. 1865, the Further Consolidated Appropriations Act, 2020 (P.L. 116-94). https://www.appropriations.senate.gov/imo/media/doc/HR%201865%20-%20SOM%20FY20.pdf (accessed February 22, 2022).

---

### BOX 1-2  STATEMENT OF TASK

An ad hoc committee of the National Academies of Sciences, Engineering, and Medicine will conduct a consensus study to examine the economic (costs), ethical, policy, regulatory, and operational issues relevant to organ allocation policy decisions involving deceased donor organs (e.g., heart, lung, liver, kidney, kidney-pancreas, intestinal, vascular composite allografts, dual and/or multi-organ organ transplants). The committee will examine the gaps, barriers, and opportunities for improving deceased donor organ procurement, allocation, and organ distribution to waiting recipients at transplant centers with a keen eye towards optimizing the quality and quantity of donated organs available for transplantation—in a cost effective and efficient, fair and equitable manner consistent with the National Organ Transplant Act and the Final Rule.

Specifically, the final consensus report will delineate the issues pertinent to organ allocation policy, modelling and simulation of anticipated policy changes for intended and unintended consequences, and the process for efficiently executing allocation policy changes in an open, trans-

**BOX 1-2   CONTINUED**

parent, fair, and equitable manner. The report will make recommendations to maximize public and professional trust in the organ donation, procurement, allocation, and distribution process. The report will also make recommendations to better align the performance metrics or incentives of various stakeholders within the Organ Procurement and Transplantation Network [specifically donor service areas (DSAs), organ procurement organizations (OPOs), and transplant centers] to maximize donor referrals, evaluations, procurement and organ placement/allocation while mini-mizing organ discard rates.

The committee will consider the following in its discussions and deliberations to address the Statement of Task:

- If deceased donor organs should be allocated to specific individuals based on need (i.e., na-tional, continuous framework) rather than groups of individuals defined by locale, zip code, or donor service area (i.e., the donor service area, geographic framework) and if measures can be taken to reduce inequities in organ allocation affecting socioeconomically disadvantaged populations;
- Relevant factors that determine transplant recipient waitlist priority (i.e., "need") for an organ;
- Best model/method(s) to ensure fairness, equity, cost effectiveness and efficiency, and reduce the reported socioeconomic and racial/ethnic disparities in the current organ allocation system;
- Challenges with current organ allocation policy development and policy change procedures and processes, including opportunities to update OPTN policies and processes to ensure organ allocation decisions consider the viewpoints of expert OPTN committees;
- Challenges involved in modeling proposed organ allocation policy changes and opportunities to improve modeling, including how costs should be factored into the modeling of organ al-location policy changes;
- Appropriate parameters, factors, and variables that should make up various transplant scoring systems (e.g., CPRA, EPTS, KDPI, LAS, MELD, etc.)* that determine organ allocation and patient prioritization to assure fair and equitable practices and reduce inequalities affecting socioeco-nomically disadvantaged patient populations;
- How to more effectively acquire needed data points to enhance transplant scoring systems (e.g., through better sharing of donor and recipient data between various federal agency databases);
- Self-reported donation metrics (e.g., "eligible deaths") and the impact on estimates of the true donor supply. Consider the development of a new, standardized, objective, and verifiable do-nation metric to permit the transplant community to evaluate DSAs and OPOs and establish best practices;
- Data sharing and optimization opportunities, revealed by the COVID-19 pandemic, via collabo-ration across Department of Health and Human Services administrative databases regarding vital statistics on transplant recipients and potential donors to better inform policy makers, the OPTN, OPOs, transplant centers, transplant healthcare workers, patients, and the public; and
- Relevant comparisons to international allocation policies and models.

* CPRA = calculated panel reactive antibody; EPTS = estimated posttransplant survival; KDPI = Kidney Donor Profile Index; LAS = lung allocation score; MELD = Model for End-Stage Liver Disease.

ago and remains relevant today. Brief summaries of previous IOM and National Academies studies on organ transplantation are in Appendix B.

## THE NATIONAL ACADEMIES STUDY PROCESS

A Statement of Task guides each National Academies study and determines what kinds of expertise are needed on a committee. A committee writes a report to answer as thoroughly as possible the questions posed in the Statement of Task.

### Committee Formation

Members of the committee that conducted this study[9] were selected from among more than 200 persons nominated during the committee-formation phase of the study. Individuals appointed to the committee were chosen for their individual expertise and the relevance of their experience and knowledge to the Statement of Task, not their affiliation with any institution. All committee members volunteer their time to serve on a study committee. Areas of expertise represented on the committee included health care system management, bioethics, population health, anthropology, transplant surgery, organ procurement, organ allocation, management science, economics, biostatistics, and law and regulation. Biographies of committee members are in Appendix C.

### Public Input and Committee Deliberations

Members of the public were invited to provide oral or written statements and information to the committee. Virtual public meetings were held in December 2020 and February, April, and July 2021 and included time for members of the public to provide comments to the committee. Public meeting agendas are in Appendix A. Recordings of the public sessions are archived on the study website.[10]

Written comments to the committee could be submitted at any point during the study process. Comments and information could be delivered to National Academies staff via the study email address and through the feedback form linked on the study website. More than 100 comments and documents were submitted to the committee, and the committee listened to or read all of them. Public submissions of comments, articles, or written testimony for the committee's consideration are available upon request from the National Academies' Public Access Records Office (paro@nas.edu). To address the Statement of Task, the committee considered information presented during public meetings. Committee members frequently requested

---

[9] Every National Academies committee is provisional until the appointed members have had an opportunity to discuss as a group their points of view and any potential conflicts of interest related to the Statement of Task. During this discussion they also determine whether the committee is missing expertise that may be necessary to answer questions in the Statement of Task. As part of their discussion, committee members consider any comments submitted by the public about the committee's composition. The discussion takes place during the first meeting of the committee. The committee is provisional until the National Academies determines that the committee has the necessary balance and composition to address the Statement of Task, and that committee members are free of unavoidable financial conflicts of interest, transparent about their relevant relationships and publications, and independent from the sponsors of the committee's work. For more information about the National Academies study process, including definitions and procedures related to composition, balance, and conflict of interest, visit https://www.nationalacademies.org/about/our-study-process (accessed January 24, 2022).

[10] The study website includes recordings of public sessions. Visit https://www.nationalacademies.org/our-work/a-fairer-and-more-equitable-cost-effective-and-transparent-system-of-donor-organ-procurement-allocation-and-distribution#sectionPastEvents (accessed January 24, 2022).

additional data or documentation from invited speakers or public commenters following their presentations. The committee also reviewed statements and articles that were submitted or referred to by speakers and thoroughly consulted the peer-reviewed scientific literature. The committee took seriously the information and passion conveyed by stakeholders throughout this study process, and some of the public comments are quoted in this report. To address the study charge, the committee deliberated virtually from December 2020 to February 2022, holding 17 closed session committee meetings in addition to the public sessions mentioned above. The committee reviewed the scientific literature on the issues identified in the Statement of Task and also commissioned seven white papers. The commissioned papers explore such topics as the use of standardized performance metrics and quality improvement in organ transplantation, algorithms used in kidney and liver allocation, challenges and opportunities in OPTN policy making, solutions to financial and policy barriers to increasing deceased donor transplantation, and the use of survival benefit in deceased donor kidney transplantation. The commissioned papers are in the study's public access file and are available upon request from the National Academies' Public Access Records Office (paro@nas.edu).

## Report Review Process

The concluding phase of a National Academies study is the report review process. When a draft report is complete, it is submitted to the National Academies' Report Review Committee (RRC). The RRC recruits a diverse and critical group of reviewers who have expertise complementary to that of the committee to ensure that critical gaps and misinformation are identified (see the Reviewers section on p. vii). The reviewers are anonymous to the committee during the review process, and their comments remain anonymous after the report is published. Reviewers are asked to assess how well a report addresses a study's Statement of Task to ensure that the report addressed the full Statement of Task but did not go beyond it, and are asked to assess whether the report includes evidence, analysis, and arguments to support the conclusions and recommendations.[11] The committee must consider and respond to, but not necessarily agree with, all reviewers' comments in a detailed "response to review" that is examined by independent report review monitors responsible for ensuring that the report review criteria have been satisfied before the report is finalized. When the RRC decides that the committee has adequately and appropriately addressed the reviewer's comments, the report is ready to be released to the public and to the sponsor.

## COMMITTEE APPROACH AND INTERPRETATION OF THE STATEMENT OF TASK

This study charge is broad and asks the study committee to address multiple longtime, vexing issues and challenges in organ procurement, allocation, and distribution. While the study charge was limited to procurement, allocation, and distribution of deceased donor organs, some of the committee's recommendations may also affect living donors and living donation policies. The committee was not asked to explore issues in tissue procurement and use.

The study charge emphasizes the importance of issues of fairness, equity, cost-effectiveness, and transparency of the organ transplantation system, concerns that were central to the committee's deliberations (see Box 1-3 for some key definitions and concepts). During the

---

[11] More information on the National Academies study process and report review process can be found on these pages: https://www.nationalacademies.org/about/our-study-process; https://www.nationalacademies.org/about/institutional-policies-and-procedures/guidelines-for-the-review-of-reports (accessed February 4, 2022).

committee's work, there were a number of activities and changes in the organ donation and transplantation system. For instance, the Centers for Medicare & Medicaid Services issued a new performance metric for OPOs. There was heightened congressional scrutiny of OPOs as well as the United Network for Organ Sharing (UNOS), the nonprofit government contractor implementing the transplantation system known as the Organ Procurement and Transplantation Network. Throughout the course of this study, UNOS, as the OPTN, continued to refine allocation policies governing how deceased donor organs are prioritized among patients on the waiting list as well as other policies related to performance metrics for transplant centers.

The committee was mindful that OPOs and UNOS were under scrutiny by Congress[12] and others,[13] and that some of these issues have become contentious among organ transplantation stakeholders who are tasked with working together.[14] Congressional scrutiny largely involves issues that this committee was not charged with addressing, nor constituted to address. The committee closely examined challenges and opportunities in deceased donor organ procurement and the variations in performance across OPOs, but some of the OPO issues that have attracted the most congressional and media attention are quite different from those this committee was tasked with addressing. For example, in addition to scrutiny of OPOs, there have been calls to formally reorganize the federal oversight responsibilities of the OPTN by moving or refocusing the current Division of Transplantation within the Health Resources and Services Administration to a new office of the Assistant Secretary of the U.S. Department of Health and Human Services.[15] The committee did not interpret its charge to include a request for recommendations on restructuring or reorganizing federal offices with oversight responsibilities for the organ transplantation system, and during the course of its work the committee did not find evidence demonstrating superiority of any particular organizational oversight structure.

The organ transplantation system has realized many amazing, lifesaving achievements in recent decades. Posttransplant outcomes remain positive and most patients see significant improvements in quality of life following transplant. In 2021, there were 41,354 transplants performed—an increase of 5.9 percent over 2020 (OPTN, 2022). Transplantation is also a multidisciplinary field, drawing on the expertise of many passionate individuals in multiple medical specialties, social work, nutrition, case management, pharmacy, surgery, primary care, nursing, home health, rehabilitation, and organ procurement. The context of this report, as requested by the study sponsor, is to discuss specific opportunities to improve the organ transplantation system. The report is written from the perspective that while much has been achieved, significant opportunities remain to improve the availability of and access to deceased donor organs for individuals needing a transplant. In some cases, the committee's recommendations may include areas where the OPTN or others are currently working to address. It is the committee's hope that even if some of these issues are already being consid-

---

[12] *Oversight subcommittee expands investigation into fraud, waste, and abuse in organ transplant industry.* May 27, 2021: https://oversight.house.gov/news/press-releases/oversight-subcommittee-expands-investigation-into-fraud-waste-and-abuse-in-organ; *Grassley, Wyden Subpoena the United Network for Organ Sharing as part of continued investigation into U.S. organ transplant system.* February 4, 2021: https://www.finance.senate.gov/ranking-members-news/grassley-wyden-subpoena-the-united-network-for-organ-sharing-as-part-of-continued-investigation-into-us-organ-transplant-system (accessed January 26, 2022).

[13] Bloom Works: The Costly Effects of an Outdated Organ Donation System: Summary of Findings. https://bloomworks.digital/organdonationreform/Introduction (accessed January 26, 2022).

[14] *As thousands wait for transplants, medical centers fight to keep livers close to home.* May 14, 2019. https://www.npr.org/sections/health-shots/2019/05/14/723371270/new-liver-donation-system-takes-effect-despite-ongoing-lawsuit (accessed January 26, 2022).

[15] For more information see https://www.healthaffairs.org/do/10.1377/forefront.20201211.229975/full (accessed February 11, 2022).

ered, that these recommendations will draw heightened attention and urgency to undertaking efforts to improve equity and fairness in the organ transplantation system.

This National Academies committee approached the Statement of Task from a systems perspective in reviewing opportunities to improve deceased donor organ procurement, allocation, and organ distribution for the benefit of patients. As this report will describe, an individual engages with the organ transplantation system and the relevant oversight systems such as the OPTN when initiating evaluation for an organ transplant. However, the upstream components—identifying patients who could benefit from transplantation, referring such patients to a transplant center for evaluating patients for their transplant suitability, and adding their names to the organ transplant waiting list—are of critical importance to ensuring that the organ transplantation system is fair and equitable.

The committee was acutely aware that the transplantation system exists within a broader health care system that falls short on delivering equitable access to care (IOM, 2013). Individuals at a disadvantage in receiving health care services in general are likely to be disadvantaged in seeking an organ transplant. The organ transplantation system may be unable to solve issues of inequity in the larger health care system, but these larger issues cannot be an excuse for those in the organ transplantation system to turn their focus away from the need to provide equitable access to the opportunity for transplantation, as well as equitable allocation of deceased donor organs among those on the waiting list. In fact, an opportunity exists for the organ transplantation system to become an example of how to manifest equity in the delivery of care and allocation of a scarce resource. The committee discusses the concepts of fairness, equity, and justice in greater detail in Chapter 3 and throughout the report. While the committee acknowledges the achievements of the organ transplantation system and the complexity of changing policies in this area to avoid unintended consequences, the committee believes the system can be fairer and more equitable.

An additional complexity and context for this study is the role of the opioid epidemic in transplantation and how much increases in organ donation over the last decade are directly attributed to the increase in opioid deaths or other factors (e.g., changes in allocation policy

---

**BOX 1-3    KEY DEFINITIONS AND CONCEPTS**

The committee reflected on the various terms used in organ transplantation and agreed upon a common lexicon for this report. The definitions and concepts below reflect the committee's choice of terminology for the purpose of presenting the committee's findings, conclusions, and recommendations as clearly and accurately as possible and not a decision to wade into standing debates over the use of particular terms and phrases. Additional definitions are included in Chapter 4.

**Organ transplantation system:** The component organizations and individuals that facilitate a patient's journey from chronic disease and organ failure to posttransplant long-term follow-up. The system includes patients, families, caregivers, donors, donor families, primary care physicians, medical specialists, organ donation and procurement professionals, policy makers, regulators, transplant coordinators, transplant surgeons, and many others. The committee believes that it is important to recognize that while federal oversight of the transplantation system currently begins when a patient is listed, the system encompasses much more and includes multiple steps earlier in the process that lead to a patient receiving, or not, a needed transplant.

*(continued)*

**BOX 1-3    CONTINUED**

**Health disparity:** This is when "a health outcome is seen to a greater or lesser extent between populations." A health disparity is

> a particular type of health difference that is closely linked with social, economic, and/or environmental disadvantage. Health disparities adversely affect groups of people who have systematically experienced greater obstacles to health based on their racial or ethnic group; religion; socioeconomic status; gender; age; mental health; cognitive, sensory, or physical disability; sexual orientation or gender identity; geographic location; or other characteristics historically linked to discrimination or exclusion (HHS, n.d.).

**Health inequities:** Health differences that are unfair, unjust, and avoidable. Inequities result when barriers keep individuals and communities who experience disparities from reaching their full health potential (Arcaya et al., 2015).

**Health equity:** The "attainment of the highest level of health for all people. Achieving health equity requires valuing everyone equally with focused and ongoing societal efforts to address avoidable inequalities, historical and contemporary injustices, and the elimination of health and health care disparities" (HHS, 2021).

**Organ nonuse rate:** This term is used to refer to the proportion of organs that are donated and procured but ultimately not transplanted. The nonuse rate is commonly referred to as the *discard* rate. However, the committee finds the term *discard* less than ideal and possibly offensive to some deceased organ donors and their families, as well as individuals waiting for an organ transplant.

**Medically complex organ:** Instead of the frequently used term *marginal organ* to describe an organ that receives lower than ideal ratings based on its quality and likelihood of being viable once transplanted, the committee uses the term *medically complex organ*. The term *marginal* has negative connotations and reflects the long-standing preferences and behaviors of professionals in the organ transplantation system that are being questioned. Many medically complex organs can be successfully transplanted, and one person's medically complex organ is another's perfect organ depending on various patient-specific factors. The committee preferred the term *medically complex* to describe organs that have medical histories deserving of special consideration in order to find the best recipient for transplant.

**System:** A group of related components that work toward a common goal. The organ transplantation system, as defined above, is composed of a number of systems. The system includes not just the professionals, patients, and families involved in organ transplantation but the incentive structures, performance metrics, and information technology involved as well.

**Systemness:** A functional state of diverse, interconnected, discrete parts that behave predictably and consistently as a coherent whole in ways that are distinct from and superior to the sum of the parts.

**Accountability:** The responsibility of an individual or organization to reach stated goals. Accountability requires a clear definition of the desired goals, the ability to measure and monitor goal achievement, and a set of consequences if the achievements are not satisfactory. Accountability also requires that the individuals or organizations are able to control the outcomes being asked of them.

**Transparency:** Within the limits of patient confidentiality, transparency refers to the public availability of information on the attributes and performance of the organ transplantation system. Transparency applies at all levels—transparency to federal regulators, Congress, and the public in the operation of organizations working in donation, procurement, and transplantation as well as transparency between patients seeking access to the waiting list or current transplant candidates and their physicians, specialists, and transplant teams about the transplant process. Transparency is also necessary for accountability—that is, not simply the obligation of the system to provide an account of its operations but also to be answerable for any deficiencies or misfeasance.

or efforts of OPOs). The drug overdose epidemic has increased deaths resulting in organ donations as these deceased individuals typically are younger and have limited medical comorbidities that would preclude them from being donors. The number of donors who died from drug overdose increased from 29 to 848, an increase of 2,924 percent, between 1994 and 2016 (Weiner et al., 2017). In 2013, there were an estimated 514 kidney donations from persons who died from drug intoxication and in 2018 this number more than doubled to 1,313 donations (Maghen et al., 2019). Disagreement exists in the transplantation system as to the degree to which the increase in deceased organ donation can be attributed to the opioid epidemic. Some authors suggest the data are indisputable that the increase in donors is due almost wholly to the opioid epidemic (Goldberg and Lynch, 2019), while others are equally passionate that this assertion is unsupported by the data given challenges in accurately categorizing "drug-related" deaths (Cmunt et al., 2020; Stewart et al., 2020). This committee was not tasked with parsing the impact of opioid overdose deaths, car accidents, or homicides on the transplantation system, though the committee recognizes that such public health trends do impact the organ donation system and affect the absolute number of potential organ donors. The committee believes that the most important takeaway is the need for the organ transplantation system to be prepared and at its most high functioning state to handle changes in the number of deaths in the United States as a result of tragedies such as the opioid epidemic or positive changes in laws related to helmet use or vehicle safety.

## WHY IS THIS STUDY NEEDED?

The foundation of the organ transplantation system is the gift of organ donation from both living and deceased donors. Every day, individuals and families throughout the United States face the critical decision to donate organs—often in moments that coincide with the loss of a loved one—for the sole purpose of saving the life of another person who is usually unknown to the donor. This study is undertaken with the goal of helping to better facilitate the transition of this valuable lifesaving resource from one person to another and to highlight the importance and challenges of doing so.

A continuous challenge for the organ transplantation system is that the number of organs transplanted each year falls below the number of patients on the waiting list, which therefore grows longer each year. For example, the more than 106,000 persons on organ transplant waiting lists in 2021 were more than double the number of transplants performed that year.

## OVERVIEW OF CHALLENGES

To address its broad charge and identify opportunities for improving deceased donor organ procurement, allocation, and organ distribution—and ultimately, downstream effects on mortality—the committee focused on three key issues that exist within the transplantation system: (1) problems of inequity in access, (2) variation and inefficiency in system performance, and (3) underuse of donated organs. In the face of these challenges, it is important to understand that organ transplantation and donation spans a complex system comprising clinics and hospitals, highly specialized transplant centers, OPOs, nonprofit government contractors, and federal oversight agencies, all of which are supported by an equally complex web of dedicated and passionate professionals. Given the complexity of the transplantation system, many of these challenges are interconnected and have the potential to benefit or harm other components within the system. However, the committee believes that for the transplantation system to be truly successful, all of these challenges must be examined within the context of known inequities and disparities.

## Challenges of Inequity in Access

The deceased donor organ procurement and transplantation system has long-standing problems of inequity in access to the organ transplant waiting list and eventual transplantation. Getting onto the waiting list (i.e., being listed) is the metaphorical gateway to gaining access to a lifesaving organ transplant. This gate may be especially hard to open for many persons who would benefit from organ transplantation, particularly persons who are racial or ethnic minorities, of lower socioeconomic status, live in rural areas, or have an intellectual disability.

One of the stated aims of the OPTN is to promote equitable access to transplantation and organ allocation; however, after examining the literature, the committee found stark health disparities in organ transplantation rates for certain subsets of the American population but also limited data on disparities for racial and ethnic groups other than those for black and white persons. Disparities are evident at different points along the complicated pathway to an organ transplant and are caused by different structural and other barriers (see Table 4-1 in Chapter 4 for a summary of key data related to health disparities in organ donation and transplantation). Illustrative of some disparities, black persons are three times more likely to develop kidney failure than whites in the United States, but they are significantly less likely to receive lifesaving kidney transplants (Saran et al., 2017). Relatively fewer black patients are referred, evaluated, and added to a transplant waiting list, and fewer living kidney donations are available to black patients compared to white patients (Gander et al., 2018; Waterman et al., 2013). The evidence of disparate access to organ transplants is not limited to black persons who need kidney transplants. As another example, women are less likely to receive a liver transplant than men, regardless of other factors including race, geography, education, body mass index, and weight (Allen et al., 2018; Darden et al., 2021).

The committee found that a rigorous and comprehensive assessment of inequities in the current transplantation system is challenging because of a lack of patient-centered data, especially for individuals not yet listed but in need of a transplant, persons with intellectual disabilities, pediatric patients, and undocumented immigrants. Reliable data on the number of patients who enter the transplant pathway (e.g., patients who might benefit from referral and transplant evaluation) are particularly lacking, and there are few—if any—ways to properly assess the effect of socioeconomic status on transplant access.

Confronting and rectifying the issues related to health inequities in organ transplantation in the United States will require a systemwide approach to prioritize equity, rethink incentive structures for the transplantation system, and collect disaggregated data to inform research on inequities and disparities. The committee's assessment of and proposed approach to this set of issues is discussed in Chapter 4.

## Variation and Inefficiency in System Performance

The performance of the component parts of the organ transplantation system is neither predictable nor consistent across the United States, especially for OPOs and transplant centers. Identifying key areas of variation in the procurement and use of deceased donor organs provides opportunities for developing and implementing quality improvement tools and standardized performance measures to reduce variation in the system. The committee focused on three critical areas of variation in system performance that affect the availability of deceased donor organs for those on transplant waiting lists: (1) the procurement of medically complex organs, in particular donation after circulatory determination of death (DCDD), (2) the acceptance rates of offered organs, and (3) nonuse of procured organs.

The percentage of total deceased donors that originate from DCDD varies widely, rang-ing from approximately 11 percent to nearly 53 percent of deceased donor organs (see Figure 6-3 and associated discussion in Chapter 6). Similar variability occurs in organ offer accep-tance rates across transplant centers. Among 65 transplant centers, acceptance of lung trans-plants varied from 9 percent to 67 percent (Mulvihill et al., 2020). This marked variability significantly affects which patients may receive a transplant on the basis of which transplant center they use. Rates of nonuse of donated organs also vary widely and are important to address because—like acceptance rates—they can advantage or disadvantage patients on the waiting list. Nonuse rates vary because of factors such as the practices of specific transplant centers and transplant teams, geographic variation in organ availability, patients' access to transplant centers, and the lack of standard donor acceptance criteria.

## Underuse of Donated Organs

While waiting lists remain long and many listed individuals die while awaiting an organ every day, too many donated organs that are procured and offered to patients at trans-plant centers are not accepted—leaving thousands of potentially lifesaving donated organs unused every year. While estimates vary, approximately 20 percent of organs procured from deceased donors are not used (i.e., the organs are not transplanted into individuals on the waiting list). The committee agreed that this issue of unused organs represents a critical need for system improvement. Evidence indicates that many, if not a large majority, of unused organs could be successfully transplanted and benefit patients. This problem is much more prominent in the United States than in many other countries. For example, the overall nonuse rate in the United States is twice that in France. In the United States, on average, patients who die waiting for a kidney had offers for 16 kidneys that were ultimately transplanted into other patients, indicating that many transplant centers refuse viable kidney offers on behalf of those on the waiting list (Husain et al., 2019).

## REFERENCES

Allen, A. M., J. K. Heimbach, J. J. Larson, K. C. Mara, W. R. Kim, P. S. Kamath, and T. M. Therneau. 2018. Reduced access to liver transplantation in women: Role of height, MELD exception scores, and renal function underes-timation. *Transplantation* 102(10):1710-1716.

Arcaya, M. C., A. L. Arcaya, and S. V. Submarinian. 2015. Inequalities in health: Definitions, concepts, and theories. *Global Health Action* 8:10. https://www.ncbi.nlm.nih.gov/pmc/articles/PMC4481045 (accessed December 21, 2021).

Cmunt, K., G. Danovitch, F. Delmonico, F. Fynn-Thompson, A. Glazier, J. Grandas, S. Gunderson, M. Jendrisak, H. K. Johnson, S. Kulkarni, G. Lipowitz, K. Meyer, D. Mulligan, H. Nathan, T. Mone, M. Moritz, K. O'Connor, W. Payne, M. Souter, and R. P. Wood. 2020. Deceased donors: Defining drug-related deaths. *Clinical Transplanta-tion* 34(3):e13800.

Darden, M., G. Parker, E. Anderson, and J. F. Buell. 2021. Persistent sex disparity in liver transplantation rates. *Surgery* 169(3):694-699.

Gander, J. C., X. Zhang, L. Plantinga, S. Paul, M. Basu, S. O. Pastan, E. Gibney, E. Hartmann, L. Mulloy, C. Zayas, and R. E. Patzer. 2018. Racial disparities in preemptive referral for kidney transplantation in Georgia. *Clinical Transplantation* 32(9):e13380.

Goldberg, D., and R. Lynch. 2019. Improvements in organ donation: Riding the coattails of a national tragedy. *Clini-cal Transplantation* 34(1). https://doi.org/10.1111/ctr.13755 (accessed January 24, 2022).

HHS (U.S. Department of Health and Human Services). Health Resources and Services Administration, Healthcare Systems Bureau. 2019. *2019 National Survey of Organ Donation Attitudes and Practices*: Report of findings. Rockville, MD: U.S. Department of Health and Human Services. https://www.organdonor.gov/sites/default/files/organ-donor/professional/grants-research/nsodap-organ-donation-survey-2019.pdf (accessed August 24, 2021).

HHS. 2021. *Healthy People 2030 questions and answers*. https://health.gov/our-work/healthy-people/healthy-people-2030/questions-answers (accessed December 17, 2021).

HHS. n.d. *Healthy People 2020*. https://www.healthypeople.gov/2020/about/foundation-health-measures/Disparities (accessed December 17, 2021).

HRSA (Health Resources and Services Administration). 2021a. *Organ donation statistics*. https://www.organdonor.gov/learn/organ-donation-statistics (accessed December 17, 2021).

HRSA. 2021b. *Patients on the waiting list vs. transplants performed by organ (2020)*. https://www.organdonor.gov/learn/organ-donation-statistics/detailed-description#fig1 (accessed December 17, 2021).

Husain, S. A., K. L. King, S. Pastan, R. E. Patzer, D. J. Cohen, J. Radhakrishnan, and S. Mohan. 2019. Association between declined offers of deceased donor kidney allograft and outcomes in kidney transplant candidates. *JAMA Network Open* 2(8):e1910312.

IOM (Institute of Medicine). 2013. *Best care at lower cost: The path to continuously learning health care in America*. Washington, DC: The National Academies Press. https://doi.org/10.17226/13444.

Maghen, A., T. D. Mone, and J. Veale. 2019. The kidney transplant waiting list and the opioid crisis. *New England Journal of Medicine* 380(23):2273-2274.

Mulvihill, M. S., H. J. Lee, J. Weber, A. Y. Choi, M. L. Cox, B. A. Yerokun, M. A. Bishawi, J. Klapper, M. Kuchibhatla, and M. G. Hartwig. 2020. Variability in donor organ offer acceptance and lung transplantation survival. *The Journal of Heart and Lung Transplantation* 39(4):353-362.

OPTN (Organ Procurement and Transplantation Network). 2022. All-time records again set in 2021 for organ transplants, organ donation from deceased donors. https://optn.transplant.hrsa.gov/news/all-time-records-again-set-in-2021-for-organ-transplants-organ-donation-from-deceased-donors (accessed January 20, 2022).

Saran, R., B. Robinson, K. C. Abbott, L. Y. Agodoa, P. Albertus, J. Ayanian, R. Balkrishnan, J. Bragg-Gresham, J. Cao, J. L. Chen, E. Cope, S. Dharmarajan, X. Dietrich, A. Eckard, P. W. Eggers, C. Gaber, D. Gillen, D. Gipson, H. Gu, S. M. Hailpern, Y. N. Hall, Y. Han, K. He, H. Hebert, M. Helmuth, W. Herman, M. Heung, D. Hutton, S. J. Jacobsen, N. Ji, Y. Jin, K. Kalantar-Zadeh, A. Kapke, R. Katz, C. P. Kovesdy, V. Kurtz, D. Lavalee, Y. Li, Y. Lu, K. McCullough, M. Z. Molnar, M. Montez-Rath, H. Morgenstern, Q. Mu, P. Mukhopadhyay, B. Nallamothu, D. V. Nguyen, K. C. Norris, A. M. O'Hare, Y. Obi, J. Pearson, R. Pisoni, B. Plattner, F. K. Port, P. Potukuchi, P. Rao, K. Ratkowiak, V. Ravel, D. Ray, C. M. Rhee, D. E. Schaubel, D. T. Selewski, S. Shaw, J. Shi, M. Shieu, J. J. Sim, P. Song, M. Soohoo, D. Steffick, E. Streja, M. K. Tamura, F. Tentori, A. Tilea, L. Tong, M. Turf, D. Wang, M. Wang, K. Woodside, A. Wyncott, X. Xin, W. Zang, L. Zepel, S. Zhang, H. Zho, R. A. Hirth, and V. Shahinian. 2017. US Renal Data System 2016 annual data report: Epidemiology of kidney disease in the United States. *American Journal of Kidney Diseases* 69(3 Suppl 1):A7-A8.

Stewart, D., A. Zehner, D. Klassen, and J. Rosendale. 2020. The drug overdose epidemic does not explain all of the rise in deceased donation. *Clinical Transplantation* 34(5):e13858.

Waterman, A. D., J. D. Peipert, S. S. Hyland, M. S. McCabe, E. A. Schenk, and J. Liu. 2013. Modifiable patient characteristics and racial disparities in evaluation completion and living donor transplant. *Clinical Journal of the American Society of Nephrology* 8(6):995-1002.

Weiner, S. G., S. M. Malek, and C. N. Price. 2017. The opioid crisis and its consequences. *Transplantation* 101(4):678-681.

# 2

# The U.S. Organ Transplantation System and Opportunities for Improvement

This chapter examines the evolution of organ transplantation policies and systems, highlighting the complexity in the overall system, the benefits of setting ambitious goals for improvement, and challenges and opportunities for improving the efficiency and effectiveness of the Organ Procurement and Transplantation Network (OPTN) policy-making process going forward.

Since solid organ transplantation began in the United States in the 1950s, the systems and policies supporting organ donation, procurement, allocation, and distribution have evolved into a highly complex network of medical organizations and professionals, federal agencies, nonprofit contractors, patients, families, and advocates. This chapter traces the evolution and current status of the nation's solid organ procurement, allocation, distribution, and transplantation system. The chapter discusses the cost-effectiveness of transplantation; the committee's recommendations for national performance goals for the system (Recommendation 1); and opportunities to improve the OPTN policy-making process (Recommendation 2).

## EVOLUTION OF NATIONAL ORGAN TRANSPLANTATION SYSTEMS, POLICIES, AND OVERSIGHT

After the first successful living donor kidney transplant between identical twin brothers in 1954, kidney transplantation was recognized as a viable medical alternative to dialysis (Tilney, 2003). With dialysis serving as a lifeboat for those awaiting transplantation and the advent of immune suppression agents to prevent organ rejection, kidney transplant operations became more commonplace by the 1960s, but donor organ procurement was primarily hospital based. Since the characteristics of donated organs could not always be matched with patients at a particular hospital, transplant programs typically relied on their informal network to facilitate the sharing of such organs with other programs. This led transplant professionals to establish more formal transplant networks in Los Angeles, Boston, and Richmond (DeVita et al., 1993).

## Legislative Milestones

In the late 1960s, improvements in mechanical ventilation and other medical measures that sustained cardiopulmonary function enabled some patients who had experienced respiratory arrest or severe brain injuries to recover. Other patients, whose injuries were more extensive or who experienced a longer period of anoxia before restoration of circulation, could remain unconscious on a ventilator indefinitely. Postmortem examinations of patients in the latter group revealed brain damage inconsistent with their ever regaining consciousness or spontaneous circulatory-respiratory functions. Physicians developed methods of diagnosing when this loss of brain function was permanent and proposed that such patients could be declared dead even while a ventilator and associated medical interventions provided circulation of oxygenated blood (Report of the Ad Hoc Committee, 1968). In the period that followed, experts further elaborated the criteria and methods for determining death based on irreversible loss of brain functions, and the traditional methods of diagnosing death based on loss of circulation were clarified (DeVita et al., 1993; Guidelines for the determination of death, 1981; Halevy and Brody, 1993). Beginning in 1981, most states adopted the Uniform Determination of Death Act, which set forth two standards under which physicians were permitted to apply accepted medical criteria to determine that death had occurred, based either on the loss of circulatory and respiratory functions or on loss of all brain functions, including the brainstem (President's Commission, 1981). For both sets of criteria, the diagnosis of death requires both the cessation of function and irreversibility (Guidelines for the determination of death, 1981). The use of neurological criteria for the determination of death has gained wide medical, legal, ethical, and public acceptance in the United States, although debates continue (Bernat, 2005; Greer et al., 2020; Laureys, 2005). During the 1970s and 1980s, organ donation in the United States involved almost exclusively brain-based determinations of death. Beginning in the early 1990s, however, protocols were developed for donation after circulatory determination of death (DCDD), and, despite some controversy, this approach has become an increasingly important source of organs from deceased donors (Domínguez-Gil et al., 2021). In some areas of the country, the practice of DCDD never went away; however, the increases in DCDD started with the advent of a 2003 national Organ Donation Breakthrough Collaborative (see Chapters 6 and 7 for greater discussion of procurement of DCDD organs and national quality improvement efforts).

## *National Organ Transplant Act (NOTA)*

In 1983, the growing demand for organ transplantation, controversies regarding the allocation of organs, and concerns about payment for organs prompted members of Congress to propose the creation of a formal, privately administered network to more effectively procure and equitably allocate deceased donor organs. This proposal became the National Organ Transplant Act (NOTA), which was adopted on October 19, 1984. NOTA authorized the creation of the OPTN to regularize and make more efficient and equitable the system for obtaining and distributing organs, based on an improved matching process (see Box 2-1).[1] NOTA specified that the OPTN would be operated by a private, nonprofit organization under federal contract. The Act also banned the purchase or sale of human organs for transplantation but allowed transplant professionals, hospitals, transporters, and organ pro-

---

[1] Organ procurement and transplantation network, 42 U.S.C. §274, https://uscode.house.gov/view.xhtml?req=granuleid%3AUSC-2020-title42-chapter6A-subchapter2-partH&saved=%7CZ3JhbnVsZWlkOlVTQy0y MDIwLXRpdGxlNDItc2VjdGlvbjI3NGU%3D%7C%7C%7C0%7Cfalse%7C2020&edition=2020 (accessed February 4, 2022).

| BOX 2-1 | FUNCTIONS OF THE ORGAN PROCUREMENT AND TRANSPLANTATION NETWORK (OPTN) |
|---------|----------------------------------------------------------------------|

The National Organ Transplant Act, as amended, now lists the following functions to be carried out by the Organ Procurement and Transplantation Network:

1. Establish in one location or through regional centers—
   (i) A national list of individuals who need organs, and
   (ii) A national system, through the use of computers in accordance with established medical criteria, to match organs and individuals included in the list, especially individuals whose immune system makes it difficult for them to receive organs;
2. Establish membership criteria and medical criteria for allocating organs and provide to members of the public an opportunity to comment with respect to such criteria;
3. Maintain a 24-hour telephone service to facilitate matching organs with individuals included in the list;
4. Assist organ procurement organizations in the nationwide distribution of organs equitably among transplant patients;
5. Adopt and use standards of quality for the acquisition and transportation of donated organs;
6. Prepare and distribute, on a regionalized basis (and to the extent practicable, among regions or on a national basis), samples of blood sera from individuals who are included on the list and whose immune system makes it difficult for them to receive organs, in order to facilitate matching the compatibility of such individuals with organ donors;
7. Coordinate, as appropriate, the transportation of organs from organ procurement organizations to transplant centers;
8. Provide information to physicians and other health professionals regarding organ donation;
9. Collect, analyze, and publish data concerning organ donation and transplants;
10. Carry out studies and demonstration projects for the purpose of improving procedures for organ procurement and allocation;
11. Work actively to increase the supply of donated organs;
12. Submit to the secretary [of HHS] an annual report containing information on the comparative costs and patient outcomes at each transplant center affiliated with the organ procurement and transplantation network;
13. Recognize the differences in health and in organ transplantation issues between children and adults throughout the system and adopt criteria, policies, and procedures that address the unique health care needs of children;
14. Carry out studies and demonstration projects for the purpose of improving procedures for organ donation, procurement, and allocation, including but not limited to projects to examine and attempt to increase transplantation among populations with special needs, including children and individuals who are members of racial or ethnic minority groups and among populations with limited access to transportation; and
15. Provide that for purposes of this paragraph, the term "children" refers to individuals who are under the age of 18.

SOURCE: 42 U.S. Code § 274 - Organ Procurement and Transplantation Network. https://uscode.house.gov/view.xhtml?req=(title:42%20section:274%20edition:prelim (accessed November 11, 2021).

curement organizations (OPOs) to receive compensation for the services they provide (HHS, 2022). NOTA also permits living donors to receive reimbursement for the costs they bear in donating (such as travel, lost income, etc.), and it encourages the honoring of an individual's documented wishes with respect to organ donation.

The Act also created the U.S. Task Force on Organ Transplantation to examine and report back to Congress on a broad range of issues including the technical, practical, and ethical limitations on sharing organs. In its April 1986 report, the Task Force concluded that "donated cadaveric organs are a national resource," whose distribution ought not to be based on "accidents of geography." This means that, to the extent technically feasible, every person in the nation in need of a transplant—not simply those who live in the area where an organ is donated—should be equally considered a potential recipient.[2] After the Task Force's report was submitted, the Secretary issued the OPTN contract to a nonprofit organization, the United Network for Organ Sharing (UNOS), based in Richmond, Virginia.

NOTA has been amended many times since 1984. In 1988 and again in 1990, the original scope of the OPTN's responsibilities—namely, to assist OPOs in distributing organs that "cannot be placed within [their] service areas"—was broadened, in line with the Task Force's conclusion, to assist OPOs "in the nationwide distribution of organs equitably among transplant patients."[3]

The Omnibus Reconciliation Act of 1986 required all hospitals performing organ transplants to be members of the OPTN and to abide by its rules to receive Medicare and Medicaid payments.[4] The Omnibus Health Amendments of 1988 required the OPTN to "establish membership criteria and medical criteria for allocating organs and provide to members of the public an opportunity to comment with respect to such criteria."[5]

On September 8, 1994, the Health Resources and Services Administration (HRSA), a unit within the Department of Health and Human Services (HHS), issued a Notice of Proposed Rulemaking for a regulation governing the operation of the OPTN. Although the public comment period was supposed to end in December 1994, the department continued to accept comments on the OPTN's operations and its policies for allocating organs.[6] Two years later, in November 1996, the department officially extended the period for public comment on the proposed rule, due to controversy over revisions in the liver allocation policies being proposed by the OPTN's board.[7] Even after HRSA published the OPTN Final Rule on April 2, 1998,[8] Congress twice delayed its going into effect.[9] HRSA finally implemented the Final Rule on March 6, 2000.[10] The OPTN board is composed of transplant physicians, recipients, candidates, family members, deceased donor families, recipient families, living donors, transplant hospitals, OPO representatives, and members of the public who are organized into various committees that are delegated with policy-making authority. In establishing the OPTN's regulatory framework, the rule instructs its board of directors to draft policies "based

---

[2] Organ Transplantation: Issues and Recommendations: Report of the Task Force on Organ Transplantation. Rockville, MD: U.S. Dept. of Health & Human Services, Public Health Service, Health Resources and Services Administration, Office of Organ Transplantation (1986), at 91.

[3] Transplant Amendments of 1990, P. L. 101-616, Title II, § 202, now codified at 42 U.S.C. 274(b)(2)(D).

[4] P. L. 99-509 (1986).

[5] P. L. 100-607 (1988).

[6] 59 Federal Register 46482 (1994), https://www.govinfo.gov/content/pkg/FR-1994-09-08/html/94-21993-2.htm (accessed February 3, 2022).

[7] 61 Federal Register 58158 (1996), https://www.govinfo.gov/content/pkg/FR-1996-11-13/pdf/96-29145.pdf (accessed February 3, 2022).

[8] 63 Federal Register 16296 (1998), https://www.federalregister.gov/documents/1998/04/02/98-8191/organ-procurement-and-transplantation-network (accessed February 3, 2022).

[9] Ticket to Work and Work Incentives Act, P. L. 106-170, §413 (1998); 1999 Consolidated Appropriations Act, P. L. 106-113 (1999).

[10] https://optn.transplant.hrsa.gov/about/final-rule (accessed February 3, 2022).

on sound medical judgment...to achieve the best use of donated organs"[11] and gives the board discretion to develop and implement these policies. But, in accordance with congressional enactments, the Final Rule also states that the Secretary of HHS must approve "significant" policies promulgated by the OPTN, such as the allocation rules for each type of organ, before they become federally enforceable.[12] OPOs, hospitals, and other entities that are members of the OPTN are expected to adhere voluntarily to the policies and bylaws adopted by the board to govern the OPTN's internal operations. These internal policies do not go through the process of Secretarial approval and are therefore not deemed to be federal rules.

## COMPLEXITY OF THE CURRENT ORGAN TRANSPLANTATION SYSTEM

"We have to make our processes more nimble. I think everyone in this system, no matter who we represent, are all extremely well intentioned. But, when we get it wrong, we have to own it and do better."

—Jayme Locke, University of Alabama at Birmingham,
testimony to the committee during July 15, 2021
public listening session

The current organ transplantation system in the United States is a complex web with multiple entities involved in various aspects of making and implementing policies, gathering data, and providing oversight. This web includes multiple agencies within HHS, including HRSA, the Centers for Medicare & Medicaid Services (CMS), Centers for Disease Control and Prevention, the Food and Drug Administration, and the National Institutes of Health. In addition, NOTA created the OPTN as an independent entity, and HRSA maintains two contracts: the OPTN and the Scientific Registry of Transplant Recipients (SRTR) to support the system (see Figure 2-1).

The OPTN is charged with developing policies for and implementing an equitable system of organ allocation, maintaining the waiting list of potential recipients, and compiling data from U.S. transplant centers. OPOs and transplant centers certified for participation in Medicare are required to participate in the OPTN. The OPTN's oversight responsibilities include solid organ donation and transplantation from deceased donors, but also include ancillary activities on living organ donation. UNOS, a nonprofit, private voluntary organization, holds the subcontract for the OPTN and has been the sole administrator of the OPTN since the initial contract was awarded by HRSA in 1986.[13]

Oversight for the OPTN contract is provided by the Division of Transplantation (DoT) in HRSA, part of HHS. DoT also administers the contract for the SRTR that provides analytical support for the OPTN's evaluation of existing allocation policies and development of new policies. For the past 12 years, the SRTR contract has been held by the Hennepin Healthcare Research Institute's Chronic Disease Research Group, which uses the data collected by the OPTN to provide HRSA with the OPTN/SRTR Annual Data Report. Section 373 of the Public

---

[11] Organ Procurement and Transplantation Network Final Rule, 42 C.F.R. §121. The current version of the Final Rule can be viewed at https://www.ecfr.gov/current/title-42/chapter-I/subchapter-K/part-121 (accessed February 3, 2022).

[12] Organ Procurement and Transplantation Network Final Rule, 42 C.F.R. § 121. The current version of the Final Rule can be viewed at https://www.ecfr.gov/current/title-42/chapter-I/subchapter-K/part-121 (accessed February 3, 2022).

[13] The OPTN board of directors are elected and simultaneously installed as UNOS Corporate Board of Directors Members, resulting in identical board memberships. However, UNOS and the OPTN are not interchangeable: UNOS is a nonprofit corporation; the OPTN is a nongovernmental body, established by law, comprised of volunteers, professionals, and other stakeholders involved in the donation and transplantation system and operated under federal contract.

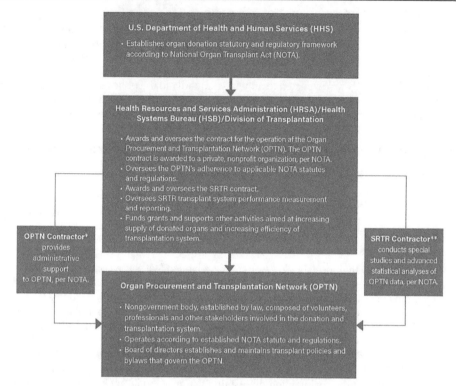

**FIGURE 2-1** Relationship between HHS, HRSA, the OPTN, the OPTN contractors, and SRTR contractors.
NOTES: HHS = Department of Health and Human Services; NOTA = National Organ Transplant Act.
*United Network for Organ Sharing (UNOS) is the current OPTN contractor. **Hennepin Healthcare Research Institute (HHRI) is the current Scientific Registry of Transplant Recipients (SRTR) contractor. The Health Resources and Services Administration (HRSA) acts as a liaison connecting the overlapping efforts of both contractors.
SOURCE: HRSA. Provided by Frank Holloman, January 31, 2022.

Health Service Act requires the SRTR operator to support ongoing evaluation of the scientific and clinical status of solid organ transplantation. It aims to present its data and analytical results in a way that facilitates their use by all constituencies in the organ transplantation community (SRTR, 2022).

The HHS Advisory Committee on Organ Transplantation (ACOT) has advised the HHS secretary on (1) enhancing organ donation, (2) ensuring that the system of organ transplantation is grounded in the best available medical science, (3) assuring the public that the system is as effective and equitable as possible, and (4) increasing public confidence in the integrity and effectiveness of the transplantation system (HRSA, 2021a). ACOT has been sporadically active since 2004. During the April 2020 ACOT meeting, recommendations were made to the HHS secretary on reexamining impediments to transplants for HIV-positive patients through the HIV Organ Policy Equity (HOPE) Act and improving testing with respect to the microbiological evaluation of organ donors and transplants (HRSA, 2021b).

## NATIONAL GOALS TO DRIVE SYSTEMATIC IMPROVEMENT

A range of federal and nonfederal actors oversees the current organ transplantation system, resulting in a complex web of responsibilities and accountabilities across stakeholders. This committee carefully considered opportunities for the federal government to set clear goals for the organ transplantation system in terms of equity and quality. The following section considers the significant successes of national efforts to improve health care quality and patient safety and sets the stage for the committee's recommendation that HHS should set national performance goals for the U.S. organ transplantation system (Recommendation 1).

Establishing clear goals at an appropriate scale is fundamental to successful quality improvement (Alyesh, 2021). For example, bold goals implemented at the national scale previously resulted in significant national increases in hospital patient safety. The IOM landmark 1999 report, *To Err Is Human*, estimated that there were between 44,000 and 98,000 deaths annually in U.S. hospitals due to medical errors (IOM, 2000). The report precipitated national, statewide, and organization-specific activities to improve patient safety, including the Institute for Healthcare Improvement 100,000 Lives Campaign, concerted and successful efforts to improve hospital patient safety in the Veterans Hospital Administration, and more.

As part of this growing movement, then HHS Secretary Kathleen Sebelius, together with CMS Administrator Don Berwick and other national leaders, launched the Partnership for Patients initiative in 2010. The partnership was grounded in a bold national goal to reduce preventable harm in all U.S. hospitals by 40 percent by 2014 (CMS, 2011). According to subsequent independent reviews by the Agency for Healthcare Research and Quality (AHRQ), safety improved in U.S. hospitals from the 2010 baseline year through 2014, resulting in 2.1 million fewer harms, an estimated 87,000 deaths prevented, and $19.9 billion in cost savings (AHRQ, 2016). U.S. hospitals achieved a 17 percent reduction in overall harm from the 2010 baseline, which equated to a 39 percent reduction in preventable harm. Based on the success of the initial 4-year Partnership for Patients initiative, CMS has continued to support hospital quality improvement in patient safety through the present.

AHRQ estimates of sustained national reductions in hospital harm rates through 2017 are summarized below in Figure 2-2 (AHRQ, 2016, 2020). The harm rate has gone from 145 harms per thousand discharges in the 2010 baseline year to 86 harms per thousand discharges in 2017. Two values are reported for 2014 to permit comparisons of rates that reflect an adjustment in AHRQ's standardized methodology for tracking hospital harm.

Bold goals implemented at the national scale also resulted in previous major national improvements in organ donation (Shafer et al., 2006). In April 2003, then HHS Secretary Tommy Thompson joined with national leaders from the Institute for Healthcare Improvement, the American Society for Minority Health and Transplant Professionals, the Association of Organ Procurement Organizations, and others to formally commit to achieving an ambitious target of a 75 percent organ donation rate in the nation's 500 largest hospitals through a Contract for Results. The goal was established based on data showing that about 15 of the nation's 200 largest trauma centers had already been able to achieve a donation rate greater than 70 percent (Shafer et al., 2006). These high-performing hospitals constituted 5 percent of the total large trauma centers targeted by the quality improvement initiative. Over the course of the next several years, all 59 of the nation's OPOs, together with many of their largest hospitals, jointly engaged in a massive quality improvement effort to learn, test, adapt, and spread the best practices of the large trauma centers and OPOs with high donation rates. This effort resulted in major increases in the numbers of the nation's largest hospitals who achieved the 75 percent donation rate goal and major increases in overall donation rates

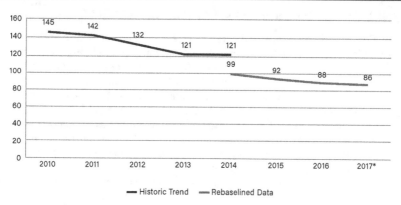

**FIGURE 2-2** Hospital-acquired conditions rate per 1,000 hospital discharges, United States, 2010–2017. SOURCE: AHRQ, 2020. AHRQ National Scorecard on Hospital-Acquired Conditions: Final Results for 2014 Through 2017.

(Shafer et al., 2006). In 2005, HRSA and HHS formally recognized teams from 184 of the nation's 500 largest hospitals and their affiliated OPOs who had achieved the 75 percent donation rate (HHS, 2005). In 2006 and 2007, 371 and 392 hospitals were recognized for achieving this rate, respectively. HHS continued various forms of recognition for increased organ donation and transplantation yield through at least 2009.

As part of this same quality improvement effort, in January 2004 HHS set an additional national goal, increasing the proportion of deceased donors whose deaths have been determined based on loss of circulatory function to 10 percent of the total. At that time, only about 4 percent of total deceased donors organs came from DCDD and only a handful of OPOs were implementing the DCDD protocol. The organ donation community of practice (i.e., donor hospitals and OPOs) achieved the 10 percent DCDD threshold in 2007. Growth in DCDD has continued since then: in 2021 approximately 30 percent of all deceased donors came from DCDD donors (4,187 DCDD donors out of the total 13,861 deceased organ donors in 2021) (OPTN, 2022).

## Approach to Establishing Ambitious Goals

In all three of the cases outlined above, the goals established by HHS were extremely ambitious, but they were also grounded in the proven practices and outcome levels already achieved by the highest performers in the system. The quality improvement goal on donation was established using the levels of performance achieved by the top 5 to 10 percent of organizations (e.g., 5 percent of the 500 largest trauma centers). After 4 years of intensive quality improvement, nearly 80 percent (392) of the 500 largest trauma hospitals in the nation were recognized by HHS for achieving the 75 percent donation rate target.

The 2003–2004 goal that 10 percent of deceased donors originate with DCDD was achieved in a similar 4-year time frame, representing a more than double increase from the original 4 percent national rate in 2003. At that time, few OPOs were pursuing DCDD donors, and only 6 of the 59 had achieved a rate where 10 percent or more of their deceased donors came from DCDD.[14] In both of these organ donation and transplant cases, and in

---

[14] https://optn.transplant.hrsa.gov/data/view-data-reports/national-data (accessed November 5, 2021).

the case of the national patient safety goal of a 40 percent reduction in preventable hospital harm within 4 years, HHS successfully used ambitious time-limited goals to substantially increase the overall performance of the system, based on the proven practices and the levels of achievement of the highest performers in the system.

When establishing ambitious goals of this nature, it is important to be mindful of potential unintended consequences. For example, in establishing a goal to increase the percentage of deceased donors coming from DCDD, it is often useful to incorporate balancing measures to ensure that the total numbers of donors coming from donation after neurological determination of death (DNDD) do not drop as a result of the ambitious DCDD goal. In recommending ambitious goals like those outlined in this report, it is the intention of the committee that the goals be pursued and obtained in ways that represent meaningful progress and true effects that benefit the patients we all serve, not as a result of gaming or manipulation of data (HRSA, 2018).

The goals recommended in this report are as ambitious as each of the prior examples detailed above. Achieving the recommended targets outlined in this report will require commitment, persistence, and focused attention to learning, testing, spread, and improvement of known best practices that are already being used by the highest performers in the system.

*Conclusion 2-1: The current organ transplantation system is unduly fragmented and inefficient. The system's component parts—physicians caring for patients with organ failure, donor hospitals, organ procurement organizations, the OPTN, transplant centers, the SRTR, CMS and other payers, among others—do not operate as a fully integrated system. Likewise, the entities with oversight responsibilities each oversee particular components, but none monitors the performance of the system as a whole in producing predictable, consistent, and equitable results.*

*Conclusion 2-2: The organ transplantation system could save additional lives and be more equitable if its component parts functioned in a more cohesive fashion and were overseen by a single entity, or by several entities operating in a coordinated fashion with common goals and unified policies and processes. Such alignment of all components and oversight responsibilities would allow the public and Congress to ascertain whether the system is fairly and efficiently maximizing the benefits provided by organ donation and transplantation.*

*Conclusion 2-3: Since deceased donor organs are a national resource, the fairest way to allocate them to patients on the waiting list is on a national, continuous basis, in accordance with the OPTN Final Rule 2000 as most recently revised by HHS. The committee recognizes that some members of the transplant community feel strongly that deceased donor organs procured in a particular geographic area should be retained for allocation to wait-listed patients in that area.*

*Conclusion 2-4: By setting ambitious goals in its prior quality improvement initiatives in organ transplantation, HHS has achieved significant progress in increasing the number of successful transplants performed nationally.*

**Recommendation 1: Develop national performance goals for the U.S. organ transplantation system.**

HHS should identify and substantially reduce or eliminate the existing variations among donor hospitals, OPOs, and transplant centers in the rates of organ donation,

DCDD procurement and transplantation, acceptance of offered organs, and nonuse of donated organs, to improve the quality of, and foster greater equity in, organ donation and transplantation. HHS should also use the proven capabilities of the highest-performing donor hospitals, OPOs, and transplant centers to establish bold goals to drive national progress toward greater equity, higher rates of organ donation, procurement and transplantation of organs from donors after circulatory determination of death, and acceptance of offered organs, along with lower rates of nonuse of donated organs, to increase the total number of organs procured and transplants performed.

These goals can inform the development and use of various levers of influence including organized programs of quality improvement, payment policies, regulations, technical assistance, and public education campaigns. The goals should be continuously reviewed (at least annually) and updated as results are obtained, and as new, higher levels of organizational performance are achieved. HHS should

- Build on the initial CMS goals established in the kidney transplant collaborative, and establish a national goal for all transplant centers to reduce donated kidney nonuse rates to 5 percent or less.
- Establish new national goals to do the following:
  - Improve donation among minority populations and disadvantaged populations, and increase transplantation rates among minority and disadvantaged populations, based on the proven practices of donor hospitals, OPOs, and transplant centers which have the highest rates in these areas.
  - Increase the number of organs procured from medically complex donors. In particular, increase DCDD donors to at least 45 percent of all deceased donors, with no reductions in the numbers of organs procured from donors from neurological determination of death.
  - Improve offer acceptance levels for each organ type to those achieved by the 5 to 10 percent highest-performing transplant centers for that organ type nationally.
  - Increase the number of transplants to at least 50,000 by 2026.

## Current OPTN Policy Development Process

The OPTN's current policy development process is lengthy and complex (see Figure 2-3).

### *Overview of Policy Development Steps*

The OPTN's policy development process begins with a proposal process informed by first gathering information from a variety of sources and stakeholders via the existing OPTN committee structure. UNOS staff leaders and the OPTN committee leadership review proposals and prioritize those that offer the greatest potential benefit for the transplant community, best align with the OPTN's strategic goals, and are within the legal and regulatory authority of the OPTN. Before proposals are released for public comment, a HRSA review for compliance is conducted. Proposals developed by committees are approved for public comment release following review by HRSA and the OPTN Board or Executive committee,[15] after

---

[15] Before the public comment period is approved, proposals are reviewed by HRSA to determine if the proposal is within the legal, regulatory, and contractual authority of the OPTN and the OPTN Policy Oversight Committee to ensure that the project engages the appropriate stakeholders and provides solutions tailored to the problem, as well as determining whether it imposes any significant fiscal burdens on the transplantation system.

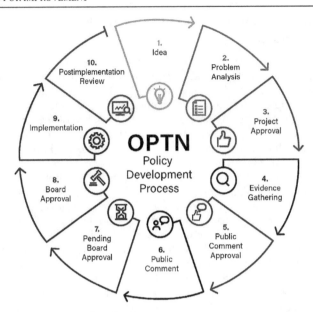

**FIGURE 2-3** The OPTN 10-step policy development process.
SOURCE: OPTN policy development process explanatory document. https://optn.transplant.hrsa.gov/media/3115/optn-policy-development-process-explanatory-document.pdf (accessed November 18, 2021).

which the arguments and concerns expressed by stakeholders are reviewed to ensure that all relevant constituencies and demographics are well represented. The sponsoring committee reviews the public comments, revises the proposal if needed (which may be subject to another round of public comments), and then votes on whether to send the policy proposal to the Board.[16] The Board considers the committees' recommended policy proposals, and receives input from Board policy groups, which are subgroups of the Board that provide initial review as part of the Board review process, consisting of stakeholders representing transplant programs, OPOs, living donors, donor families, and members with specific policy-relevant competencies. The Board policy group review is an operational process; only the OPTN Board approves policies.

To approve a policy, the Board requires evidence that the proposal addresses the stated problem, complies with NOTA and the Final Rule, and is aligned with the OPTN strategic plan. Rejected proposals are returned to the appropriate committee for further consideration. When the board adopts a policy proposal, it is officially designated as the "OPTN policy." UNOS staff regularly review the effectiveness and potentially negative effects of implemented policies by collecting and analyzing relevant data, then report their findings to the board and the sponsoring committees. These continuous review activities may result in new projects to further refine a policy. Similarly, the Membership and Professional Standards Committee's monitoring of member compliance with policies may also lead to new policy projects.

---

[16] During this time, UNOS staff also prepares an estimate of the resources that the OPTN will need to implement and maintain the new policy, including the costs of monitoring member compliance, as well as a review by subject matter experts of the proposal's fiscal effect on the OPTN members.

## Advantages and Disadvantages of the OPTN Policy Development Approach

The OPTN's current policy development process has advantages and disadvantages. Its advantages include transparency, collaboration, and centralization. For instance, to ensure ample stakeholder involvement throughout the policy development process, multiple stakeholder individuals and organizations are encouraged to collaborate with the responsible OPTN committee(s) in the development of national transplant policies and medical criteria. During the public comment period feedback is solicited from those closely aligned within the organ transplantation system, and most importantly, the overall public who are outside the system. Following the close of the public comment period, the relevant OPTN committee addresses the issues raised by publishing written responses. Stakeholder and public engagement with the policy-making process is an advantage of the OPTN approach, providing important feedback and direction for policy-making and strengthening public trust in the process. A recent change was made to enhance the role of the Policy Oversight Committee, which is responsible for harmonizing and prioritizing policy-making work and timelines across OPTN committees. Additionally, centralized rulemaking enables OPTN policy makers to focus on a set of predetermined policy objectives.[2]

The disadvantages of the process relate to its length, complexity, and challenges in implementation. Because the OPTN's rulemaking process seeks engagement and input from a broad range of passionate stakeholders, the policy process requires multiple committee reviews to avoid possible unintended consequences across the OPTN. Although rare, additional public comment periods may also be necessary if substantial policy revisions are made as a result of public comment. As an operating committee of the OPTN, the Policy Oversight Committee advises the OPTN Board of Directors and Executive Committee in the development of strategic policy priorities, prioritization and coordination of policy and committee projects with broad implications for the OPTN, evaluation of policy and committee proposals prior to public comment, assessment of the impact of proposed policies, and confirmation that the OPTN committees justify proposals in compliance with policy development requirements. The Policy Oversight Committee has helped to avoid situations in which committee projects are placed on hold and started again, sometimes multiple times. The consensus-driven nature of the OPTN policy development process can create slowness and policy implementation challenges can further delay the process, such as when stakeholders are in disagreement about how best to allocate organs and categorize patient prioritization on the waiting list. Recently, this already lengthy process has been further exacerbated by litigation.[17]

The steps in the OPTN policy-making process are also complex and variable in the time allotted for public comment periods, as well as the overall time taken from committee project approval to OPTN board approval. For example, a federal study of the similarities and differences in the processes the OPTN used to change the liver and lung allocation policies revealed variations in public comment periods for informing the policy development process. The current liver allocation policy included a 25-day public comment period; the 2017 liver allocation policy included two separate 62-day and 64-day public comment periods; and the current lung allocation policy had a retroactive 61-day public comment period (GAO,

---

[17] An April 2019 press release posted to the OPTN website explained that "implementation of both the liver and intestinal organ distribution policy based on acuity circles and the National Liver Review Board (NLRB) will be deferred" as a result of a pending federal lawsuit challenging this new OPTN-approved liver distribution policy, which had been under development for years. https://optn.transplant.hrsa.gov/news/liver-distribution-policy-nlrb-implementation-deferred-until-may-14 (accessed April 12, 2022).

2020). Significant variability exists in terms of the average time it takes from committee project approval to final board approval. For example, as presented during the virtual public session of the OPTN's December 6, 2021, Board meeting,[18] between 2009 and 2021 the longest period of policy development was 9.6 years for the revised kidney allocation system in 2013 (see Figure 2-4). A project on liver distribution redesign modeling in 2017 took 6.4 years from committee project approval to board approval. Since 2019, project timelines have shown a downward trend with the 2021 continuous distribution policy for lungs taking 2.6 years. Implementation time for each policy was not included in the presented analysis.

There is limited information and analyses of the overall performance of the policy-making process in meeting the stated goals of the OPTN. Based on the evidence of variability in overall OPTN policy development timelines and challenges in maintaining stakeholder agreement on contentious issues in patient prioritization and organ allocation, the committee believes there is an opportunity for the OPTN to draw on previously untapped external organizations with expertise in managing complex stakeholder involvement through a transparent and collaborative process.

> *Conclusion 2-5: The OPTN policy-making process includes extensive committee reviews that aim to involve all stakeholders, but the nature of the reviews contributes to variability and a general slowness in policy development and implementation. Identifying and prioritizing strategic objectives through process changes in committee responsibilities and implementing continuous distribution as the uniform policy model have been effective in the last 2 years in decreasing the time for policy approval by the OPTN Board of Directors; however, opportunities for improvement in policy development and implementation timelines exist.*

---

[18] https://unos.org/news/optn-board-adopts-new-transplant-program-performance-metrics (accessed January 26, 2022).

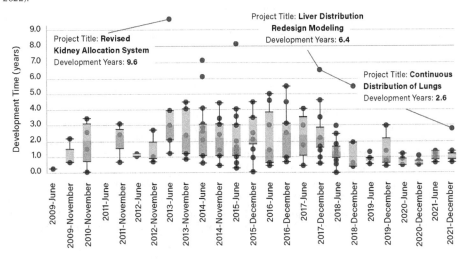

**FIGURE 2-4** Average time from committee project approval to board approval.
SOURCE: "OPTN Contract Requirement 3.3.2.: Policy Development Process Metrics – Metric 9: Average Time from Committee Project Approval to Board Approval." OPTN Policy Oversight Committee Chair Report to the OPTN Board of Directors. 6 December 2021. Provided by: Chelsea Haynes, UNOS.

*Conclusion 2-6: Organizations such as the National Quality Forum (NQF) are skilled in the development and use of timely, multistakeholder, consensus-based developmental processes, like the Measure Applications Partnership (MAP). The work of the NQF MAP is tied to, and guided by, specific regulatory and payment timelines of participating HHS agencies and their associated rulemaking processes. The experience and expertise of the NQF and/or other similar organizations can provide valuable insights to inform improvements in speed and agility, as well as stakeholder engagement and consensus of OPTN policy development work.*

**Recommendation 2: Improve the OPTN policy-making process.**

**HHS should hold the OPTN and HRSA accountable for developing a more expedient and responsive policy-making process including increasing racial, ethnic, professional, and gender diversity on the boards and committees responsible for developing OPTN policies. HHS should use the agreed on policy priorities established by the OPTN Policy Oversight Committee to establish contractual deadlines for completion of these policy-making priorities. HHS should consider requiring the OPTN to work with and receive support from an external organization, such as the NQF or the National Academy of Public Administration, with expertise in guiding federal programs through unique challenges in leadership and stakeholder collaboration. HHS should require the OPTN to consider the following elements of the policy-making process:**

- Proven approaches by others, such as the NQF Measure Applications Partnership, for meeting aggressive timelines with intensive, consensus-based, multistakeholder policy development processes;
- Optimal board size and stakeholder balance;
- Continuous and concurrent versus sequential policy-making processes;
- Managing strategic priorities and ensuring priority items have sufficient momentum, institutional memory, and timelines;
- Alternative governance models; and
- Appropriate tools and processes for evaluating the effectiveness of the policy-making process.

## DECEASED DONOR ORGAN USE AND ECONOMICS TODAY[19]

This section briefly summarizes data and trends pertaining to deceased donor organ use that are relevant to the committee's charge, including statistics on wait-listing (see Table 2-1), deceased organ donation, transplantation, and resource use metrics such as initial hospital length of stay and hospital readmission rates. Although the organ system writ large is greatly affected by living donor donation, this study's scope is limited to deceased donation after brain death or circulatory death. Living donation has the potential to increase the number of organs available for transplantation, shorten waiting times, improve morbidity, improve quality of life, and address inequity and unfairness in distribution systems (Gruessner and Gruessner, 2018; Humar et al., 2019; Kazley et al., 2019; Levy et al., 2016; Mathur et al.,

---

[19] This section draws heavily from the 2019 SRTR/OPTN Annual Data Report (released February 2021). The 2019 SRTR/OPTN Annual Data Report includes data from 2008–2019 and was the most recent summary publication available at the time this committee's report was published. Wherever possible, the committee uses 2021 data on the number of individuals on the waiting list and the number of transplants performed from the OPTN website: https://optn.transplant.hrsa.gov/data (accessed January 26, 2022).

**TABLE 2-1** Overview of Waiting Lists and Transplants from Living and Deceased Organ Donors in the United States (2021)

| | U.S. waiting list candidates (n) | Living donor organ transplants in 2021 | Deceased donor organ transplants in 2021 |
|---|---|---|---|
| Kidney | 90,293 | 5,970 | 18,699 |
| Pancreas | 838 | 0 | 143 |
| Liver | 11,489 | 569 | 8,667 |
| Intestine | 201 | 0 | 96 |
| Heart | 3,458 | 0 | 3,817 |
| Lung | 1,055 | 0 | 2,524 |
| Kidney / Pancreas | 1,815 | 0 | 820 |
| Heart / Lung | 35 | N/A | 45 |

SOURCE: OPTN https://optn.transplant.hrsa.gov/data/view-data-reports/national-data (accessed January 25, 2022). U.S. waiting list candidates for each organ as of February 1, 2022. Total waiting list candidates are 106,557; organ totals are less than the sum because of patients in multiple categories. Living donor and deceased donor organ transplants are totals for 2021.

2020; Pena, 2016; UNOS, 2021). Neither tissue transplantation nor vascularized composite allotransplantation were a significant focus of the committee.

The nonuse rates provided for each organ, which are based on the number of organs recovered for transplant but not transplanted, are particularly important in informing efforts to optimize the use of deceased donor organs (Figure 2-5). Over the past decade in the United States, there have been increases in the numbers of both deceased organ donors and deceased donor organ transplants, which reached all-time highs of 13,861 and 41,354 in 2021, respectively (OPTN, 2022). However, the percentage of organs recovered for transplant but not transplanted has continued in an upward trend. For each type of organ, the rates of nonuse also increased in 2019 over 2018 (Figure 2-5). In addition to issues of organ nonuse, some argue that after controlling for the impact of public health crises and trends, organ donation rates have not kept pace with population growth, as they should (Karp et al., 2021).

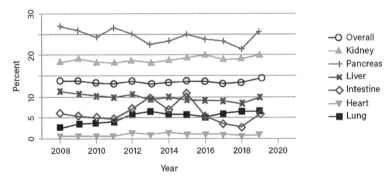

**FIGURE 2-5** Organs recovered for transplant and not transplanted (2019).
NOTE: Percentages are calculated as the difference between the number of organs recovered and the number of organs transplanted, divided by the number of organs recovered. Pancreata recovered for islet transplant are excluded.
SOURCE: Israni et al., 2021.

## Vascularized Composite Allotransplantation

Vascularized composite allotransplantation (VCA) is a form of solid organ transplantation involving the transplantation of multiple structures that may include skin, bone, muscles, blood vessels, nerves, and connective tissue as a functional unit in patients with major tissue loss or injury. A VCA may provide an alternative treatment option when reconstructive surgery is not feasible or effective. VCA transplants are performed to improve functional outcomes and quality of life and thus intend to be life enhancing, and are not considered lifesaving. For example, some recipients received a VCA organ after traumatic injury or limb loss through trauma (e.g., war-related exposure to explosive devices or traffic accidents).

In the United States, the first unilateral upper extremity transplant was performed in 1999. In the past decade, more than 90 individuals have received a VCA (American Society of Transplantation, 2021). HHS redefined VCAs as organs, as opposed to tissue, in 2014, which enabled the OPTN to assume oversight of policies pertaining to authorization for deceased donation, allocation, and distribution of VCA organs. CMS redefining VCA as an organ would allow increased alignment across performance metrics in the transplantation system. VCA transplants include upper extremity, face, uterus, penis, larynx, abdominal wall, and others. Most VCA organs are donated by deceased donors; however, uterus donors may also be living donors.

The field of VCA is growing. The surgical procedures themselves are generally no longer construed as experimental procedures, considering the mastery of microsurgical techniques and immunosuppressive approaches have placed reconstructive surgery at the highest rung in the surgical ladder (Cetrulo et al., 2017; Kaufman et al., 2019). However, the determination of whether VCA is a standard of care is a complex matter. Some countries consider certain forms of VCA as being a standard of care (Kaufman et al., 2019).

In the United States, all transplant programs have traditionally been required to obtain institutional review board (IRB) oversight to perform VCA. However, some VCA programs are no longer functioning under IRB oversight. Currently, VCA costs are covered by transplant programs. Insurance companies do not currently pay for VCA because they view VCA as not being the standard of care. A major challenge to becoming a standard of care is the small number of patients undergoing each type of VCA procedure. Without enough information on long-term functional outcomes among enough recipients to control for demographic and clinical variables, it is unclear whether the procedure is effective and worth the risks (ethically) and resources (financially). Insurance companies are awaiting long-term outcomes data before covering these procedures.

For reasons delineated, the broad scope of the study task and the limited time frame for this study, the committee did not conduct an in-depth analysis of VCA transplantation. The committee considered the implications that increased use of VCA could have on organ donation including some of the challenges that may arise as the public increasingly confronts difficult questions of whether they, as individuals, would approve donation of their organs (e.g., face, uterus, or penis) upon their death. Public opinion is generally supportive of VCA donations from deceased donors (Rodrigue et al., 2017); however, given the limitations of educational materials on VCA (Rasmussen et al., 2020), the transplant community will need to develop efforts to educate the public about how to make informed decisions about donating VCA organs and explain how VCA organs will be procured and used.

# Key Use Statistics and Trends by Organ[20]

The landscape of kidney transplantation in the United States is characterized by promising trends and ongoing challenges. The overall number of kidney transplants has continued to increase over the past 6 years, reaching 24,273 in 2019—more than 70 percent of which were deceased donor organ transplants. However, the number of available donor kidneys is far surpassed by the number of patients awaiting kidney transplant, and the extent of the shortage is far greater than other organs. From 2014 to 2019, only approximately 25 percent of patients on the waiting list received a deceased donor kidney transplant within 5 years, and this varies significantly based on donation service area—from 15.5 to 67.8 percent. In 2019, the nonuse rate for deceased donor kidneys was 20.1 percent overall (Israni et al., 2021). As will be described in Chapter 6, the probability of receiving a deceased donor kidney transplant within 3 years of waiting list placement varies across transplant centers in the United States, with 16-fold variance between centers. Waiting patients at transplant centers with low offer acceptance rates have only a 4 percent chance of getting a transplant within 3 years. Conversely, patients waiting at transplant centers with high offer acceptance rates have a 65 percent chance of getting a transplant within 3 years (King et al., 2020).

Of note, the rate of nonuse of hepatitis C virus (HCV)-positive kidneys has been declining since 2014 and by 2019, the rate was nearly equivalent to that of HCV-antibody-negative kidneys. In terms of resource use, the average length of hospital stay after transplant for kidney recipients was 7.4 days in 2019, a slight decline since 2008. The rate of reported hospital readmission during the first year posttransplant was 48.1 percent in 2018.

More than 1,000 pancreas-alone and kidney-pancreas transplants were performed in 2019—a number that remained relatively stable compared to 2018, as did the number of wait-listed patients awaiting transplant. The number of deceased organ pancreas transplants has increased marginally since the 2014 revision of the Pancreas/Kidney-Pancreas Allocation System. However, a concerning issue is the high rate of nonuse for deceased donor pancreata—25.4 percent in 2019—compared to other organs; this may be related to relatively short pancreas transplant wait times and the current state of the art for pancreas transplantation. For pancreas recipients, the average length of transplant hospitalization in 2019 was 11.5 days and the rate of hospital readmission during the first year posttransplant was almost 62 percent; both of these have declined in recent years.

Almost 8,900 liver transplants were performed in 2019, 94 percent of which were deceased donor transplants. HCV-positive donor organs have continued to increase since 2008, representing 9.7 percent of deceased donor livers in 2019. Both the number of new waiting list registrations and the number of transplants performed have been on the rise, while both the median waiting time for candidates with a Model for End-Stage Liver Disease (MELD) score of 15–34 and the number of transplants performed for patients with exception points decreased.[21] The nonuse rate for deceased donor livers was 9.6 percent in 2019 compared to 8.6 percent in 2018, likely driven by an increase in nonused organs from donors aged 55 years or more. For liver recipients, the average length of transplant hospitalization in 2019 was 20.8 days and the rate of hospital readmission during the first year posttransplant

---

[20] This section reflects information in the 2019 SRTR/OPTN Annual Data Report (https://www.srtr.org/reports/srtroptn-annual-data-report [accessed January 26, 2022]) which was the most recent summary publication available at the time this committee's report was published.

[21] These changes may have been related to the policy changes that took effect in May 2019, which increased waiting list priority for candidates without exception status.

was almost 60 percent among those who received a transplant in 2018; both of these have remained relatively stable since 2008.

Intestine transplants represent the smallest proportion of solid organ transplants performed in the United States.[22] Intestine transplantation is a maturing field, and advances in intestine failure therapies have resulted in fewer patients being added to the waiting list for intestine transplant alone or for intestine transplant in combination with other organs. Just 81 deceased donor intestine transplants were performed in 2019. The nonuse rate for deceased donor intestines was relatively low, at about 6 percent. For intestine recipients, average length of transplant hospitalization in 2019 was about 61 days, which has varied substantially over the past decade. The rate of hospital readmission during the first year posttransplant was almost 96 percent among those who received a transplant in 2018—far higher than any other organ.

Around 3,600 heart transplants were performed in 2019—a slight increase over the previous year—but the number of candidates on the waiting list continued to increase.[23] The number of donor hearts increased by almost 64 percent between 2008 and 2019, when the number reached an all-time peak. The nonuse rate for deceased donor hearts was less than 1 percent, the lowest of all organs, although this rate has fluctuated over the past decade. For heart recipients, the average length of transplant hospitalization in 2019 was about 49 days, trending upward in recent years. The use of some preoperative devices or days of requiring extracorporeal membrane oxygenation as a bridge to transplantation could account for the lengthier hospital stay for some heart transplant recipients. Heart transplant patients without these interventions have much shorter hospital stays (e.g., less than 10 days). The rate of hospital readmission during the first year posttransplant was just under 40 percent, which was also the lowest rate of all organs.

The number of lung transplants performed each year in the United States is continuing to rise, increasing by 52.3 percent over the past decade and reaching an all-time peak of almost 2,800 transplants in 2019. This trend is likely attributable to increasing numbers of wait-listed candidates as well as the number of donors, which has increased by 62 percent in the last 10 years. The mortality rate for individuals on the lung waiting list decreased 14.6 percent in 2019, which is an important positive trend given the increasingly older and sicker lung candidate population. The nonuse rate for deceased donor lungs was more than 6 percent in 2019. For lung recipients, average length of transplant hospitalization in 2019 was around 34 days, which has generally increased in recent years. The rate of hospital readmission during the first year posttransplant was close to 52 percent.

From 2013 to 2017, 8,246 multiorgan transplants (MOTs) were performed in the United States, with 1,853 occurring in 2017 (OPTN, 2019). The most frequent type of MOT across this 4-year period were kidney–pancreas, kidney–liver, and kidney–heart, respectively. Additionally, the rate of MOT has been increasing over the last 2 decades (OPTN, 2019). MOTs, however, create issues of inequities, given that each combination of organs has its own allocation strategies and prioritization of those awaiting a MOT has not been standardized across the different organs. For example, some organ combinations require a candidate to join a single, combined, or multiple organ waiting lists. Confusion has arisen because of the varying levels of OPO discretion regarding their ability to "choose which MOT combinations get allocated if there are multiple MOT combinations possible from the same donor" (OPTN, 2019). Additionally, across the United States the current prioritization according to Policy

---

[22] Intestine transplants may be performed alone, with a liver transplant, or as part of a multivisceral transplant including combinations of liver, stomach, pancreas, colon, spleen, and kidney.

[23] A new adult heart allocation policy was approved in 2016 and implemented in October 2018; 2019 data may illustrate early effects of this policy.

5.10: Allocation of Multi-Organ Combinations is that a MOT is typically prioritized above single organ transplant at the local level, which can also affect equity differently across the country depending on the volume of MOTs in the differing geographic areas.

## Cost-Effectiveness of Transplantation by Organ

This section provides an overview of recent studies that have estimated the cost-effectiveness of kidney, liver, heart, and lung transplantation. It should be noted that even though the *OPTN/SRTR's Annual Data Report* releases data suitable for use in cost-effectiveness modeling of solid organ transplantation, up-to-date cost-effectiveness studies are not always available for all organs. Although cost-effectiveness analyses provide important information, they are only one element among others guiding health policy. There is debate about methodological and ethical shortcomings of the "quality-adjusted life year" (QALY), the most typically used measure of health gains in cost-effectiveness assessments of medical interventions (Rand and Kesselheim, 2021).

## Cost-Effectiveness of Kidney Transplantation

Kidney transplantation is associated with a significant improvement in patient survival and quality of life across the spectrum of organ quality compared with maintenance dialysis (Axelrod et al., 2018; Massie et al., 2014; Whiting et al., 2000; Wolfe et al., 1999, 2009). Recent estimates (Axelrod et al., 2018) indicate that end-stage kidney disease (ESKD) patients who receive a living donor kidney transplantation (LDKT) or deceased donor kidney transplantation (DDKT) experience significantly longer expected survival than ESKD patients who receive dialysis therapy in terms of derived QALYs: 10 years with dialysis therapy, 4.03 QALYs; LDKT (human leukocyte antigen [HLA]-compatible, well-matched living donor [LD]), 6.34; LDKT (ABO-incompatible LD), 6.12; LDKT (HLA-incompatible LD), 5.47; DDKT (KDPI[24] < 85), 6.07; DDKT (Public Health Service [PHS] increased risk), 5.91; DDKT (KDPI > 85), 5.20. Kidney transplants are also the most cost-effective treatment for ESKD,[25] although the extent of the cost savings varies by quality of the donor organ.

Axelrod et al. (2018) estimate that from the payer's (i.e., Medicare's) perspective, low-to-moderate KDPI (≤ 85) DDKTs are cost saving over 10 years compared to dialysis ($49,017 vs. $72,476 per QALY), as are high-KDPI (> 85%) DDKT compared to dialysis ($63,531 vs. $72,476 per QALY). Despite the additional therapeutic procedures needed to facilitate complex transplants such as ABO-incompatible LDKT, they also represent cost savings ($59,564 per QALY) compared to remaining on dialysis. Compared to DDKT, HLA-compatible LDKT was more cost effective for compatible donors with up to three HLA mismatches ($39,939 per QALY) and for compatible donors with four to six HLA mismatches ($41,016 per QALY). Consistent patterns were found upon repeat analysis using a 20-year time horizon; all transplantation options resulted in cost-effectiveness ratios lower than the commonly cited willingness-to-pay threshold of $100,000 per QALY (Neumann et al., 2016).

---

[24] For deceased donor kidneys, the Kidney Donor Profile Index (KDPI) provides a measure of organ quality by summarizing the likelihood of graft failure after DDKT.

[25] Organ transplantation cost-effectiveness studies typically compare the cost of achieving one additional QALY between alternative treatments. A payer perspective is usually adopted, implying that direct medical care costs are considered. Direct health care cost comparisons, however, underestimate the potential overall societal benefit, which ought to include both the productivity gains from returning to employment and associated tax revenue, which are higher for transplant recipients. Held et al. (2016) estimate that the full value of a transplant to a patient on the waiting list is $937,000.

## Cost-Effectiveness of Liver Transplantation

Recent studies found liver transplantation to be cost effective (less than $100,000 per QALY). For instance, Dageforde et al. (2013)[26] studied the cost-effectiveness of liver transplantation with DNDD organs and DCDD organs by considering two waiting list strategies: (1) only DNDD organs and (2) both DNDD and DCDD organs (DNDD + DCDD). Over a 10-year horizon, the DNDD + DCDD waiting list strategy was more cost effective (5.6 QALYs; cost of $69,000/QALY) than the DNDD-alone strategy (6.0 QALYs; cost of $61,000/QALY) because of the decreased waiting list mortality and pretransplant morbidity associated with the former strategy.

In the United States, the current practice is for HCV-negative patients only to accept HCV-negative livers. Bethea et al. (2019) compared the cost-effectiveness of this current strategy versus a strategy of accepting any HCV-negative or HCV-positive livers, with recipients of HCV-positive livers receiving preemptive direct-acting antiviral therapy. For patients with a MELD score of 28,[27] it was cost effective for them to accept any liver. The incremental cost-effectiveness ratio of accepting any liver versus accepting only HCV-negative livers was $62,600/QALY. Incremental cost-effectiveness ratios of receiving any liver were less than $100,000 for patients with a MELD score of 22 or greater; the strategy was also cost effective for patients with low MELD scores that may not accurately reflect disease severity.

Sarasin et al. (2001) study found that in the United States, LDLT can be cost effective for patients with early hepatocellular carcinoma when waiting times for transplantation exceed 7 months.[28] A study using more recent data[29] found that over a 10-year period, both LDLT and deceased donor liver transplantation are cost effective compared to no transplant (i.e., medical management of cirrhosis) (Northup et al., 2009). Being on a waiting list with possible deceased donor liver transplant (DDLT) versus being on a waiting list with possible DDLT or LDLT were associated with 4.4 and 4.9 QALYs, respectively. The DDLT or LDLT strategy had an incremental cost-effectiveness ratio of $106,788 over DDLT only.

## Cost-Effectiveness of Heart Transplantation

The 2013 *OPTN/SRTR Economics Annual Data Report* presented a cost-effectiveness analysis of heart transplantation—the most expensive of the major transplants—that compared transplant recipients who had received a ventricular assist device (VAD) procedure with those who had not (Schnitzler et al., 2015). The total expected discounted cost of care from 1 year prior to the transplant through 20 years posttransplant was lower for a patient with a VAD ($505,000) than patients without a VAD ($525,000). However, patients with a VAD gained fewer discounted QALYs (5.53) than patients without a VAD (6.28). Thus, the cost per QALY was greater for patients with a VAD ($91,000) than those without a VAD ($84,000), although both are within the conventional willingness-to-pay threshold (less than $100,000).

---

[26] The study (Dageforde et al., 2013) adopted a societal perspective, including direct medical costs and indirect cost such as lost earnings and out-of-hospital expenses.

[27] The median MELD score at transplant centers in the United States (Bethea et al., 2019).

[28] For short waiting times, the gains from LDLT were only marginal and were outweighed by the losses in life-years caused by the donor operation.

[29] From the Adult to Adult Living Donor Liver Transplantation Cohort Study.

## Cost-Effectiveness of Lung Transplantation

Schnitzler et al. (2014) used Medicare data linked to SRTR data to examine the effect of allocation based on the lung allocation score (LAS) on the cost-effectiveness of a lung transplant compared with medical management of end-stage pulmonary disease, finding that the relative cost-effectiveness of a lung transplant is correlated with LAS. Specifically, incremental cost-effectiveness ratios—measuring additional costs per QALY gained from a transplant—increased with LAS. Even at the highest LAS scores, the cost-effectiveness of lung transplants is within the conventionally cited limits.[30]

> *Conclusion 2-7: Transplantation, independent of organ type, is a cost-effective intervention overall. Although SRTR has been releasing current data on pre- and posttransplant costs suitable for cost-effectiveness modeling, there is a need for up-to-date cost-effectiveness analyses for all organs to ensure that current data on effectiveness and costs are taken into account. There is debate about methodological and ethical shortcomings of cost-effectiveness analyses. In particular, cost-effectiveness may fail to capture features relevant to equity. Cost-effectiveness analyses are only one factor among others guiding health care policy choices.*

## INNOVATION CHALLENGES AND OPPORTUNITIES

Recommendations made in this report could change some of the OPTN's operations and processes; thus it is important to identify challenges related to innovation and consider how health care systems can evolve to improve. A robust understanding of health care delivery and innovation science can inform the profession with a specific focus on organ donation and transplantation. Nonetheless, it is a daunting task to change a massive and complicated system with multiple elements and complex interactions. With that in mind, the goal is to create a fairer, more equitable, cost-effective, and transparent system of donor organ procurement, allocation, and distribution.

One successful model for health care systems operationalizing and upscaling innovations is the Veterans Health Administration's Innovation Ecosystem (VHA IE), which is predicated on multiple pillars that are critical to support the development and implementation of the types of health care innovation suggested in this report (Vega and Kizer, 2020).

1. The target workforce must have the capacity to adopt and actualize any innovation.
2. The organization infrastructure and leadership must be integrated, practice systemness, and be able to develop repeatable procedures for change.
3. An engaging and supportive culture of innovation and resulting change is necessary.
4. Collaborations with strategic external partnerships are needed.
5. The infrastructure must align with financial resources and incentives, obtain clinical and administrative championship, and appropriate allocation of resources to enable change.

As part of this model's success, the various innovative health care delivery approaches initiated through the model positively affected more than a million caregivers and veterans, with over 25,000 employees participating, and resulted in $40 million in direct cost avoid-

---

[30] The cost of 1 QALY gained was $46,472 for LAS scores < 35, $73,053 for LAS scores between 35 and 50, and $103,448 for LAS scores > 50.

ance for the system. The success of the VHA IE approach to innovation, program evolution, and change deserves consideration for the OPTN, OPOs, and transplant centers in prioritizing innovation.

Of course, the complexities of the United States organ procurement and transplant enterprise are not the only challenges to innovative practice implementation and change. External pressures from a variety of professional, political, health care, insurance, and patient advocacy groups will likely present opposition to some suggested changes; these entities may also have their own agendas and recommendations.

While it is critical to improve organ recovery and organ use, addressing the organ shortage and improving the available organs for transplantation can be modified greatly through innovation. For example, the HOPE Act has provided increased transplantation opportunities for transplant candidates with HIV who are willing to accept organs from donors identified as HIV positive. Since the HOPE Act became law in 2013, 170 kidneys and 53 liver transplants have taken place (UNOS, 2020). Similarly, the release of direct acting antiviral medications for the curative treatment of HCV in 2014 has facilitated improved use of HCV-antibody-positive and viremic organs to be transplanted into recipients without HCV with curative posttransplant treatment. This has further increased accessibility and use of organs for transplant. Recently, the use of normothermic perfusion has improved use of physiologically stressed organs, most commonly DCDD organs, with improved outcomes.

Ongoing innovation will be needed in the organ transplantation system. Innovations to improve organ availability and accessibility include all aspects of research, including but not limited to

- Developing novel organ sources (e.g., organoids, printed organs, artificial organs, xenotransplantation);
- Rehabilitating organs not currently being transplanted (e.g., defatting of livers);
- Creating novel organ distribution and transport mechanisms (e.g., using drones, transporting kidneys while on a pump);
- Minimizing immunosuppression posttransplant in order to improve posttransplant outcomes;
- Maximizing both deceased and living donation through improving understanding and outreach to diverse communities;
- Conducting patient-centered research to understand patient priorities for the transplantation system;
- Improving education initiatives for providers, potential donors, and potential transplant recipients; and
- Applying health care delivery and implementation science in the field of organ transplantation, specifically in regards to advancing health equity.

# REFERENCES

AHRQ (Agency for Healthcare Research on Quality). 2016. *Saving lives and saving money: Hospital-acquired conditions update: Final data from national efforts to make care safer, 2010–2014.* https://www.ahrq.gov/sites/default/files/wysiwyg/professionals/quality-patient-safety/pfp/2014finalhacreport-cx.pdf (accessed October 15, 2021).
AHRQ. 2020. *AHRQ National Scorecard on Hospital-Acquired Conditions: Final results for 2014 through 2017.* https://www.ahrq.gov/sites/default/files/wysiwyg/professionals/quality-patient-safety/pfp/Updated-hacreport FInal2017data.pdf (accessed October 15, 2021).

Alyesh, A. Z. 2021 (unpublished). *Quality improvement lessons from health care and applications to the United States organ donation and transplantation system.* Paper commissioned by the Committee on a Fairer and More Equitable, Cost-Effective, and Transparent System of Donor Organ Procurement, Allocation, and Distribution, National Academies of Sciences, Engineering, and Medicine, Washington, DC.

American Society of Transplantation. 2021. *Vascularized composite allotransplantation (VCA) research.* https://www.myast.org/public-policy/vascularized-composite-allotransplantation-vca-research (accessed November 16, 2021).

Axelrod, D. A., M. A. Schnitzler, H. Xiao, W. Irish, E. Tuttle Newhall, S. H. Chang, B. L. Kasiske, T. Alhamad, and K. L. Lentine. 2018. An economic assessment of contemporary kidney transplant practice. *American Journal of Transplantation* 18(5):1168-1176.

Bernat, J. L. (2005). The concept and practice of brain death. *Progress in Brain Research* 150:369-379. https://doi.org/10.1016/S0079-6123(05)50026-8.

Bethea, E. D., S. Samur, F. Kanwal, T. Ayer, C. Hur, M. S. Roberts, N. Terrault, R. T. Chung, and J. Chhatwal. 2019. Cost effectiveness of transplanting HCV-infected livers into uninfected recipients with preemptive antiviral therapy. *Clinical Gastroenterology and Hepatology* 17(4):739-747.

Cetrulo, C. L., Z. Y. Ng, J. M. Winograd, and K. R. Eberlin. 2017. The advent of vascularized composite allotransplantation. *Clinics in Plastic Surgery* 44(2):425-429. https://doi.org/10.1016/j.cps.2016.12.007.

CMS (Centers for Medicare & Medicaid Services). 2011. *Partnership for patients to improve care and lower costs for Americans.* https://www.cms.gov/newsroom/press-releases/partnership-patients-improve-care-and-lower-costs-americans (accessed October 28, 2021).

Dageforde, L. A., I. D. Feurer, C. W. Pinson, and D. E. Moore. 2013. Is liver transplantation using organs donated after cardiac death cost-effective or does it decrease waitlist death by increasing recipient death? *International Hepato-Pancreato-Biliary Association* 15(3):182-189.

DeVita, M. A., J. V. Snyder, and A. Grenvik. 1993. History of organ donation by patients with cardiac death. *Kennedy Institute of Ethics Journal* 3(2):113-129.

Domínguez-Gil, B., N. Ascher, A. M. Capron, B. Gardiner, A. R. Manara, J. L. Bernat, E. Miñambres, J. M. Singh, R. Porte, J. F. Markmann, K. Dhital, D. Ledoux, C. Fondevila, S. Hosgood, D. Van Raemdonck, S. Keshavjee, J. Dubois, A. McGee, G. V. Henderson, A. K. Glazier, S. G. Tullius, S. D. Shemie, and F. L. Delmonico. 2021. Expanding controlled donation after the circulatory determination of death: Statement from an international collaborative. *Intensive Care Medicine* 47(3):265-281.

GAO (U.S. Government Accountability Office). 2020. *Organ transplants: Changes in allocation policies for donated livers and lungs.* https://www.gao.gov/assets/gao-21-70.pdf (accessed January 24, 2022).

Greer, D. M., S. D. Shemie, A. Lewis, S. Torrance, P. Varelas, F. D. Goldenberg, J. L. Bernat, M. Souter, M. A. Topcuoglu, A. W. Alexandrov, M. Baldisseri, T. Bleck, G. Citerio, R. Dawson, A. Hoppe, S. Jacobe, A. Manara, T. A. Nakagawa, T. M. Pope, W. Silvester, D. Thomson, H. Al Rahma, R. Badenes, A. J. Baker, V. Cerny, C. Chang, T. R. Chang, E. Gnedovskaya, M. K. Han, S. Honeybul, E. Jimenez, Y. Kuroda, G. Liu, U. K. Mallick, V. Marquevich, J. Mejia-Mantilla, M. Piradov, S. Quayyum, G. S. Shrestha, Y. Y. Su, S. D. Timmons, J. Teitelbaum, W. Videtta, K. Zirpe, and G. Sung. 2020. Determination of brain death/death by neurologic criteria: The World Brain Death Project. *Journal of the American Medical Association* 324(11):1078-1097.

Gruessner, R. W. G., and A. C. Gruessner. 2018. Solid-organ transplants from living donors: Cumulative United States experience on 140,156 living donor transplants over 28 years. *Transplant Proceedings* 50:3025-3035.

Guidelines for the determination of death: Report of the medical consultants on the diagnosis of death to the President's Commission for the Study of Ethical Problems in Medicine and Biomedical and Behavioral Research. 1981. *Journal of the American Medical Association.* 246(19):2184-2186.

Halevy, A., and B. A. Brody. 1993. Brain death: Reconciling definitions, criteria, and tests. *Annals of Internal Medicine* 119:519-525.

Held, P. J., F. McCormic, F. Ojo, and J. P. Roberts. 2016. A cost-benefit analysis of government compensation of kidney donors. *American Journal of Transplantation* 16(3):877-885.

HHS (U.S. Department of Health and Human Services). 2005. *HHS Honors 184 hospitals for increasing their donation rate to 75%.* https://www.thefreelibrary.com/HHS+honors+184+hospitals+for+increasing+their+donation+rate+to+75%25.-a0134175445 (accessed October 28, 2021).

HHS. 2022. *History & NOTA.* https://optn.transplant.hrsa.gov/about/history-nota (accessed February 1, 2022).

HRSA (Health Resources and Services Administration). 2018. *White paper on manipulating waitlist priority.* https://optn.transplant.hrsa.gov/governance/public-comment/white-paper-on-manipulating-waitlist-priority (accessed November 17, 2021).

HRSA. 2021a. *Advisory Committee on Organ Transplantation.* https://www.hrsa.gov/advisory-committees/organ-transplantation (accessed November 16, 2021).

HRSA. 2021b. *Summary of Advisory Committee on Organ Transplantation (ACOT) consensus recommendations to the secretary of Health and Human Services (HHS)*. https://www.hrsa.gov/advisory-committees/organ-transplantation/recommendations (accessed October 1, 2021).

Humar, A. H., S. Ganesh, D. Jorgensen, A. Tevar, A. Ganoza, M. Milinari, and C. Hughes. 2019. Adult living donor versus deceased donor liver transplant (LDLT versus DDLT) at a single center—Time to change our paradigm for liver transplant. *Annals of Surgery* 270(3):444-451.

IOM (Institute of Medicine). 2000. *To err is human: Building a safer health system*. Washington, DC: National Academy Press.

Israni, A. K., D. Zaun, J. D. Rosendale, C. Schaffhausen, W. McKinney, and J. J. Snyder. 2021. OPTN/SRTR 2019 annual data report: Deceased organ donors. *American Journal of Transplantation* 21(S2):567-604.

Karp, S. J., G. Segal, and D. J. Patil. 2021. Using data to achieve organ procurement organization accountability—reply. *JAMA Surgery* 156(1):99-100.

Kaufman, C. L., N. Bhutiani, A. Ramirez, H. Y. Tien, M. D. Palazzo, E. Galvis, S. Farner, T. Ozyurekoglu, and C. M. Jones. 2019. Current status of vascularized composite allotransplantation. *The American Surgeon* 85(6):631-637. https://doi.org/10.1177/000313481908500628.

Kazley, A. S., E. Johnson, L. Holland-Carter, S. Mauer, J. Correll, N. Marlow, K. Chavin, and P. Baliga. 2019. The non-directed living kidney donor: Why donate to strangers? *Journal of Renal Care* 45(2):102-110.

King, K. L., S. A. Husain, J. D. Schold, R. E. Patzer, P. P. Reese, Z. Jin, L. E. Ratner, D. J. Cohen, S. O. Pastan, and S. Mohan. 2020. Major variation across local transplant centers in probability of kidney transplant for wait-listed patients. *Journal of the American Society of Nephrology* 31(12):2900-2911.

Laureys, S. 2005. Death, unconsciousness and the brain. *Nature Reviews Neuroscience* 6:899-909. https://doi.org/10.1038/nrn1789.

Levy, G. A., N. Selzner, and D. R. Grant. 2016. Fostering living donor liver transplantation. *Current Opinion in Organ Transplantation* 21:224-230.

Massie, A. B., X. Luo, E. K. Chow, J. L. Alejo, N. M. Desai, and D. L. Segev. 2014. Survival benefit of primary deceased donor transplantation with high-KDPI kidneys. *American Journal of Transplantation* 14(10):2310-2316.

Mathur, A. K., Z. A. Stewart-Lewis, P. H. Warren, M. C. Walters, K. A. Gifford, J. Xing, N. P. Goodrich, R. Bennett, A. Brownson, J. Ellefson, G. Felan, G. Barrett, R. E. Hays, C. Klein-Glover, S. Lagreco, N. Metzler, K. Provencher, E. Walz, K. Warmke, R. M. Merion, and A. O. Ojo. 2020. Best practices to optimize utilization of the National Living Donor Assistance Center for the financial assistance of living organ donors. *American Journal of Transplantation* 20:25-33.

Neumann, P. J., G. D. Sanders, L. B. Russell, J. E. Siegel, and T. G. Ganiats, eds. 2016. *Cost-effectiveness in health and medicine*. Oxford University Press.

Northup, P. G., M. M. Abecassis, M. J. Englesbe, J. C. Emond, V. D. Lee, G. J. Stukenborg, L. Tong, C. L. Berg, and Adult-to-Adult Living Donor Liver Transplantation Cohort Study Group. 2009. Addition of adult-to-adult living donation to liver transplant programs improves survival but at an increased cost. *Liver Transplantation* 15(2):148-162.

OPTN (Organ Procurement and Transplantation Network). 2019. *Ethical implications of multi-organ transplants*. https://optn.transplant.hrsa.gov/media/2989/ethics_boardreport_201906.pdf (accessed November 18, 2021).

OPTN. 2022. *All-time records again set in 2021 for organ transplants, organ donation from deceased donors*. https://optn.transplant.hrsa.gov/news/all-time-records-again-set-in-2021-for-organ-transplants-organ-donation-from-deceased-donors (accessed January 26, 2022).

Pena, A. 2016. Wanted: Living organ donor. *Transplantation* 100(11):2239-2243.

President's Commission for the Study of Ethical Problems in Medicine and Biomedical and Behavioral Research. 1981. *Defining death: A report on the medical, legal and ethical issues in the determination of death*. Washington, DC: U.S. Government Printing Office.

Rand, L. Z., and A. S. Kesselheim. 2021. Controversy over using quality-adjusted life-years in cost-effectiveness analyses: A systematic literature review: Systematic literature review examines the controversy over the use of quality-adjusted life-year in cost-effectiveness analyses. *Health Affairs* 40(9):1402-1410.

Rasmussen, S., J. Uriart, N. Anderson, B. Doby, A. Ferzola, H. Sung, C. Cooney, G. Brandacher, E. Gordon, D. Segev, and M. Hendersen. 2020. Public education materials about vascular composite allotransplantation and donation in the United States: Current scope and limitations. *Clinical Transplantation* 34(11). https://doi.org/10.1111/ctr.14066.

Report of the Ad Hoc Committee of the Harvard Medical School to Examine the Definition of Brain Death. A definition of irreversible coma. 1968. *JAMA*. 205(6):337-340. https://doi.org/10.1001/jama.1968.03140320031009.

Rodrigue, J., D. Tomich, A. Flieshman, and A. Glazier. 2017. Vascularized composite allograft donation and transplantation: A survey of public attitudes in the United States. *American Journal of Transplantation* 17:2687-2695.

Sarasin, F. P., P. E. Majno, J. M. Llovet, J. Bruix, G. Mentha, and A. Hadengue. 2001. Living donor liver transplantation for early hepatocellular carcinoma: A life-expectancy and cost-effectiveness perspective. *Hepatology* 33(5):1073-1079.

Schnitzler, M., M. Skeans, A. Israni, and M. Valapour. 2014. Incremental cost-effectiveness of lung transplant by lung allocation score: Abstract 1386. *Transplantation* 98:192.

Schnitzler, M. A., M. A. Skeans, D. A. Axelrod, K. L. Lentine, J. E. Tuttle-Newhall, J. J. Snyder, A. K. Israni, and B. L. Kasiske. 2015. OPTN/SRTR 2013 annual data report: Economics. *American Journal of Transplantation* 15(S2):1-24.

Shafer, T. J., D. Wagner, J. Chessare, F. A. Zampiello, V. McBride, and J. Perdue. 2006. Organ donation breakthrough collaborative: Increasing organ donation through system redesign. *Critical Care Nurse* 26(2):33-48.

SRTR (Scientific Registry of Transplant Recipients). 2022. *Mission, vision, and values.* https://www.srtr.org/about-srtr/mission-vision-and-values (accessed February 1, 2022).

Tilney, N. L. 2003. *In transplant: From myth to reality.* New Haven, CT: Yale University Press. Pp. 199-216.

UNOS (United Network for Organ Sharing). 2020. *HOPE Act impact continues at five-year milestone.* https://unos.org/news/in-focus/hope-act-impact-continues-at-five-year-milestone (accessed November 16, 2021).

UNOS. 2021. *Living donation.* https://unos.org/transplat/living-donation (accessed March 14, 2021).

Vega, R. J., and K. W. Kizer. 2020. VHA's innovation ecosystem: Operationalizing innovation in health care. *NEJM Catalyst* 1(6). https://doi.org/10.1056/CAT.20.0263.

Whiting, J. F., R. S. Woodward, E. Y. Zavala, D. S. Cohen, J. E. Martin, G. G. Singer, J. A. Lowell, M. R. First, D. C. Brennan, and M. A. Schnitzler. 2000. Economic cost of expanded criteria donors in cadaveric renal transplantation: Analysis of Medicare payments. *Transplantation* 70(5):755-760.

Wolfe, R. A., V. B. Ashby, E. L. Milford, A. O. Ojo, R. E. Ettenger, L. Y. C. Agodoa, P. J. Held, and F. K. Port. 1999. Comparison of mortality in all patients on dialysis, patients on dialysis awaiting transplantation, and recipients of a first cadaveric transplant. *New England Journal of Medicine* 341(23):1725-1730.

Wolfe, R. A., K. P. McCullough, and A. B. Leichtman. 2009. Predictability of survival models for waiting list and transplant patients: Calculating LYFT. *American Journal of Transplantation* 9(7):1523-1527.

# 3

# Foundations for a Trustworthy Deceased Donor Organ Transplantation System

A s described in Chapter 1, the committee's charge is to address the doubts expressed by many members of the public about the efficiency, equity, fairness, and transparency of the organ transplantation system and their resulting lack of trust in the system. For example, the 2019 survey data presented in Box 1-1 show that while two-thirds of the respondents affirmed that the system "uses a fair approach to distribute organs," about half do not trust the system to provide "minority patients" and "poor persons" with an equal chance of receiving an organ transplant as other patients.

The present chapter discusses how the individual and societal trust that the organ transplantation system needs to succeed depends on health care professionals fulfilling their ethical duties to do good and not to harm, to respect patients' autonomy, and to strive for justice and utility in organ allocation decisions. Additionally, such trust is contingent on other institutions—the organ procurement organizations (OPOs), the Organ Procurement and Transplantation Network (OPTN), and agencies of the federal government—upholding these same values. The chapter pays special attention to the concept of justice as it relates to two important points in the committee's charge, namely, the "equity" and "fairness" of transplant processes and outcomes, and the relationship of equity and fairness to another objective of the system, namely, "optimizing the quality and quantity of donated organs available for transplantation," in the words of the committee's charge (see Box 3-1). The chapter also reflects on the role of transparency as an instrumental value in shaping public beliefs and attitudes about the trustworthiness of the organ transplantation system.

## WHY IS TRUSTWORTHINESS IMPORTANT?

"Trust underlies the entire organ and tissue donation and transplantation environment, and everyone must act to obtain, sustain, and nurture that trust among those directly and indirectly affected."

—Kenneth Moritsugu, testimony to the committee
during February 5, 2021 public workshop

61

---

**BOX 3-1**  **KEY COMMITTEE MESSAGES ON JUSTICE, FAIRNESS, AND EQUITY IN ORGAN TRANSPLANTATION**

The committee's report overall, and particularly Chapter 3, contains a number of reflections related to justice, fairness, and equity in the organ transplantation system. Key messages include

- Even when policies are premised on all people being treated alike, measurable—in fact, often very large—disparities exist which are not explained by medical differences, but rather arise from historical patterns of discrimination.
- Historical patterns of discrimination are embedded in social institutions (including in health care) and are perpetuated by conscious prejudices as well as unexamined practices.
- In a just society, people whose physical and psychological needs are roughly similar have comparable access to appropriate, timely care, and all are treated as equally deserving of respect in their interactions with the health care system.
- Justice demands fair processes when policies are adopted that could result in medically similar patients experiencing significantly different access to particular, needed resources. This means that any factor used to differentiate among people not only is relevant (i.e., it pertains to the right or interest affected by the policy) but also accounts for the effects of drawing the distinction on the groups thus differentiated and on other persons or institutions affected by the policy.
- Justice demands that access to health care be equitable, meaning that persons in equivalent medical circumstances actually receive equivalent medical care, free from irrelevant considerations such as their sex, race, ethnicity, religion, socioeconomic condition, physical and mental capabilities, geographic residence, and other personal attributes.
- Disparities in the ways that certain historically disadvantaged groups are treated or in the outcomes that the transplantation system produces for them are signals that an injustice exists.
- To the extent that such disparities are avoidable, an equitable system will take the steps necessary to eliminate them.
- To be perceived as being trustworthy and deserving of the public's trust, the organ transplantation system must be open and honest in communicating its values, methods, and outcomes in ways that are comprehensible to a wide range of stakeholders with different needs and various levels of interest in, and understanding of, organ transplantation.

---

For organ transplantation to succeed, people—individually and as a society—must trust that the transplantation system operates in an ethical, just, and efficient manner (Boulware et al., 2007; HHS, 2013). Indeed, transplantation stands out as a part of health care where "public trust is utterly indispensable" (IOM, 2006, p. 81). When public trust declines, so too do deceased donation rates (Boulware et al., 2007; Wachterman et al., 2015). Fewer organs being donated can result in medical burdens and loss of life among patients awaiting a transplant. The committee is therefore troubled that many members of the public do not fully trust our current organ transplantation system, and even more troubled that good reasons exist for this lack of trust, particularly for some groups of patients awaiting a transplant. Some of these reasons are specific to transplantation and others are broader, such as having been treated poorly by health care providers and the history of such abuses in society. Barriers to public trust must be overcome if organ transplantation is going to fulfill its lifesaving and life-enhancing potential.

As vital as public trust is to the success of the organ transplantation system, it is at least as essential that such trust be justified. To be worthy of trust, the transplantation system needs a firm foundation: all parts of the system must adhere to clear, coherent, and justified ethical principles and must obtain and use donated organs efficiently and effectively. This chapter begins by examining the role that ethical theories and principles play in creating a system for obtaining and distributing organs from deceased donors that is worthy of the public's trust. In addition to health care professionals' usual ethical obligations—to act beneficently and to respect persons—the chapter gives special attention to the ethical principle of justice because it is, as John Rawls maintains, "the first virtue of social institutions" (Rawls, 1999, p. 3), such as the government agencies and health care organizations that play central roles in transplantation. In addition to the theory that right action depends on health care professionals and institutions fulfilling their ethical duties to organ donors, recipients, and their families, the chapter also develops the implications of consequentialist theories, including those such as utilitarianism that equate a right action with that which maximizes total well-being. An organ transplantation system that is cost effective and efficient as well as fair and equitable would deserve the trust of the public and transplant professionals.

Besides deserving the public's trust, the organ transplantation system must also be seen as being trustworthy. Perception depends on the system operating transparently, which means that it is open and honest in communicating its values, methods, and outcomes in ways that are comprehensible to a wide range of stakeholders with different needs and varied levels of interest in, and understanding of, organ transplantation. After discussing the relevant ethical principles, this chapter turns to the important role that the principle of transparency plays in achieving trustworthiness, and explores opportunities for overcoming barriers to achieving trust.

The concepts and arguments developed here are then applied in the chapters that follow. Chapters 4 analyzes current disparities in organ transplantation, such as the lower rates at which poorer patients, patients of color, and women are listed as transplant candidates and often the longer time it takes for them to receive a transplant once listed. The chapter explains why such disparities constitute inequities that can—and must—be eliminated, and recommends practical steps to overcome the barriers to equitable treatment. Chapter 5 examines justice in organ allocation policies, looking first at inequities and then turning to the task of enhancing the fairness of a number of policies. Chapter 6, which examines ways to improve the number and quality of organs donated and increase their use, shows how consequentialism is significant in transplant ethics, and offers a way of combining the goal of maximizing the benefits transplantation provides with the goal of a fair and equitable system.

## ETHICAL PRINCIPLES AND THEORIES FOR A TRUSTWORTHY SYSTEM

What principles and theories support an ethical system of organ transplantation? The usual starting point in contemporary health care ethics—namely, an analysis of physicians' duties to their patients—is well suited for organ transplantation, since the care of organ donors and recipients is at heart a medical activity. But our country's transplantation system encompasses more than individual patients and their physicians. It depends not only on a multidisciplinary team but also on generous individuals who donate organs. The system also depends on many large private and governmental institutions that handle the process by which donated organs are identified, recovered, allocated, and transported to particular recipients; that fund and oversee this process; and that adopt and administer laws and regulations that make this all possible. For this reason, in addition to looking at the duties of physicians and other professionals, this chapter gives special attention to justice as an obligation not just in medicine, but especially in collective activities such as organ transplantation. In addition to drawing on deontology (from the Greek for "duty"), we examine consequentialist ethics since the perception that the organ transplantation system is inefficient or wasteful can also undermine trust. After outlining the basic concepts, the chapter applies them to the issues that arise in the procurement and distribution of organs from deceased donors.

## The Ethical Duties of Health Care Professionals and Institutions

The utility of an ethical theory in guiding a field of endeavor depends on whether the theory will prove useful in resolving the conflicts that create the need for ethical guidance in the first place. In transplantation, guidance is particularly needed about how donors should be treated in organ procurement and the basis on which donated organs should be allocated. Certain traditions, such as virtue ethics, which focus on the character traits of ethical practitioners rather than on the morality of their actions, offer little that is helpful in addressing the central issues of transplantation (Veatch, 2000). Those issues are, however, well addressed by the dominant approach in contemporary health care ethics, which combines the philosophical traditions of consequentialism and deontology. This approach originated with the Belmont Report, a report of the federal commission empaneled in 1974 to examine and propose responses to revelations of unethical medical research over the preceding four decades, which found that the "codes" crafted by jurists and physicians to govern human subjects research were inadequate to cover ethical complex cases (National Commission for the Protection of Human Subjects of Biomedical and Behavioral Research, 1979). Instead, the commissioners offered three ethical principles—beneficence, respect for persons, and justice—that they drew from "our cultural tradition" as the most relevant to the task of providing an analytic framework for resolving the ethical problems that arise in research. Since its conclusions were situated at the level of principles rather than rules, the Belmont Report has proved influential across health care ethics, not just for research (Beauchamp and Childress, 2019). The principles—along with others, such as utility—have been relied upon by the OPTN (through its Ethics Committee) in elaborating the ethical underpinnings of the National Organ Transplant Act (NOTA) and the Final Rule,[1] have been developed by scholars addressing ethical challenges in organ transplantation (Veatch and Ross, 2015), and have been employed in prior National Academies reports on organ transplantation (see Appendix B).

### Doing Good and Not Doing Harm

The health care professions are grounded in a set of ethical obligations to patients. Since ancient times, medical practitioners and their patients have realized that the trust necessary for therapeutic relationships would not exist if the profession operated under the norms that govern commercial activities such as caveat emptor ("let the buyer beware"). Therefore, two related moral duties have long been central to medical ethics: nonmaleficence, the obligation not to harm others, and beneficence, the obligation to act to benefit others. These duties are often associated with a commandment attributed to Hippocrates, primum non nocere ("Above all, do no harm"). The Hippocratic Oath expresses this obligation through the promise that the physician will both use treatments "which, according to my ability and

---

[1] In "Ethical Principles in the Allocation of Human Organs," first adopted in 1992 (Burdick et al., 1992) and revised in 2010 (OPTN Board, 2010), the OPTN Ethics Committee concluded that the Final Rule's "regulatory requirements" for the operation of the OPTN "embody the familiar ethical principles of utility (doing good and avoiding harm), justice, and respect for persons" but that the OPTN needed a policy statement to provide the ethical guidance that is lacking in the Final Rule. In equating "doing good and avoiding harm" with the principle of utility, the committee departed from the prevailing description of utility as the maximization of net welfare and of doing good and avoiding harm as the principles of beneficence and nonmaleficence.

judgment, I consider for the benefit of my patients" and "abstain from whatever is deleterious and mischievous" (Hippocrates, n.d.).

Beneficence sounds like a consequentialist concept: Which action will create the greatest benefit? But in the Hippocratic tradition, this duty is framed in terms of intention rather than consequences, and generates a commitment to the primacy of patients and their interests. In ordinary life, behaving beneficently generally connotes acting in a kind or generous fashion, beyond what one is required to do. In health care, however, beneficence—physicians' duty to put the interests and welfare of their patients before those of others, including their own—is not supererogatory, or beyond the call of duty, but obligatory. This commitment to placing the patient's best interests first and acting to help the patient, not only by promoting good, but also by preventing harm, is at the heart of medical deontology, that is, the ethical theory that judges whether an action is right or wrong based on physicians' adherence to their duties to patients rather than solely on the consequences of the actions. Consequences may still be relevant, however, since fidelity to the patient's best interests usually means trying to maximize the particular patient's welfare. Health care professionals typically conceptualize welfare in terms of bodily functioning, absence of disease or disability, length of life, and the like, but other aspects of well-being, such as happiness, feelings of security, and the protection of other interests, such as reputation and financial welfare, are also aspects of patient-centered assessments of welfare. These are in turn manifested in specific rules that are derived from physicians' basic duties of beneficence and nonmaleficence, such as duties to keep confidential information about their patients and not to take advantage (financially, sexually, or otherwise) of patients' vulnerability. A major limitation of the principle of beneficence as it is usually understood in a clinical context is that the welfare being sought is solely that of an individual patient, rather than encompassing the consequences for, or duties, to others in the health care system.

## Respect for the Patient's Autonomy

While the ancient precepts of nonmaleficence and beneficence remain central to medical care—and hence to achieving an ethical system of organ transplantation—the second principle of contemporary bioethics, respect for persons, is intended to correct another limitation in the traditional precepts, namely, the equation of benefit with physicians' judgment about what they believed will best serve their patients' interests. The Belmont Report described respect for persons as having two facets, treating competent adults as autonomous agents and protecting persons with diminished competence (National Commission for the Protection of Human Subjects of Biomedical and Behavioral Research, 1979). Attention usually focuses on the first facet and the principle is condensed to "respect for autonomy" (Beauchamp and Childress, 2019), leaving the second facet to be addressed under the principles of beneficence and nonmaleficence, with ethical concern directed at who may make decisions, and on what grounds, for persons who are not autonomous agents, such as minors and individuals with intellectual disabilities.

The concept of autonomy, or self-rule, has deep roots in Western philosophy, especially as regards the spheres of law and government. People expect that their permission is needed before someone intrudes on their private property or touches their body; even governments, whose authority rests on the consent of the governed, can interfere with someone's property or person without their approval only as is needed to protect the public from serious harm, such as through public health or traffic laws or court orders.

With the growth of scientific medicine in the twentieth century, treatments became more elaborate and hospital based, and the formality of consent, if not its substance, grew (Capron,

1974). Change was also driven by revelations of vulnerable persons being used in medical experiments without their consent, from European orphanages and charity hospitals at the beginning of the previous century through the Nazi concentration camps during World War II, and from elderly, debilitated patients at the Jewish Chronic Disease Hospital in Brooklyn in the early 1960s to poor black farmers in the United States Public Health Service Syphilis Study at Tuskegee between 1932 and 1972. As the first requirement of ethical medical research, the tribunal that passed judgment on the Nazi doctors after the war stated, "The voluntary consent of the human subject is absolutely essential" (Nuremberg Code [1947], 1996). The judges held that the conditions for an "understanding and enlightened decision" include the person having "the legal capacity to give consent," being "able to exercise free power of choice," free of fraud or coercion, and having "sufficient knowledge and comprehension of the elements of the subject matter" (e.g., the nature, duration, and purpose of the experiment; how it will be conducted; what hazards it entails). While medical societies attempted to maintain a wider sphere of discretion in treatment settings,[2] the principle of autonomous choice—which requires an act that is intentional, with understanding, and free of controlling influences (Beauchamp and Childress, 2019)—came to be recognized as an ethical (and legal) requirement in diagnosis and treatment as well as in biomedical and behavioral research (Faden and Beauchamp, 1986).

Respect for persons includes manifesting a respectful attitude, but it also requires respectful actions: for example, by acknowledging that people may make choices based on their beliefs and values, which others will accept even when they think a different choice would be better. In contemporary terms, autonomy is the ethical bedrock on which patient-centered care is built. Patient autonomy supplants physicians making medical decisions for their patients, a practice which often extended to medical paternalism, that is, the tradition of physicians overriding medical choices made by patients that the physicians believed would not be in the patients' best interests. Although often thought of as a relic of a medical custom that came to an end in the previous century, the impulse to protect patients from bad choices remains and can lead to subtle and sometimes unnoticed forms of paternalism, including in organ transplantation.

Four aspects of the principle of autonomy deserve special attention. First, the negative version of autonomy—that is, competent patients withholding consent to proposed medical interventions—is much stronger and more absolute than the positive version—that is, patients designing their own treatment. During the 1960s and 1970s, some patients' rights advocates, in aiming to supplant physicians' dominant position in health care, sought to assign patients full responsibility for and control over all decisions about their own care. This position—sometimes called "patient sovereignty"—in effect flips medical paternalism on its head, making physicians the servants of their patients, using their technical skills as patients direct and refraining from trying to influence them. Today, it is generally agreed that neither extreme is ethically defensible or even sensible; instead, physicians and patients—each with their own personality, attitudes, and values—should strive for shared decision making, based on mutual respect and joint participation in the process (President's Commission for the Study of Ethical Problems in Medicine and Biomedical and Behavioral Research, 1982). The principle of respect for autonomy—and its legal counterpart, informed consent—holds that ultimately, the choice among possible medical options (including, of course, no treat-

---

[2] As originally adopted by the World Medical Association in 1964, the Declaration of Helsinki differentiated between research on normal volunteers, for which "free" and "fully informed" consent was necessary, and "clinical research combined with professional care" for which "the doctor must be free to use a new therapeutic measure, if in his judgment it offers hope of saving life, reestablishing health, or alleviating suffering," with the informed consent of the patient, "if at all possible, consistent with patient psychology" (WMA, 1964).

ment) belongs to the patient, but health care providers are not obligated to provide medical interventions that have no basis in medical science and practice or that violate their own deeply held moral beliefs.

Second, the principle of autonomy does not imply that patients are, or ever could be, self-directed in the sense of being totally independent of other persons or free from interior or exterior influences. This speaks to the concept of relational autonomy, which rejects traditional understandings of autonomy as both too atomistic and unrealistically rational, and insists instead that autonomy arises from relationships with others, such as parents, teachers, friends, and loved ones (Nedelsky, 1989). In various individualized ways, patients are situated within families, communities, and other social institutions; they have personal histories that shape their understanding of the world and the view of what is possible for them going forward; they have real and perceived social, moral, and financial obligations—or what may feel like obligations—to others, including the health care professionals who provide them with care. Everyone involved in decision making—especially members of the medical team who will implement whatever medical choice the patient makes—should endeavor to help patients in making choices which are consistent with their lives and values as persons within relationships, which can entail assisting them not only cognitively, by providing comprehensible information about the medical options and their benefits and risks, but psychologically and emotionally as well (Walter and Ross, 2014). Since relational autonomy not only rejects the conception of autonomy as complete independence from others but also recognizes that some "choices" actually reflect domination by others or by societal expectations, health care professionals may need to protect patients from coercion, manipulation, or other attempts by third parties to control their choice. Yet it will rarely, if ever, be possible to free the patient from all external influences, or indeed, to identify where a line can be drawn between factors that are external and those that are internal, wherever the latter may have originated. The fact that patients are enmeshed in relationships that strongly influence their medical choices is not inconsistent with the proposition that their "autonomous choices" should be respected; indeed, such relationships are often very helpful in supporting patients in making decisions that are true reflections of their individual selves and the ends they seek to achieve.

Third, while physicians who foster shared decision making can thereby adhere to the principle of autonomy, the principle does not require that all physician–patient relationships take a single form. Certain minimal requirements—disclosure to the patient of material information about the medical options and ensuring the patient has the ability and opportunity to participate in the decision-making process and the right to accept or reject medical interventions—must always be met. Still, each physician and patient can shape their specific search for successful treatment in ways that fit their own abilities and objectives, questions, and hopes as well as their particular situation (e.g., a long-standing primary care relationship versus a one-time consultation with a specialist; preventive care versus life-sustaining treatment; and so forth). Ideally, the nature of the relationship will grow organically, influenced by the personalities and needs of each party as they exchange information and respond to issues that arise. Parties outside the physician–patient dyad, such as the institution where the physician practices and the insurer that pays for some or all of the care, will also affect the contours of the relationship. A variety of arrangements are all consistent with respecting an autonomous exercise of choice about medical care.

Finally, the well-known theory of deontological ethics developed by Immanuel Kant places rational choice of autonomous moral agents at its center. In Kantian ethics, the moral worth of an action depends on its being autonomously chosen based on a universally valid rule, rather than for some other motive. The criterion for judging the validity of a rule is termed the categorical imperative, which says that rules must be universalizable and consistent, that is, not contradict themselves. The most familiar formulation of the categorical imperative is, "One must act to treat every person as an end and never as a means only" (Kant, 1959). In situations where what is being done to a patient is not solely for that person's benefit, such as when a patient is enrolled in a clinical trial, Kantian deontology holds that such an act is permissible only if the patient had a choice whether or not to take part, thus embracing the objectives of the clinical trial as his or her own end, not solely that of the physician–investigator.[3]

## Justice

Contemporary accounts of health care ethics include justice as an important obligation of physicians and other health care professionals (National Commission for the Protection of Human Subjects of Biomedical and Behavioral Research, 1979). But the principle of justice has its greatest effect when applied at a higher level in health care, from institutions (such as hospitals) to broader systems (such as the organ transplantation system) to society as a whole (such as tax and expenditure policies related to the financing of health care). Adjusting policies and practices to make access to health care—and the distribution of its benefits—more just is not a new goal, but it is a matter of particular urgency today.

The concept of justice applies in a number of ways to social institutions, including health care.[4] Justice concerns the processes and procedures by which decisions are reached and actions are taken, as well as to the policies that guide those processes. Justice has been articulated in various ways, among which equality, fairness, and equity receive attention here, since each has implications for the goal of achieving justice in the organ transplantation system.

*Equality*: "Justice" can connote procedural justice, which is usually expressed as equality, namely that people must be treated equally, both by the institutions of government (such as the courts) and in settings open to the general public (such as stores and restaurants). Equality means that all persons will receive equal respect and concern, have equal access to decision makers, and will have their rights and interests equally protected.

What implications does the principle of human equality have for health care policies? Given the huge variation in human health and the wide range of diseases and injuries that

---

[3] The categorical imperative is often cited as an ethical foundation for informed consent, even though not all instances of a person consenting to a medical intervention (or to any other act by a third party) would meet Kant's definition of autonomy, which is much narrower than the way the term is used here or generally in medical ethics. Kant limits "autonomy of the will" to actions taken knowingly in accord with a universally valid principle that accords with the categorical imperative, rather than a knowing, voluntary choice made for any reason that is sufficient in the patient's eyes.

[4] In treating health care as an activity that should adhere to the requirements of justice, the committee is not suggesting that all policies or practices in society must be judged by their adherence to this principle. Many things in our society are distributed in other ways, such as by inheritance or through the market. While health care is in part a market good, our society does not leave it entirely to the market for several reasons: it is not a free market, it generates large externalities, and, most important, it provides the means for obtaining relief from the burdens of disease and disability which restrict people's chance to attain a state of well-being or a fair share of the normal range of opportunities (Daniels, 2008; Powers and Faden, 2006). In sum, health care is different because it is closely connected to health which is a basic good that is valued by all people however much they may differ in their other preferences because it is a basic requisite not just for survival but for living a full life, with an opportunity to achieve one's goals. Thus, for many years, access to the means for attaining and maintaining health has been described as a basic human right (President's Commission, 1953) or an ethical obligation of a just society (President's Commission for the Study of Ethical Problems in Medicine and Biomedical and Behavioral Research, 1982). Recognizing that few people can be certain that they could afford all the medical care they need, most people obtain health insurance, either in the marketplace or as a benefit of employment, while some groups, particularly the elderly, veterans, some children, and other poor people, rely on public insurance or public providers of care.

people experience, justice does not demand that all people receive the same amount of health care services, much less that they are guaranteed to be equally healthy. Indeed, most individuals experience different levels of health—and hence have very different needs for health care—at different times across their life. But in a just society, people whose physical and psychological needs are roughly similar have comparable access to appropriate, timely care, and all are treated as equally deserving of respect in their interactions with the health care system.

*Fairness*: A maxim attributed to Aristotle—treat like cases alike, and unlike cases differently—suggests that the goal of justice is to avoid arbitrariness or favoritism.[5] The first precept reiterates the principle of equality, but the second recognizes the inevitability of relevant differences among people. That is, we may be equal before the law in our rights, but the ways in which we differ can legitimately lead to differences in the way we are treated.

One must look beyond the maxim itself to posit which characteristics may be relied on when determining who is similar or dissimilar. Thus, the fairness of a policy that treats certain people in one way and others in a different way depends upon three conditions. First, the right or interest addressed by the policy cannot not be one that must always be based on equality but rather must be one where it is ethically acceptable to treat people differently. Second, the process for arriving at the policy must be fair, meaning that the decision maker is free of bias and all interested parties have an opportunity to present their views. Third, the factors relied upon in distinguishing among people and placing them into groups is ethically justified and supported by the best evidence to the extent possible. Aside from characteristics that antidiscrimination laws exclude from being considered, it is often challenging to determine which features may legitimately be taken into account and which are factually or ethically irrelevant, especially when the features arise from the system itself, such as the jurisdictional or geographic division of activities or authority, or relate to other objectives that the policy is intended to advance, such as maximizing total welfare or redressing past injustices. Justice demands fair processes when policies are adopted that could result in medically similar patients experiencing significantly different access to particular, needed resources, meaning that any factor used to differentiate among people not only is relevant (i.e., it pertains to the right or interest affected by the policy) but also accounts for the effects of drawing the distinction on the groups thus differentiated and on other persons or institutions affected by the policy.[6]

*Equity*: If questions of fairness arise when debating whether to take certain factors into account in framing a policy, the question of equity comes to the fore when measurable—in fact, often very large—disparities exist among identifiable groups in access to needed services and in health outcomes even though on paper the policies in question entitle all people in the various groups to equal treatment. Justice demands that access to health care be equitable, meaning that persons in equivalent medical circumstances actually receive equivalent

---

[5] Justice, which assumes individuals are members of groups who have interests and claims that compete with other members, provides a possible corrective for the individualistic focus of the principle of beneficence, under which physicians are expected to favor the interests of their own patients over other interests.

[6] Despite the requirement of fairness that medically similar patients have similar access to resources, it is sometimes suggested that a "coin flip" or a lottery would be the fairest way of distributing a scarce resource since such a method gives all parties an equal chance. Yet for officials to consciously choose to distribute something important, such as potentially lifesaving treatment, in a random fashion can appear disrespectful of the individuals who will be affected. Moreover, it can seem a dereliction of the expectation that such officials will work to identify the factors that are both ethical and scientifically relevant to a fair allocation. On the other hand, adopting a distribution policy that relies on factors that align with membership in an identifiable group (e.g., one defined by age or sex) can be taken as a judgment that the lives of people in the groups that are placed further back in the queue for the resource are worth less than the lives of other people.

medical care, free from irrelevant considerations such as their sex, race, ethnicity, religion, socioeconomic condition, physical and mental capabilities, and similar personal attributes.

For many years, the concept of health equity has been an explicit part of efforts to improve the overall level of population health in our country and strengthen quality improvement efforts (IOM, 2001). Among such disparities, those that are "closely linked with social, economic, and/or environmental disadvantage" are of particular concern (HHS, 2021a). In a just society, such disparities must be regarded as health inequities that are morally unacceptable, not only because they demonstrate a failure in our proclaimed commitment to the equal worth of all people but also because they result from historical and contemporary injustices, many of which are embedded in social institutions (including in health care) and are perpetuated not only by conscious prejudice but also by unexamined practices. To the extent that such disparities are avoidable, then an equitable system will take the steps necessary to eliminate them (see Box 3-2).

A just society is thus one characterized by equality, fairness, and equity. In this report, the committee gives particular attention to the latter two terms (which appear often in our charge), and has chosen to consider them separately. The committee's decision to do so is pragmatic rather than epistemological, since equity and fairness are—along with "justice" itself—often used as synonyms. But by distinguishing the two terms, the committee can examine the somewhat different ways that the principle of justice—or its absence—can arise in the organ transplantation system. Just as "equity" provides a way to ascertain when justice is manifestly absent because the organ transplantation system treats groups of people very differently for reasons that are unconnected to their medical needs but that align with their membership in a group that is subjected to discrimination, "fairness" is useful in choosing the most just policy from among alternatives, each of which is defended by reasonable people.

## Efficiently Maximizing Welfare: Utilitarian Ethics

While the ethics of medical practice and research is typically framed in terms of physicians' duties, deciding what is the right thing to do in a particular circumstance sometimes

---

**BOX 3-2**  **DEFINITIONS OF HEALTH DISPARITY, HEALTH INEQUITIES, AND HEALTH EQUITY**

**Health disparity:** This is when "a health outcome is seen to a greater or lesser extent between populations." A health disparity is "a particular type of health difference that is closely linked with social, economic, and/or environmental disadvantage. Health disparities adversely affect groups of people who have systematically experienced greater obstacles to health based on their racial or ethnic group; religion; socioeconomic status; gender; age; mental health; cognitive, sensory, or physical disability; sexual orientation or gender identity; geographic location; or other characteristics historically linked to discrimination or exclusion" (HHS, 2021a).

**Health equity:** "Attainment of the highest level of health for all people. Achieving health equity requires valuing everyone equally with focused and ongoing societal efforts to address avoidable inequalities, historical and contemporary injustices, and the elimination of health and health care disparities" (HHS, 2021b).

**Health inequities:** Health differences that are unfair, unjust, and avoidable. Inequities result when barriers keep individuals and communities who experience disparities from reaching their full health potential (Arcaya et al., 2015).

is guided by comparing the potential good and bad results of the available courses of action. This version of consequentialism is therefore consistent with—indeed, inherent in—physicians' duties of beneficence and nonmaleficence, since it recognizes that serving a patient's interests usually entails offering the preventive, diagnostic, or therapeutic intervention that is most likely to provide the maximum benefit for the patient. To decide whether a physician's duty of beneficence has been fulfilled, a consequentialist would thus ask whether the recommended medical intervention will probably produce the greatest benefit for the patient.

When making collective rather than individual (that is, patient-focused) choices and rules, the best known consequentialist theory is utilitarianism. As formulated by Jeremy Bentham and John Stuart Mill, utilitarian ethics holds that the right action is the one that produces the greatest net utility for a population, by impartially giving equal consideration to the legitimate interests of the affected parties (Beauchamp and Childress, 2019). Utility—that is, what is being maximized—has been described in various ways; Bentham, for example, favored happiness. Today, most utilitarian accounts include a diverse set of values, which can be summed up as welfare. In the context of medicine, maximum welfare can be thought of in terms of the value of the population's health and well-being less the cost of achieving it. In this way, ethical theory supports attending to the efficiency of the health care system, which is one aspect of a trustworthy system of organ transplantation, namely, that the available resources are being used efficiently to maximize welfare.

Utilitarianism faces some objections that are internal to the theory. First, doubts are raised as to whether an "impartial" assessment of individual interests is even possible. Second, how can those interests be combined to calculate net utility? Many of the resources involved in health care are readily monetized (such as facilities, equipment, personnel, and supplies) which facilitates their being brought into a net-cost calculus. But other costs are intangible, such as the anxiety and suffering experienced by patients and their families from illness as well as in efforts to alleviate it. The same is true of the benefits: the restoration of health allows people to return to work and engage in other productive activities, but some of the benefits that people value the most—relief from pain and suffering, return of the ability to form and carry on relationships, and the like—do not have a ready market price. Further, any calculation of net benefit also needs to take into consideration the value of alternative goods that could have been produced using the same resources elsewhere in health care. Given the inherently subjective nature of many of the interests involved, how could one say which is a greater contribution to net social utility, the value to 16,000 people of not having a severe, day-long migraine or the value to one person of not dying suddenly but painlessly at age 25 (with the loss of about 16,000 days of life expectancy)?

Utilitarianism faces other problems when it conflicts with non-consequentialist theories, such as medical deontology, which produce divergent conclusions about what should be done. In particular, utilitarian policies can produce results that appear unjust, particularly when they are framed against an existing set of circumstances that incorporate manifest inequities. Suppose, for example, that when the resources available to treat a potentially fatal condition are limited, more lives could be saved if they were used to treat patients in urban hospitals because the treatment can be provided more efficiently there—each hospital has a large number of patients in need of care and possesses adequate staff expertise and infrastructure to apply the treatment well—compared to using some of the resources in small rural facilities that lack the necessary expertise and infrastructure and that each have only a few patients. While utilitarian theory would direct using the resources only at the urban hospitals, that would challenge the principle of justice if the patients who seek care at the small rural hospitals come from the poorest sector of the population and already bear a much heavier burden of chronic diseases. Just as decisions that are grounded in justice must take into account utilitarian—or, more broadly, consequentialist—concerns, by giving preference among equitable alternatives to those that use resources most efficiently, so too decisions made using a utilitarian calculus are subject to a justice constraint. The result is that sometimes a choice that would maximize welfare must be rejected in favor of an alternative that creates less utility but avoids creating, or perpetuating, an existing distribution of benefits and burdens that is inequitable.

## THE RELEVANCE OF ETHICAL PRINCIPLES FOR THE ORGAN TRANSPLANTATION SYSTEM

To what extent are the ethical expectations generated by the foregoing theories and principles manifested in the policies and practices of our nation's organ transplantation system? Asked another way, does the system adhere to ethical standards in a way that should inspire people most directly involved to regard organ transplantation as a system worthy of their trust? This section applies the summary of ethics presented above, principle by principle, to a number of policies and practices to illustrate the ways that the system may or may not meet ethical obligations to organ recipients and donors. The chapter aims to show how ethics is relevant to the system, but leaves to subsequent chapters a detailed examination of the ways that organ donation, procurement, allocation, and transplantation policies and practices affect donors and recipients and their families as well as the health care professionals involved with these persons and thereby may create or undermine trust in the system. While most of the issues that the committee was asked to study, such as organ allocation policies and maximizing the use of donated organs, focus on patients who need a transplant, transplantation begins with organ donors and even deceased donors also begin as patients, to whom ethical obligations are owed not only by the health care professionals who care for them, but also by other individuals and institutions within the organ transplantation system with whom they never personally interact.[7]

## Beneficence and Nonmaleficence

For patients who experience organ failure, transplantation offers a route back to health and long-term survival. Yet the obvious benefits of a system that provides organ recipients something of such great value does not end all doubts about beneficence and nonmaleficence. To begin, some unique features of the system create dual loyalties among transplant professionals, who have to be both an advocate for individual patients and a steward of a scarce resource that needs to be used to maximize overall welfare (Griffin, 2002; Khazanie and Drazner, 2019; OPTN, 2018). For example, a transplant center may be offered a kidney but then declines it on behalf of the transplant candidate to whom it was first offered. Does this situation entail a failure—or only an appearance of failure—to "put the patient's interests first" as to those patients for whom the organ would have been medically suitable but who were not selected to receive it? Without knowing the full context of clinical decision making, potential recipients may feel that their trust has been breached upon learning that a kidney that was suitable for them had been given to another patient. If choices of this sort are inevitable for transplant centers and transplant teams, trust might be better protected if this situation were explained in advance.

To say that the organ transplantation system treats potential recipients ethically requires more than individual professionals fulfilling their duty of beneficence. The system as a whole

---

[7] The ethical duties owed to living organ donors (Ross and Thistlethwaite, 2021) overlap with but also differ significantly from those owed to deceased donors.

must do so as well, from the time that a patient develops a medical condition for which transplantation is the best treatment through to the posttransplant phase, when the patient needs continued follow-up and care to maintain a functioning organ. One example is access to the immunosuppressive medication needed to prevent rejection of a transplant. Until recently, the End-Stage Renal Disease program paid up to 80 percent of the cost of antirejection medicines for only 3 years, which placed financial strain on transplant recipients, and in some cases, led to organ failure in transplant recipients who could not afford to buy the medication. The Beneficiary Improvement and Protection Act of 2000 extended coverage of immunosuppressants for the life of the kidney for patients who qualify for Medicare coverage because they are disabled or 65 years or older (Gordon et al., 2008). A further change in the law approved in December 2020 expanded Medicare payment for the antirejection drugs to all kidney recipients who lack other insurance.[8] The amendment does not, however, extend other Medicare benefits for kidney recipients, including for other transplant-related medications. Failing to provide all care needed to preserve the function of transplanted kidneys is not beneficent—and not efficient, as well—since recipients whose transplant fails will need a second transplant and, in the meantime, dialysis.

The issue of a potential dual loyalty, which can compromise physicians in fulfilling their duty of beneficence, also arises in the care of deceased organ donors, where it is recognized and dealt with directly in the law. Since deceased donation obviously does not occur until the prospective donor has died, a trustworthy organ transplantation system needs to ensure that death will not be declared prematurely and never by anyone involved in transplanting the organs or taking care of the patients who receive them.[9]

## Autonomy

### Donors

The respect shown for donors' choices provides a solid basis for trust in the U.S. organ transplantation system. All U.S. states endorsed an autonomy-based donation policy, by enacting the Uniform Anatomical Gift Act (UAGA) in 1968. Further, the UAGA made the deceased person the "giver." Prior to the UAGA, the common law put disposition of dead bodies in the hands of the legal next of kin. The Act changed that, allowing potential donors to decide during their lifetime, and it made it easy for them to document that choice; only if the deceased had not done so would the decision fall to the legal next of kin. On the federal level, the NOTA of 1984 made explicit that donated organs must be voluntary gifts, neither seized by the state nor purchased. The 1987 revision of the UAGA retreated slightly from autonomy by allowing a state medical examiner or other public health official to authorize the removal of a part from a deceased body in their possession without permission of the family when attempts to contact next of kin had failed. But that authority was removed when the UAGA was amended again in 2006 to emphasize respect for donor's autonomy by ensuring that a donor's decision "is to be honored and implemented" even when a family member objects (Sadler and Sadler, 2018).

Since 1993, the Health Resources and Services Administration (HRSA) has contracted with the Gallup organization to conduct four nation-wide public opinion surveys (1993,

---

[8] H.R. 5334, the Comprehensive Immunosuppressive Drug Coverage for Kidney Transplant Patients Act of 2020, was incorporated in and passed as part of the Consolidated Appropriations Act, 2021. The bill was signed into law on December 27, 2020. For the full text see https://www.congress.gov/bill/116th-congress/house-bill/133/text (accessed November 5, 2021).

[9] Uniform Determination of Death Act (1980); Revised Uniform Anatomical Gift Act (2006).

2005, 2012, 2019) on the nation's attitudes and practices toward organ donation. Across the nearly 30 years of survey data, support for organ donation has been high and sustained at over 90 percent (HHS, 2019). This long-standing public support was the basis of the increased focus on personal autonomy in the donation process, and resulted in the Revised UAGA (2006). The revisions simplified the document of gift process to allow individuals to make the personal choice to donate anatomic gifts at the time of their death using the driver's license documents as the state donor registry. Another key element of the 2006 UAGA was establishing two separate legal avenues to arrive at a "yes" to donation—an individual can make a gift before death, known as first-person authorization, or a surrogate can authorize a gift at the time of the donor's death (Glazier, 2018). The UAGA also strengthened an individual's right not to donate by permitting signed refusals.

Donor registries proliferated in all 50 states, plus the District of Columbia and Puerto Rico as a result of the revisions to the UAGA. State donor registries are managed through each individual state's department of motor vehicles (DMV) in close collaboration with the OPO, tissue and eye procurement entities within a donor service area. In the years since the 2006 UAGA, donor registries have matured, and over 90 percent of the public surveyed who indicated that they had signed up as organ donors stated they joined a donor registry through their state DMV (HHS, 2019). To address the challenges of a mobile population and the limitations of accessing donor registry information when death occurs outside the state of residency, Donate Life America launched the National Donate Life Registry in 2015 as a way to make donor registration an easy and secure process across the country.[10] When a death occurs in a hospital, the OPO accesses the state of residence donor registry and the national donor registry to determine if the individual has made a first-person authorization for donation.

Given the variety of databases, there have been challenges in knitting together nonstandardized data from 52 independent state agencies to better understand the individual registry rates by state and by demographic. Donate Life America notes that 55 percent of all organ donors in the United States have been authorized by first-person authorization via a donor registry (Donate Life America, 2021); with better data, it is estimated the number could be higher. Despite the data challenges, the number of donors registered has grown from 156 million in 2019 to 169 million in 2021 (Donate Life America, 2021). Improved data would also show the gaps in registries—that is, which groups are joining donor registries at rates well below the general population, an important factor in better understanding inequities in the organ donation process. Another area not well understood is how the donor's autonomy is respected if a surrogate decision maker "at the bedside" expresses opposition to donating organs from a patient whose wish to donate appears in the donor registry.

Accurate knowledge of organ donation and transplantation is fundamental to the success of the transplant enterprise (see Box 3-2). Misinformation and public distrust can lead to reduced rates of organ donation. At the individual level, members of the public vary in their awareness and knowledge of transplantation. Despite efforts to educate the public about organ donation and transplantation, many members of the public report being unaware of organ donation. Making information about organ and tissue donation more readily available to, and comprehensible by, the public, including how to sign a donor registry, is an important part of respecting personal autonomy. Such information can increase people's awareness of their right to decide for themselves about organ transplantation, including the value of using the registry and how it relates to other aspects of the process, as well as help them to

---

[10] For information on the Donate Life Registry see https://www.donatelife.net/national-donate-life-registry (accessed January 28, 2022).

understand how and when donation occurs. Information programs need to take account of differences among the audience being addressed. Targeted interventions have shown promise in increasing black donor registry rates (DuBay et al., 2018). Further research about the attitudes of racial and ethnic groups toward donation is needed if educators are to tailor the information content and manner of presentation to different audiences, whether through DMV offices or by other means that take into account each group's cultural and religious traditions and beliefs (Craig et al., 2021).

## Recipients

If the ethical principle of autonomy is clear as to organ donors, what about for recipients? Like any patient, potential organ recipients receive respect when the transplant professionals who provide their care involve them as informed decision makers in the treatment process from being evaluated and listed for, to then undergoing, a transplant. Respect for autonomy is typically equated with obtaining informed consent, but a good deal can be lost in translation from ethical principle into legal necessity, especially when the latter is reduced to getting a patient's signature on a consent form before surgery may commence.

Studies have repeatedly shown that many barriers exist to achieving informed consent. Some arise on the patient side: a lack of basic understanding of the illness and its treatment, an inability to process complex information (short of mental incapacity), and anxiety or wishful thinking, which can lead to denial of facts or to false beliefs. A major issue on the doctors' side is that their busy schedules may not offer time for in-depth discussions with patients, for which they are in any case poorly compensated. Further, they may lack either the maturity or in-depth education needed to navigate such conversations comfortably and productively or to discern the degree to which patients want to be true partners in shared decision making. Instead, clinicians' main objective is usually to obtain approval for what they genuinely regard as the best course of treatment; this aim can lead to selective disclosure of information on potential harms and benefits and on the relative merits of therapeutic alternatives (Hall et al., 2012).

Transplant professionals are mandated by the OPTN to deliver education to patients initiating transplant evaluation (as well as to potential living donors at the time of donor evaluation). However, the format for delivering transplant education varies from videos to one-on-one education by a nurse to group discussions led by surgeons or nurses; such education may not be available in Spanish or languages other than English (Gordon et al., 2010). Further, dialysis facilities are mandated by the Centers for Medicare & Medicaid Services to inform dialysis patients about the option of transplantation when the patient begins their dialysis treatment,[11] though compliance with this policy is not 100 percent (Waterman et al., 2015).

If, as research has shown (Braddock et al., 1999; Hudak et al., 2008), informed consent processes typically fall short in health care generally, might the ethical ideal of autonomous decisions be more achievable for transplant patients? Patients awaiting a transplant typically have considerable time to learn about their disease and its expected progression, to realize how it affects them and how they feel about that, to learn about the different ways it can be treated as well as what is likely to occur if these options are rejected, and to form a therapeutic relationship with the team of professionals managing their care. Thus, assuming that they have, and retain, decision-making capacity and that the decision to have a transplant is voluntary, potential recipients would seem to be in a good position to participate in a process of shared decision making with a surgeon and other members of the transplant team. Yet a

---

[11] Condition: Patients' Rights, 42 C.F.R. §494.70 (2021), https://www.ecfr.gov/current/title-42/chapter-IV/subchapter-G/part-494/subpart-C/section-494.70 (accessed November 18, 2021).

number of features of organ transplantation pose barriers to shared decision making (Gordon et al., 2013). Indeed, some of these features—such as transplant centers' ongoing responsibility for a large set of patients waiting for deceased donor organs, the fragmented relationships that occur when patients have to interact with a variety of professionals in multiple settings (e.g., their primary physician's office; a dialysis center; the transplant center, which they may visit only once a year, or less), and the unpredictable timing of deceased donor offers—can make clinicians' typical shortage of time for detailed discussions with patients even more pronounced.

Nevertheless, programs need to be forthcoming with organ transplant candidates about the decisions that will need to be made and to find out the extent to which patients want to be involved in those decisions. As noted above, respect for autonomy can manifest through any number of different arrangements between physician and patient; even shared decision making can take many different forms, as chosen by the people involved, with no expectation that patients must exercise their autonomy in a particular way (Hall et al., 2012). But certain ethical requisites must be met—especially disclosure of central, material information about the process and discussion of the choices entailed—if potential recipients are to regard organ transplantation as a trustworthy process.

As discussed in Chapter 6, when an organ has been offered for a particular patient on the waiting list, the patient's surgeon has little time to decide whether or not to recommend to the patient to accept the organ; yet, if the surgeon concludes that the offer should be declined, the patient may not be alerted. Many factors go into the decision, such as the type of organ (e.g., kidney versus other organs), the patient's situation (e.g., hospitalized versus outpatient), and technical factors about the organ, its medical suitability for the patient, and why it was declined. Since the decision ultimately turns on whether the probable benefit to the patient of receiving the particular organ outweighs the probable benefit of rejecting the organ and waiting for another, the decision should reflect the patient's values and goals, and if the surgeon believes that the moment when an organ is offered is not the right time to discuss this topic, then the transplant program must find another time for this conversation in order to meet the expectation that decision making will be patient centered. For example, at the time patients are placed on the list for a transplant and periodically thereafter, members of the transplant team can have conversations with patients about their view of their current situation and about what they hope for, about how they cope with adversity, about their understanding of what is entailed in transplantation, and about similar topics as a means not only of responding to patients' doubts and confusions but also of learning about their goals and values (Gordon et al., 2013). Once an individual patient's preferences have been revealed and he or she has reached an understanding with the transplant team about the goals of care, the professionals will be able to carry out their fiduciary duty to make technical decisions (such as whether to accept an organ offer) in a fashion that is informed by, and aligned with, that particular patient's goals under the circumstances (Joffe and Truog, 2010).

Another opportunity for transplant programs to make sure that prospective recipients are adequately informed about the transplant process is to discuss how decisions are made regarding the allocation of organs that become available to the program. Such disclosure and discussion would enable patients to ascertain whether the reasons are acceptable and pertinent factors have been considered (Emanuel et al., 2008). It may, for example, be material to some patients' understanding of their status to know how many organs have been offered to and declined by their center in order to gauge their own likelihood of receiving an organ; this can promote a process of shared decision making as to whether the patient wants to reconsider accepting organs that the center would otherwise decline (Mohan and Chiles, 2017).

Discussions about patients' goals need to include frank consideration of the attendant uncertainties, especially if the patient's condition is likely to be more emergent by the time an organ is offered, as is the case, for example, with most lung transplants. The progress of disease prior to transplantation can necessitate long periods in intensive care posttransplant, with the resulting complications and debilities, and it is important for these to be discussed (Courtwright et al., 2019).

Likewise, when several alternative approaches are possible and vary in the way they combine probable benefits and harms, assessing the patient's preferences for these outcomes can be informative. Such conversations need to be repeated with patients who are awaiting a transplant for months or years, since their views on what risks are worth taking may change over time. Finally, transplant teams need to remember that voluntariness is an essential component of informed consent, which means that patients must be able not only to give but to withdraw consent. Remaining patient centered is essential if the organ transplantation system hopes to be worthy of the trust of patients and their families.

## Justice

The lack of complete data on health inequities means that the first step in improving justice in the organ transplantation system is to approach data gathering and analysis in a manner that is both broad and deep. Scrutiny of comprehensive, longitudinal data about which patients with organ failure receive transplants and which do not should reveal which disparities in rates reflect inequities. This monitoring and analysis needs to extend to all aspects of the transplant process. For example, as instructed by §121.8 of the Final Rule, the OPTN board has looked closely at the ethical and policy aspects of equitable access to donated organs among patients on a transplant waiting list. Yet, although the "primary barrier" for socioeconomically disadvantaged people in getting a transplant is "gaining access to a waiting list" (IOM, 1999), the OPTN has given only sporadic attention to policies that reduce the inequities in access to transplant services resulting from socioeconomic status, such as policies providing for listing of all patients in need without regard to ability to pay or source of payment, or "procedures for transplant hospitals to make reasonable efforts to make available" themselves or to obtain from others, "financial resources for patients unable to pay" such that they have the opportunity to obtain a transplant.[12] At the heart of this problem is the unacceptable reality that "Many uninsured Americans give organs, but they rarely receive them" (Herring et al., 2008, p. 641). The purview of the OPTN begins when an individual patient is added to the waiting list for a deceased donor organ. As stated throughout this report, the committee finds that this gap in oversight presents a significant challenge to ensuring fairness and equity in the organ transplantation system (Patzer et al., 2012).

While disparities that arise from the discrimination or implicit bias against people based on their color, sex, religion, socioeconomic status, or the like, or from the general effects of racism, ableism, ageism, or sexism, are unquestionably inequitable, other policies that generate claims of unfairness are harder to resolve. For example, some people believe that sending organs donated at a hospital to recipients in distant cities is unfair to patients awaiting an organ at a transplant center located in the same city as the donor hospital; others claim that certain methods of prioritizing potential recipients are unfair because they either neglect important criteria or include irrelevant ones. Such complaints may either be objections to the process by which the algorithm for allocating a type of organ is carried out or objections to the factors that are incorporated into rules that emerge from the process. Both

---

[12] OPTN Final Rule, 42 C.F.R. §121.4(a)(3).

types of objections should be considered; a justification is owed whether or not the process of rule development is modified or otherwise enlarged to encompass more stakeholders, or whether or not other factors are incorporated. Achieving health care justice is such a central concern that the next two chapters are devoted to disparities in organ transplantation and when and why they amount to health inequities, as well as how the deceased donor organ allocation system can be made more fair.

> Conclusion 3-1: The organ transplantation system lacks sufficient oversight from the U.S. Department of Health and Human Services (HHS). Specifically, there is no oversight beginning when individuals are diagnosed with end-stage organ failure until being wait-listed. Without such oversight, inequities are more likely to arise throughout this initial phase of access to transplantation. Allowing inequities to arise without any monitoring is unjust.

## TRANSPARENCY: AN INSTRUMENTAL VALUE FOR A TRUSTWORTHY SYSTEM

The ethical principle of respect for individual autonomy requires that health care providers disclose to patients the information they need or want to understand their choices and make an informed decision. Making relevant information available to patients is thus part of what makes the organ transplantation system trustworthy to them. Transparency about the system—that is, its policies and outcomes—is also essential to achieving trust among members of the general public as well as authorities who exercise oversight of the system for the public. This aspect of transparency is an instrumental precept (i.e., a means toward a trustworthy system) rather than a bioethical precept. Indeed, the ethical principle of nonmaleficence imposes on professionals the duty of keeping information about patients confidential, so that the data made available to others to achieve "transparency" is always limited to what the patient permits to be disclosed or what can be disclosed without breaching confidentiality. Within such limits, everyone involved in organ transplantation is well served by erring toward disclosing rather than withholding information, given the relationship between transparency and public trust.

Like many aspects of health care, the organ transplantation system faces increasing demands to provide information beyond existing regulatory and statutory obligations (which began with NOTA because the public has such a substantial stake in whether the process of obtaining and distributing lifesaving materials of human origin is operating fairly and efficiently). Besides trust, transparency is necessary for accountability as well—which is to say, not simply the obligation of the system to provide an account of its operations but also to be answerable for any deficiencies or misfeasance. Only by having access to information about how decisions are made, by whom, and with what premises and goals; about what decision makers are doing or plan to do; and about the results of their policies and practices can outsiders, including the public and its representatives in government, hold the system's operators accountable. Accountability in transplantation signifies requiring the professionals and bureaucrats involved to explain and accept responsibility for meeting their primary obligations, not merely complying with regulations or meeting managerial performance targets (O'Neill, 2004). Some have posited that trust could be fostered throughout all phases of the transplantation system by respecting family wishes and individual autonomy (Sadler and Sadler, 2018).

When the duty to be transparent is framed in terms of primary obligations, it is important to remember that—as noted earlier—the organ transplant "system" has many components that operate with different degrees of interrelation but that lack a single director who can be held accountable. At a national level, the policies developed by the OPTN are published by the HRSA, the federal agency which oversees the OPTN contract. Thus, accountability comes from having to explain and justify those policies publicly before they may be implemented. By contrast, when individual transplant programs or donor hospitals, and the professionals who practice in those facilities, develop their own policies, the public is usually not consulted and may be unaware of their content or reasoning.

A different type of transparency exists for data about transplant waiting lists, organs donated and used, and transplant outcomes because of the requirements of law and regulations for annual reports on a national basis. Data from the Scientific Registry of Transplant Recipients and other sources are not only carefully scrutinized by regulators, congressional oversight committees, and advocacy organizations but also sometimes covered by the press. The complexity of the process means that many matters remain obscure to the public. Some situations suggest that decision makers or organizations are motivated by personal interests or are otherwise conflicted.[13] Thus, while greater transparency of the features of the national, regional, and local arrangements could help to prevent adverse response to media disclosures, some problems are unlikely to be solved by disclosure alone.

When the World Health Assembly updated the World Health Organization (WHO) Guiding Principles on Human Cell Tissue and Organ Transplantation in 2010, it added Guiding Principle 11:

> The organization and execution of donation and transplantation activities, as well as their clinical results, must be transparent and open to scrutiny, while ensuring that the personal anonymity and privacy of donors and recipients are always protected (WHA, 2010, p. 419).

As WHO explained:

> Transparency can be summarized as maintaining public access to regularly updated comprehensive data on processes, in particular allocation, transplant activities and outcomes for both recipients and living donors, as well as data on organization, budgets and funding (WHA, 2010, p. 419).

The Guiding Principles further state that the objective of transparency goes beyond providing data for scholarly study and government oversight to identifying risks and facilitating their correction "in order to minimize harm to donors or recipients" (WHA, 2010, p. 419).

For the goals of transparency to be met, the information provided must not only be accurate and timely but also readily accessible and easily understood by all segments of the intended audience. The views of relevant stakeholders must be considered when determining the limits of transparency and what information is needed by whom in order to maximize the utility and fairness of transplantation. Yet transparency cannot be achieved simply by making information available to the public (Kass and Faden, 2018). Some members of the public may not have the time, desire, or capacity to read and comprehend complex information or even the ability to access it. Data on performance indicators can be simplified by providing it in numeric or tabular form (i.e., graft survival rates over various periods of time, such as 1 year or 5 years). Still, simplification to improve comprehension can risk losing subtlety or being misleading. For example, were a color-coding method (red, yellow, green) used to indicate whether transplant centers meet graft survival targets, the display of the results may denote that a center's survival rate is very deficient (red) even though the actual difference

---

[13] See https://oversight.house.gov/news/press-releases/oversight-subcommittee-launches-investigation-into-poor-performance-waste-and (accessed November 18, 2021).

between it and a center designated in yellow is less than 1 percent. More basically, numeric information may lack a narrative for readers to discern the point of the message or they may not put the data in context. If data are disclosed in a way that grades actors against each other—for example, by color-coding, as just described—then people seeing such reports will not be made aware if all the actors are failing to perform as expected. It is, however, possible to provide simplified interactive—yet narrative—information, as shown by the 2021 Annual Data Report of the U.S. Renal Data System. Box 3-3 contains information on public education efforts in organ donation and transplantation.

---

**BOX 3-3    PUBLIC EDUCATION IN ORGAN DONATION AND TRANSPLANTATION**

Public education efforts about organ donation and transplantation vary. Public education campaigns have been sponsored by U.S. states, Donate Life America, the Department of Transportation, and by OPOs. For example, the State of Illinois includes information about organ donation in license renewal documents mailed to its residents. The call to action in many OPO public education campaigns is for the public to sign up on their state's donor registries. While some OPOs educate the public about organ donation and transplantation, most OPO-sponsored education focuses on deceased organ donation, and transplant centers are more likely to engage in public education efforts on living donation. Public education is delivered in different formats such as public awareness news and social media campaigns that can reach large population groups, but are infrequent, brief in message, and last a short duration owing to the high costs of running news media campaigns.

Public education campaigns have been shown to be effective in increasing knowledge about organ donation and organ donation registration rates (Anker et al., 2016). Such campaigns have included peer-to-peer campaigns (Feeley et al., 2009), OPO-sponsored challenge campaigns (Feeley and Kruegler, 2015), use of voter registration forms (Feeley et al., 2020), social media campaigns (Stefanone et al., 2012), direct mail campaigns (Feeley et al., 2016), and culturally targeted campaigns for Hispanics (Alvaro et al., 2010). However, having a point of decision at the offices of the Departments of Motor Vehicles is not effective for increasing donation registration (Feeley et al., 2017).

However, research suggests that people are more responsive to state-sponsored public education campaigns. As an example, Quick and colleagues (2016) found that direct mail campaigns that were authored by state officials (e.g., Iowa Department of Public Health, Illinois Secretary of State) resulted in higher registration rates than by campaigns sponsored by local OPOs.

Based on these findings, state governments could achieve higher donor registration rates by working with research scientists and other transplantation experts to develop and publish accurate and appropriate educational materials.

However, as with any public health activity, it is essential that public education campaigns be evaluated for both outcome and process measures. Process measures are key to evaluating whether the intervention (the campaign) is implemented with fidelity (adherence to the protocol). By measuring processes, evaluators can determine whether an ineffective campaign was caused by implementation with low fidelity, or by a poor campaign message or the delivery itself. Key factors to consider when developing process measures should include dosage (number, duration, and frequency) of campaign exposures delivered, type of exposure (e.g., news media, social media, direct postal mailing), number of people exposed to the campaign (e.g., metadata on number of people visiting donation website; see Gordon et al., 2016, for example), satisfaction with the campaign, and whether targeted campaigns increase registry rates. Ideally, process measures are built into the intervention throughout its implementation, when feasible, rather than being evaluated at the end of intervention implementation. Moreover, it is critical that campaign messaging and delivery approaches be driven by a theoretical framework to foster greater scientific rigor.

Transplant experts vary in the clarity and comprehensiveness with which they communicate to the public about organ donation and transplantation. Even though available education materials about organ donation and transplantation may be publicly available, they may not be publicly accessible. Studies document that organ transplant and donation educational consent research used by transplant centers are prepared at college reading levels (Gordon and Wolf, 2009; Zhou et al., 2018). Little is known about the reading grade levels of OPO or other public education materials. Health literacy refers to "the degree to which individuals have the capacity to obtain, process, and understand basic health information needed to make appropriate health decisions" (HRSA, 2019). In 2003, nearly 80 million Americans (36 percent) had limited functional health literacy and thus poor knowledge and ability to understand health-related information (Berkman et al., 2011). Limited health literacy is associated with numerous adverse health consequences including poor medication adherence, increased hospitalizations, and higher mortality (Berkman et al., 2011; Dore-Stites et al., 2020; Taylor et al., 2016; Warsame et al., 2019). Further, limited health literacy is significantly more common among minorities, individuals with less than high school education, the poor, and the elderly (Kutner et al., 2006; Ricardo et al., 2014). Limited health literacy is common among dialysis patients and kidney transplant recipients (up to 30 percent) (Devraj et al., 2015; Muscat et al., 2018; Ricardo et al., 2014; Taylor et al., 2018) and liver transplant recipients (Bababekov et al., 2019; Serper et al., 2015), but there are limited data on health literacy in lung transplant recipients (Lennerling et al., 2018). Thus, given the prevalence of limited health literacy in the population of patients in need of organ transplantation, and the fact that current materials are prepared at a high reading grade level, the committee recommends that health information be communicated and prepared in a simple, accessible fashion.

*Conclusion 3-2: Transparency throughout the transplant process is key. The transplant team has an ethical obligation to ensure that transplant candidates stay well informed about the organ transplant evaluation and allocation process. Professionals can engage candidates in a conversation about when organs become available and provide evidence-based information about the risks and potential benefits of accepting or declining different types of medically complex organs. Although engaging in the informed consent discussions at the time of the organ offer is feasible, the committee recognizes that logistical and timing factors can make the informed consent process challenging.*

*Conclusion 3-3: Public knowledge about organ transplantation remains lower than desired to optimize trust in the transplantation system. Many people hold beliefs about organ transplantation and donation that are not accurate and that, if corrected, could increase the trustworthiness of the system.*

# REFERENCES

Alvaro, E. M., J. T. Siegel, W. D. Crano, and A. Dominick. 2010. A mass mediated intervention on Hispanic live kidney donation. *Journal of Health Communication* 15(4):374-387.

Anker, A. E., T. H. Feeley, B. McCracken, and C. A. Lagoe. 2016. Measuring the effectiveness of mass-mediated health campaigns through meta-analysis. *Journal of Health Communication* 21(4):439-456.

Arcaya, M. C., A. L. Arcaya, and S. V. Subramanian. 2015. Inequalities in health: Definitions, concepts, and theories. *Global Health Action* 8:10. https://www.ncbi.nlm.nih.gov/pmc/articles/PMC4481045 (accessed December 21, 2021).

Bababekov, Y. J., Y. C. Hung, C. G. Rickert, F. C. Njoku, B. Cao, J. T. Adler, A. G. Brega, J. J. Pomposelli, D. C. Chang, and H. Yeh. 2019. Health literacy burden is associated with access to liver transplantation. *Transplantation* 103(3):522-528.

Beauchamp, T. L., and J. F. Childress. 2019. *Principles of biomedical ethics,* 8th ed. New York: Oxford University Press.

Berkman, N. D., S. L. Sheridan, K. E. Donahue, D. J. Halpern, A. Viera, K. Crotty, A. Holland, M. Brasure, K. N. Lohr, E. Harden, E. Tant, I. Wallace, and M. Viswanathan. 2011. Health literacy interventions and outcomes: An updated systematic review. *Evidence Report/Technology Assessment* (199):1-941.

Boulware, L. E., M. U. Troll, N. Y. Wang, and N. R. Powe. 2007. Perceived transparency and fairness of the organ allocation system and willingness to donate organs: A national study. *American Journal of Transplantation* 7(7):1778-1787.

Braddock, C. H. III, K. A. Edwards, N. M. Hasenberg, T. L. Laidley, and W. Levinson. 1999. Informed decision making in outpatient practice: Time to get back to basics. *Journal of the American Medical Association* 282:2313-2320.

Burdick, J. F., J. G. Turcotte, and R. M. Veatch, eds. 1992. Principles of organ and tissue allocation and donation by living donors. *Transplantation Proceedings* 24(5):2226-2237.

Capron, A. M. 1974. Informed consent in catastrophic disease research and treatment. *University of Pennsylvania Law Review* 123:340-438.

Courtwright, A. M., E. Rubin, E. M. Robinson, S. ElChemaly, D. Lamas, J. M. Diamond, and H. J. Goldberg. 2019. An ethical framework for the care of patients with prolonged hospitalization following lung transplantation. *Healthcare Ethics Committee Forum* 31:49-62.

Craig, M., M. Quinn, M. R. Saunders, and A. I. Padela. 2021. Muslim Americans' views on making organ donation decisions in the Department of Motor Vehicles setting. *Progress in Transplantation* 31(4):323-329.

Daniels, N. 2008. *Just health: Meeting health needs fairly.* New York: Cambridge University Press.

Devraj, R., M. Borrego, A. M. Vilay, E. J. Gordon, J. Pailden, and B. Horowitz. 2015. Relationship between health literacy and kidney function. *Nephrology (Carlton)* 20(5):360-367.

Donate Life America. 2021. *2021 Annual Update.* https://www.donatelife.net/wp-content/uploads/2022/01/2021DonateLifeAmericaAnnualUpdate.pdf (accessed January 28, 2022).

Dore-Stites, D., M. J. Lopez, J. C. Magee, J. Bucuvalas, K. Campbell, V. Shieck, A. Well, and E. M. Fredericks. 2020. Health literacy and its association with adherence in pediatric liver transplant recipients and their parents. *Pediatric Transplant* 24(5):e13726.

DuBay, D. A., N. V. Ivankova, I. Herbey, D. T. Redden, C. Holt, L. Siminoff, M. N. Fouad, Z. Su, T. A. Morinelli, and M. Y. Martin. 2018. A quantitative appraisal of African Americans' decisions to become registered organ donors at the driver's license office. *Clinical Transplant* 32(10):e13402.

Emanuel, E. J., D. Wendler, and C. Grady. 2008. An ethical framework for biomedical research. *The Oxford textbook of clinical research ethics.* New York: Oxford University Press. Pp. 123-135.

Faden, R. R., and T. L. Beauchamp. 1986. *A history and theory of informed consent.* New York: Oxford University Press.

Feeley, T. H., and J. Kruegel. 2015. Promoting organ donation through challenge campaigns. *Progress in Transplantation* 25(2):176-181.

Feeley, T. H., A. E. Anker, B. Watkins, J. Rivera, N. Tag, and L. Volpe. 2009. A peer-to-peer campaign to promote organ donation among racially diverse college students in New York City. *Journal of the National Medical Association* 101(11):1154-1162.

Feeley, T. H., B. L. Quick, and S. Lee. 2016. Using direct mail to promote organ donor registration: Two campaigns and a meta-analysis. *Clinical Transplantation* 30(12):1564-1569.

Feeley, T. H., A. E. Anker, M. Evans, and T. Reynolds-Tylus. 2017. A department of motor vehicle-based intervention to promote organ donor registrations in New York State. *Progress in Transplantation* 27(3):273-280.

Feeley, T. H., M. A. Evans, A. K. O'Mally, and A. Tator. 2020. Using voter registration to increase enrollment into the organ and tissue registry in New York State. *Progress in Transplantation* 30(3):208-211.

Glazier, A. K. 2018. Organ donation and the principles of gift law. *Clinical Journal of the American Society of Nephrology* 13(8):1283-1284.

Gordon, E. J., and M. S. Wolf. 2009. Health literacy skills of kidney transplant recipients. *Progress in Transplantation* 19(1):25-34. https://doi.org/10.7182/prtr.19.1.qnj8621040488u52.

Gordon, E. J., T. R. Prohaska, and A. R. Sehgal. 2008. The financial impact of immunosuppressant expenses on new kidney transplant recipients. *Clinical Transplantation* 22(6):738-748.

Gordon, E. J., J. C. Caicedo, D. P. Ladner, E. Reddy, and M. M. Abecassis. 2010. Transplant center provision of education and culturally and linguistically competent care: A national study. *American Journal of Transplantation* 10(12):2701-2707.

Gordon, E. J., Z. Butt, S. E. Jensen, A. L.-M. Lehr, J. Franklin, Y. Becker, L. Sherman, W. J. Chond, N. Beauvais, J. Hanneman, D. Penrod, M. G. Ison, and M. M. Abecassis. 2013. Opportunities for shared decision making in kidney transplantation. *American Journal of Transplantation* 13:1093-1158.

Gordon, E. J., J. Shand, and A. Black. 2016. Google analytics of a pilot mass and social media campaign targeting Hispanics about living kidney donation. *Internet Interventions* 6:40-49.

Griffin, L. 2002. Retransplantation of multiple organs: How many organs should one individual receive? *Progress in Transplantation* 12(2):92-96.

Hall, D. E., A. V. Prochazka, and A. S. Fink. 2012. Informed consent for clinical treatment. *Canadian Medical Association Journal* 184(5):533-540.

Herring, A. A., S. Woolhandler, and D. U. Himmelstein. 2008. Insurance status of US organ donors and transplant recipients: The uninsured give, but rarely receive. *International Journal of Health Services* 38(4):641-652.

HHS (U.S. Department of Health and Human Services). 2013. *2012 National Survey of Organ Donation Attitudes and Behaviors*. Rockville, MD: Healthcare Systems Bureau.

HHS. 2019. *2019 National Survey of Organ Donation Attitudes and Practices: Report of findings*. Rockville, MD: U.S. Department of Health and Human Services.

HHS. 2021a. *Healthy People 2020*. https://www.healthypeople.gov/2020/about/foundation-health-measures/Disparities (accessed November 18, 2021).

HHS. 2021b. *Healthy People 2030*. https://health.gov/our-work/healthy-people/healthy-people-2030/questions-answers (accessed November 18, 2021).

Hippocrates. n.d. The oath and law of Hippocrates. Vol. 38, Part 1. *The Harvard Classics*. New York: P.F. Collier & Son. Pp. 1909-1914. https://www.bartleby.com/38/1 (accessed November 5, 2021).

HRSA (Health Resources and Services Administration). 2019. *Health literacy*. https://www.hrsa.gov/about/organization/bureaus/ohe/health-literacy/index.html (accessed January 28, 2022).

Hudak, P. L., R. M. Frankel, C. Braddock III, R. Nisenbaum, P. Luca, C. McKeever, and W. Levinson. 2008. Do patients' communication behaviors provide insight into their preferences for participation in decision making? *Medical Decision Making* 28:385-393.

IOM (Institute of Medicine). 1999. *Organ procurement and transplantation: Assessing current policies and the potential impact of the DHHS Final Rule*. Washington, DC: National Academy Press.

IOM. 2001. *Crossing the quality chasm: A new health system for the 21st century*. Washington, DC: National Academy Press.

IOM. 2006. *Organ donation: Opportunities for action*. Washington, DC: The National Academies Press.

Joffe, S., and R. Truog. 2010. Consent to medical care: The importance of fiduciary context. In *The ethics of consent: Theory and practice*, edited by F. Miller and A. Wertheimer. New York: Oxford University Press. Pp. 347-373.

Kant, I. 1959. *Foundations of the metaphysics of morals*. Translated by L. W. Beck. Indianapolis: Bobbs-Merrill.

Kass, N. E., and R. R. Faden. 2018. Ethics and learning health care: The essential roles of engagement, transparency, and accountability. *Learning Health Systems* 2(4):e10066.

Khazanie, P., and M. H. Drazner. 2019. The blurred line between gaming and patient advocacy: Heart transplant listing decisions in the modern era. *Circulation* 140(25):2048-2050.

Kutner, M., E. Greenberg, Y. Jin, and C. Paulsen. 2006. *The health literacy of America's adults: Results from the 2003 National Assessment of Adult Literacy*. Washington, DC: National Center for Education Statistics.

Lennerling, A., A. M. Kisch, and A. Forsberg. 2018. Health literacy among Swedish lung transplant recipients 1 to 5 years after transplantation. *Progress in Transplantation* 28(4):338-342.

Mohan, S., and M. C. Chiles. 2017. Achieving equity through reducing variability in accepting deceased donor kidney offers. *Clinical Journal of the American Society of Nephrology* 12(8):1212-1214.

Muscat, D. M., R. Kanagaratnam, H. L. Shepherd, K. Sud, K. McCaffery, and A. Webster. 2018. Beyond dialysis decisions: A qualitative exploration of decision-making among culturally and linguistically diverse adults with chronic kidney disease on haemodialysis. *BMC Nephrology* 19(1):339.

National Commission for the Protection of Human Subjects of Biomedical and Behavioral Research. 1979. *The Belmont report: Ethical principles and guidelines for the protection of human subjects of research*. Washington, DC: U.S. Government Printing Office.

Nedelsky, J. 1989. Reconceiving autonomy: Sources, thoughts and possibilities. *Yale Journal of Law and Feminism* 1:7-36.

Nuremberg Code (1947). 1996. *BMJ* 313:1448.

O'Neill, O. 2004. Accountability, trust and informed consent in medical practice and research. *Clinical Medicine* 4(3):269-276.

OPTN (Organ Procurement and Transplantation Network). 2018. *Manipulation of the organ allocation system waitlist priority through the escalation of medical therapies*. https://optn.transplant.hrsa.gov/media/2500/ethics_white paper_201806.pdf (accessed November 17, 2021).

OPTN Board. 2010. *Ethical principles to be considered in the allocation of human organs* (approved on June 22, 2010). http://optn.transplant.hrsa.gov/resources/ethics (accessed January 24, 2022).

Patzer, R. E., J. P. Perryman, J. D. Schrager, S. Pastan, S. Amaral, J. A. Gazmararian, M. Klein, N. Kutner, and W. M. McClellan. 2012. The role of race and poverty on steps to kidney transplantation in the southeastern United States. *American Journal of Transplantation* 12(2):358-368.

Powers, M., and R. Faden. 2006. *Social justice: The moral foundations of public health and health policy.* New York: Oxford University Press.

President's Commission on the Health Needs of the Nation. 1953. *Summary report.* Washington, DC: U.S. Government Printing Office.

President's Commission for the Study of Ethical Problems in Medicine and Biomedical and Behavioral Research. 1982. *Making health care decisions: The ethical and legal implications of informed consent in the patient-practitioner relationship.* Washington, DC: U.S. Government Printing Office.

Quick, B. L., T. Reynolds-Tylus, A. E. Fico, and T. H. Feeley. 2016. Source and message framing considerations for recruiting mature adults as organ donors through direct mail campaigns. *Progress in Transplantation* 26(4):309-313.

Rawls, J. 1999. *A theory of justice: Revised edition.* Cambridge, MA: The Belknap Press of Harvard University Press.

Ricardo, A. C., W. Yang, C. M. Lora, E. J. Gordon, C. J. Diamantidis, V. Ford, J. W. Kusek, A. Lopez, E. Lustigova, L. Nessel, S. E. Rosas, S. Steigerwalt, J. Theurer, X. Zhang, M. J. Fischer, and J. P. Lash. 2014. Limited health literacy is associated with low glomerular filtration in the Chronic Renal Insufficiency Cohort (CRIC) study. *Clinical Nephrology* 81(1):30-37.

Ross, L. F., and J. R. Thistlethwaite. 2021. *The living organ donor as patient: Theory and practice.* New York: Oxford University Press.

Sadler, B. L., and A. M. Sadler. 2018. Organ transplantation and the Uniform Anatomical Gift Act: A fifty-year perspective. *Hastings Center Report* 48(2):14-18.

Serper, M., R. E. Patzer, P. P. Reese, K. Przytula, R. Koval, D. P. Ladner, J. Levitsky, M. M. Abecassis, and M. S. Wolf. 2015. Medication misuse, nonadherence, and clinical outcomes among liver transplant recipients. *Liver Transplantation* 21(1):22-28.

Stefanone, M., A. E. Anker, M. Evans, and T. H. Feeley. 2012. Click to "like" organ donation: The use of online media to promote organ donor registration. *Progress in Transplantation* 22(2):168-174.

Taylor, D. M., J. A. Bradley, C. Bradley, H. Draper, R. Johnson, W. Metcalfe, G. Oniscu, M. Robb, C. Tomson, C. Watson, R. Ravanan, P. Roderick, and ATTOM Investigators. 2016. Limited health literacy in advanced kidney disease. *Kidney International* 90(3):685-695.

Taylor, D. M., S. Fraser, C. Dudley, G. C. Oniscu, C. Tomson, R. Ravanan, and P. Roderick. 2018. Health literacy and patient outcomes in chronic kidney disease: A systematic review. *Nephrology, Dialysis, Transplantation* 33(9):1545-1558.

Veatch, R. M. 2000. *Transplantation ethics.* Washington, DC: Georgetown University Press.

Veatch, R. M., and L. F. Ross. 2015. *Transplantation ethics, second edition.* Washington, DC: Georgetown University Press.

Wachterman, M. W., E. P. McCarthy, E. R. Marcantonio, and M. Ersek. 2015. Mistrust, misperceptions, and miscommunication: A qualitative study of preferences about kidney transplantation among African Americans. *Transplant Proceedings* 47(2):240-246.

Walter, J. K., and L. F. Ross. 2014. Relational autonomy: Moving beyond the limits of isolated individualism. *Pediatrics* 133:S16-S23.

Warsame, F., C. E. Haugen, H. Ying, J. M. Garonzik-Wang, N. M. Desai, R. K. Hall, R. Kambhampati, D. C. Crews, T. S. Purnell, D. L. Segev, and M. A. McAdams-DeMarco. 2019. Limited health literacy and adverse outcomes among kidney transplant candidates. *American Journal of Transplantation* 19(2):457-465.

Waterman, A. D., J. D. Peipert, C. J. Goalby, K. M. Dinkel, H. Xiao, and K. L. Lentine. 2015. Assessing transplant education practices in dialysis centers: Comparing educator reported and Medicare data. *Clinical Journal of the American Society of Nephrology* 10(9):1617-1625.

WHA (World Health Assembly). 2010. *WHO guiding principles on cell, tissue, and organ transplantation.* https://www.who.int/transplantation/Guiding_PrinciplesTransplantation_WHA63.22en.pdf (accesed December 28, 2021).

WMA (World Medical Association). 1964. *Declaration of Helsinki. Recommendations guiding doctors in clinical research.* https://www.wma.net/what-we-do/medical-ethics/declaration-of-helsinki/doh-jun1964 (accessed February 17, 2022).

Zhou, E. P., E. Kiwanuka, and P. E. Morrissey. 2018. Online patient resources for deceased donor and live donor kidney recipients: A comparative analysis of readability. *Clinical Kidney Journal* 11(4):559-563.

# 4

# Confronting and Eliminating Inequities in the Organ Transplantation System

The preceding chapter established that a trustworthy organ transplantation system must adhere to ethical principles and have transparent processes and results. The committee concluded that the principle of justice is central for the system's success, and that one essential measure of justice is the equity[1] of the system's processes and patient outcomes. This chapter presents evidence that factors such as patients' race, ethnicity, socioeconomic circumstances, and similar attributes do affect the way patients are treated at multiple points along the transplantation journey, from referral for evaluation at a transplant center to the speed with which a transplant occurs. Not surprisingly, the differences in the way that various patient populations are treated result in marked disparities[2] in the outcomes they experience, ranging from longer, better lives for some and early deaths for others. Further, existing data-gathering practices leave gaps concerning processes and outcomes for other groups, such as women, the elderly, and people with disabilities or hereditary disorders. Additionally, there are major gaps in our knowledge about those with failing organs who never enter the transplant pathway in the first place, but who would otherwise be eligible or interested in receiving a transplant. These gaps in data, along with the complex way diverse factors—socioeconomic, racial and ethnic, federal and state policies, various features of health systems, and individual-level characteristics—interact makes it difficult to describe the true scope of the disparities in transplantation. Nonetheless, the existence of such disparities is undeniable.

---

[1] Health equity is the "attainment of the highest level of health for all people. Achieving health equity requires valuing everyone equally with focused and ongoing societal efforts to address avoidable inequalities, historical and contemporary injustices, and the elimination of health and health care disparities" (HHS, 2021b).

[2] As discussed in Chapter 1, the committee adopted the following definition for *health disparities* in the context of this report: "a particular type of health difference that is closely linked with social, economic, and/or environmental disadvantage. Health disparities adversely affect groups of people who have systematically experienced greater obstacles to health based on their racial or ethnic group; religion; socioeconomic status; gender; age; mental health; cognitive, sensory, or physical disability; sexual orientation or gender identity; geographic location; or other characteristics historically linked to discrimination or exclusion" (HHS, 2021a).

Structural problems in society, including injustices in the provision and financing of health care, lie behind the disparities associated with chronic disease care and the health care system more broadly; these also affect processes and outcomes in organ transplantation. However, some of the causes for disparities are specific to the current system of organ transplantation, which are discussed further in this chapter. Organizations working on organ transplantation have multiple aims, such as increasing the number and quality of deceased donor organs and advancing scientific knowledge about, and techniques to prevent, the rejection of organs by transplant recipients' immune system. These aims affect organizations' interactions with transplant candidates, health care providers and researchers, and the public and its elected representatives. When equity is not one of the key aims, instances of inequitable treatment are less likely to be noticed, much less to become a focus for the organization's efforts to improve the system. For example, the object of principal concern for the Organ Procurement and Transplantation Network (OPTN) has been individuals who are on the waiting lists for each type of organ—that is, patients who have been referred to and evaluated and accepted by a transplant center—rather than all patients diagnosed with organ failure. Although more data are needed concerning patients who are not referred for evaluation, enough is known to conclude that members of groups that experience subordination and exclusion in many aspects of their lives are more heavily represented among patients diagnosed with organ failure than on transplant waiting lists. Further study is needed to understand how and why such disparities occur, but the evidence examined in this chapter makes clear the harmful effects of the disparities in terms of the greater likelihood for some populations of not being listed for a needed transplant and of dying prematurely.

The transplantation system's commitment to justice does not mean that the principle of justice always takes priority over all other objectives. As Chapter 3 explained, the various values being sought—not only justice but also respect for the choices of organ donors and recipients, minimizing harm, and maximizing benefits, especially for the least well off—can sometimes pull in different directions. This tension is explored further in Chapter 5 in the assessment of alternative allocation policies. A just organ transplantation system could resolve this conflict between maximizing utility and acting fairly by adopting one policy or the other or some combination of the two. In contrast, when the transplantation system produces glaringly worse results for certain groups of patients—especially those defined by perceived race, ethnicity, sex, religion, socioeconomic status, disability status, geographic location of residence, or the like—a just system would seek the roots of such inequities and take whatever steps are needed to remove them because the benefits experienced by historically favored groups do not justify the imposition of harm on the victims of transplant disparities.

The Statement of Task for the study, found in Box 1-2, has specific charges to the committee for considering equity and fairness throughout the procurement, allocation, and distribution processes. Specifically, the committee was asked to consider whether measures could be taken to reduce inequities in organ allocation affecting socioeconomically disadvantaged populations. This chapter details what is currently known about inequities in access to organ transplants in the United States as well as related aspects including referral to specialists, access to the transplant waiting list, and posttransplant outcomes, and it proposes a recommendation for addressing root causes of inequities in the transplantation system. Other issues examined in this chapter include structural challenges and data gaps that contribute to health inequities in the organ transplantation system in the United States.

## PRIORITIZING HEALTH EQUITY IN THE TRANSPLANTATION SYSTEM— WHY IS THIS IMPORTANT?

The National Organ Transplant Act of 1984 created the Task Force on Organ Transplantation charged with, among other duties, providing recommendations for ensuring equitable access to and allocation of donated organs. Ensuring equity in transplantation requires recognizing inequities that persist across the transplantation system. Removing inequities is vital for creating a system that ensures that all people who need care achieve their best possible health outcomes. Addressing disparities within the system is also vital for building a trustworthy and transparent system (discussed further in Chapter 3). For too long, acknowledgments of individual-level health disparities have taken priority over attention to structural and systemic solutions to inequities (the definitions used by the committee throughout this report can be found in Box 1-3). By not addressing the structures that perpetuate inequities, the system has not adapted to care for patients who may experience more barriers to receiving an organ transplant.

As the focus on promoting health care and social equity in the larger national discussion increases, it is important that the transplantation community commit to working toward equity in both stated policies and practices. Recent years have seen more attention directed toward issues of equity in organ transplantation. For example, the OPTN's strategic plan for 2018–2021 again included providing equity in access to transplant as a strategic goal, and the 2021–2024 strategic plan includes the same goal with a specific initiative focused on identifying and addressing ethnic, socioeconomic status, and geographic disparities.[3] Some professional groups in the transplant community have also more recently included equity as strategic initiatives or explicit goals, though this is not consistent across the community. When equity is not one of the key aims, instances of inequitable treatment may not be noticed, much less become a focus for the organization's efforts to improve the system. While equity has been a long-standing goal of the transplantation system as a whole, stated goals and intentions have not always matched the actions of the stakeholders within the system and translated into change for communities who have been disadvantaged by policies and practices (including racial and ethnic minorities, individuals with disabilities, and the poor). As a result, achieving equity has not been realized.

Current practices of the organ transplantation system lie downstream from earlier, and often times compounding issues, in the health care system (e.g., unequal access to primary care physicians, chronic disease inequities, uneven referral to specialists). However, stakeholders within the organ transplantation system can take many actions to improve equity, including increasing access to the waiting list. Dialysis providers and others caring for patients with end-stage organ failure can establish more systematic referral pathways to transplant centers. Transplant centers can improve their inclusiveness and approaches to the evaluation and listing of referred patients. Organ procurement organizations (OPOs) can promote training and efforts to better meet the needs of minority donor families. Stakeholders within the system need to be held accountable for working to eliminate inequities in organ transplantation, and should be incentivized to do so. The system should also be nimble enough to move quickly in identifying and mitigating unintended consequences that may arise as new policies are implemented. The committee's conclusions and recommendation that follow describe the current state of inequities in transplantation and identify actions that should be taken as the organ transplantation system works to eliminate inequities.

*Conclusion 4-1: Although equity in access and allocation has been a proclaimed principle of the organ transplantation system for decades, and appears in federal regulations directing allocation policy, equity has, until recently, been absent as a stated goal or vision in the strategic plans of many organizations working in organ transplantation. While the stated priorities and plans of organizations involved in*

---

[3] For information on the OPTN Strategic Plan (2021–2024) see https://optn.transplant.hrsa.gov/media/2546/optn_unos_strategic_plan.pdf (accessed January 26, 2022).

*the transplantation system may now include equity, current policies and practices do not always reflect this commitment to equity.*

## STRIVING FOR HEALTH EQUITY AND FAIRNESS IN ORGAN TRANSPLANTATION

"As a medical and scientific community, it is time for our actions to move beyond describing and acknowledging inequities. Rather, we must commit to enacting solutions that rectify inequity through multidimensional approaches that address fundamental causes."
—Boulware and Mohottige, 2021, p. 816
Presented by Kimberly Jacob Arriola, Emory University,
testimony to the committee during February 5, 2021 public workshop

It is well documented that various populations in the United States experience health disparities at specific steps along the pathway to an organ transplant. Table 4-1 and Figure 4-1 provide a sampling of data on health disparities in the context of organ donation and transplantation and the groups that are advantaged and disadvantaged as a result. The committee wanted to highlight these areas of health disparities at various points in the organ donation and transplantation pathway. The committee's overall goal was to use a broader lens and bring attention to structural causes of inequities that drive these disparities in the transplantation system and propose solutions to further health equity.

*Conclusion 4-2: The current organ transplantation system in the United States is demonstrably inequitable. Certain groups of patients (e.g., racial and ethnic minority populations, lower socioeconomic status, female gender, older patients, individuals with intellectual and developmental disabilities, or inheritable diseases such as cystic fibrosis) receive organ transplants at a disproportionately lower rate and in some cases after longer wait times than other patients with comparable need.*

### Inequities Among Racial and Ethnic Groups

Flawed assumptions about trends according to race pervade the clinical literature on organ transplantation and undermine efforts to understand and address inequities in access to transplantation (Harding et al., 2021). Moreover, much transplant research, following U.S. government and National Institutes of Health requirements, fails to disaggregate data, and instead uses categorical race descriptors (e.g., black, Latino, Hispanic, Asian, white, Alaska Native, American Indian, nonblack) that conflate the categories of race and ethnicity and preclude meaningful comparisons across and within diverse ethnic groups (see Box 4-1). As highlighted in Table 4-1, much of the existing data on disparities in organ transplantation focus on race and ethnicity in kidney transplantation, mainly between black and white populations.

### Limitations of the Literature

While most research has focused on black patients, a major limitation of the extant literature on disparities in transplantation is that relatively little attention has focused on Latinx and Hispanic patients, American Indian patients, Asian, or ethnic groups within European American patients. Another limitation of the literature is that authors do not provide definitions of race or ethnicity and do not disaggregate groups for refined analysis (Boyd et al., 2020; Fontanarosa and Bauchner, 2018); in some cases, this is attributable to small sample sizes.

**TABLE 4-1** Data on Health Disparities Related to Steps in the Organ Donation and Transplant Pathway

| Step in the Organ Donation and Transplant Pathway | Organ | Adult vs. Pediatric | Population(s) Affected | Key Outcomes |
|---|---|---|---|---|
| Registration for organ donation | n/a | n/a | Black, Asian American | • Self-reported donor registration rates among black and Asian Americans were lower compared to other racial/ethnic groups (HHS, 2019; p. 25, Table 3). |
| Organ donation authorization | n/a | n/a | Black, American Indian/Alaska Native | • While deceased organ donation rates have improved over time for individuals who are black or American Indian/Alaska Native, those individuals donated at 69% and 28%, respectively, the rate of individuals who are white (Kernodle et al., 2021).<br>• Black families often experience differences in the donation process. For example, one study found that OPO representatives met with a larger proportion of white families of potential donors (66.1%) than black families (50.8%) (Siminoff et al., 2003).<br>• Compared to black families authorizing donation, black families who were approached about donation but ultimately refused were more likely to report feeling pressured, had less comprehensive discussions about donation, and generally rated the OPO requesters' communication skills lower (Siminoff et al., 2020) |
| Primary care physician/ specialist assessment of suitability for transplant[a] | Kidney | Adult | Black | • White patients are more likely than black patients to be rated as appropriate candidates for organ transplantation (20.9% vs. 9.0%) (Epstein et al., 2000). |
| | Kidney | Adult | Patients over age 65, women | • Older hemodialysis patients are less likely to have had discussions with medical professionals about the potential of transplantation as a treatment option (Salter et al., 2014).<br>• Women undergoing hemodialysis were 1.45 times less likely to have had discussions about transplantation with medical professionals (Salter et al., 2014). |
| Referral to transplant center[a] | Kidney | Adult | Black | • Black patients have 37% lower odds of being preemptively referred for transplant evaluation than white patients (Gander et al., 2018). |
| Completing pretransplant evaluation[a] | Kidney | Adult | Black | • Black patients are less likely than white patients to complete pretransplant medical evaluation (Waterman et al., 2013; Weng et al., 2005) |
| Preemptive placement on transplant waiting list | Kidney | Adult | Black, Hispanic | • White candidates are more often preemptively listed for kidney transplant vs. black and Hispanic candidates (39.4% vs. 17.5% vs. 18.5%) (Nissaisorakarn et al., 2021). |

*(continued)*

| Step in the Organ Donation and Transplant Pathway | Organ | Adult vs. Pediatric | Population(s) Affected | Key Outcomes |
|---|---|---|---|---|
| Access to the waiting list | Kidney | Adult | Women | • Men have greater access to the kidney transplant waiting list compared to women and also have increased access to a deceased donor kidney transplant (Ahearn et al., 2021). |
| | All organs | Pediatric | Individuals with an intellectual disability | • Transplant centers and providers factor neurodevelopmental issues into their decision-making process for placement on the waiting list in a nontransparent and inconsistent manner. A survey of pediatric transplant program staff found that 71% of heart programs, 30% of kidney programs, and 33% of liver programs would "always" or "usually" consider neurodevelopmental status in their decision (Richards et al., 2009). |
| Time from waiting list to transplant | Kidney | Adult | Black | • White patients had a lower median number of days from placement on the waiting list to kidney transplant compared to black patients (374 days compared to 727 days, respectively) (Patzer et al., 2012). |
| Access to advanced therapies for organ disease and waiting list outcomes | Heart | Adult | Women, black | • Advanced therapies for heart failure, such as continuous flow left ventricular assist devices (CF-LVADs) are used more in men compared to women, and those women who received CF-LVADs were less likely to have a heart transplant and more likely to die on the waiting list (DeFilippis et al., 2019). |
| | Heart | Pediatric | Female, black | • Pediatric patients on the waiting list who are black and female have higher waiting list mortality (Bhimani et al., 2020). |
| | Liver | Adult | Hispanic | • Hispanic individuals were more likely to be removed from the transplant waiting list due to death or deterioration compared to white individuals (Thuluvath et al., 2020) |
| Living organ donation[b] | Kidney | Adult | Black | • There is a lower rate of living kidney donation among the black population (0.4 per 100 patient-years) vs. whites (1.4 per 100 patient-years) (Arriola, February 2021 workshop).<br>• Black patients are almost 60% less likely to receive a living donor kidney (USRDS, 2020). |
| | Kidney | Adult | Lower socioeconomic status (SES), black | • Transplant recipients in communities with a lower Social Vulnerability Index (SVI)[c] were more likely to receive a living donor kidney transplant than individuals in communities with higher SVI (Killian et al., 2021). |
| Deceased donor organ transplant | Liver | Adult | Undocumented immigrants | • Approximately 3% of deceased donor organs come from undocumented immigrants (Glazier et al., 2014), while disproportionately fewer undocumented immigrants (0.4 percent) receive liver transplants (Lee and Terrault, 2020). |

| | | | |
|---|---|---|---|
| Kidney | Adult | American Indian or Alaska Native, black, Pacific Islander, Hispanic | • American Indian or Alaska Native, black, Hispanic, and Pacific Islander individuals initiating dialysis had lower annual deceased donor transplantation rates compared to white and Asian individuals (Hall et al., 2011). |
| Kidney | Adult | Lower SES | • Patients in the highest SES quartile had greater access to organ transplants than those in the lowest SES quartile and were more likely to be able to travel between donor service areas (Axelrod et al., 2010). |
| Heart | Adult | Lower SES (inadequate funds or health insurance) | • Having health insurance (or another funding source) is necessary for patients with end-stage heart failure to be eligible for cardiac transplantation but is not required for deceased donation, and 23% of organ donors are uninsured (King et al., 2005); this lack of reciprocity—that poor, uninsured individuals can give but not receive a cardiac transplant—creates an injustice in the organ transplantation system. |
| Liver | Adult | Women | • Women are less likely to receive a liver transplant than men, and adjusting for factors such as race, geography, education, body mass index, and weight reduces the difference, but the disparity remains consistent across the 11 OPTN allocation regions (Darden et al., 2021). |
| Posttransplant outcomes | | | |
| Heart | Adult | Black | • Black patients experience a higher risk of rejection and death postheart transplant (Morris et al., 2016). |
| Kidney | Pediatric | Uninsured or underinsured | • McEnhill et al. (2016) looked at pediatric outcomes in 289 children (48 undocumented and 241 permanent resident or citizen) and found that early graft survival rates were similar between the two groups, owing in part to insurance access. Of the 24 pediatric patients who reached the age of 21 over the study period (the age at which California state-sponsored transplant funding ends), 19 had stable graft function and access to insurance; the remaining 5 patients were unable to pay for immunosuppressive medication and lost grafts as a result. |

NOTES: The data displayed in this table do not reflect all disparities in the U.S. organ transplantation system but rather a sampling of the scientific literature reviewed by the committee. SES = socioeconomic status; SVI = Social Vulnerability Index; CF-LVAD = continuous flow left ventricular assist device; OPTN = Organ Procurement and Transplantation Network.
[a] The steps highlighted in this section occur prior to a patient being placed on a transplant waiting list and therefore fall outside of the scope of the OPTN's data collection. Disparities that occur within these steps affect downstream access to transplantation and are noted here as measures contributing to the overall equity or inequity of the transplantation system.
[b] Although the Statement of Task for this consensus study is focused on deceased donor organ transplants, the health disparities related to living donation are critical and have an effect on the overall transplantation system and therefore are highlighted above.
[c] The Centers for Disease Control and Prevention Social Vulnerability Index (SVI) uses U.S. census data to determine which communities may be more vulnerable based on social factors.

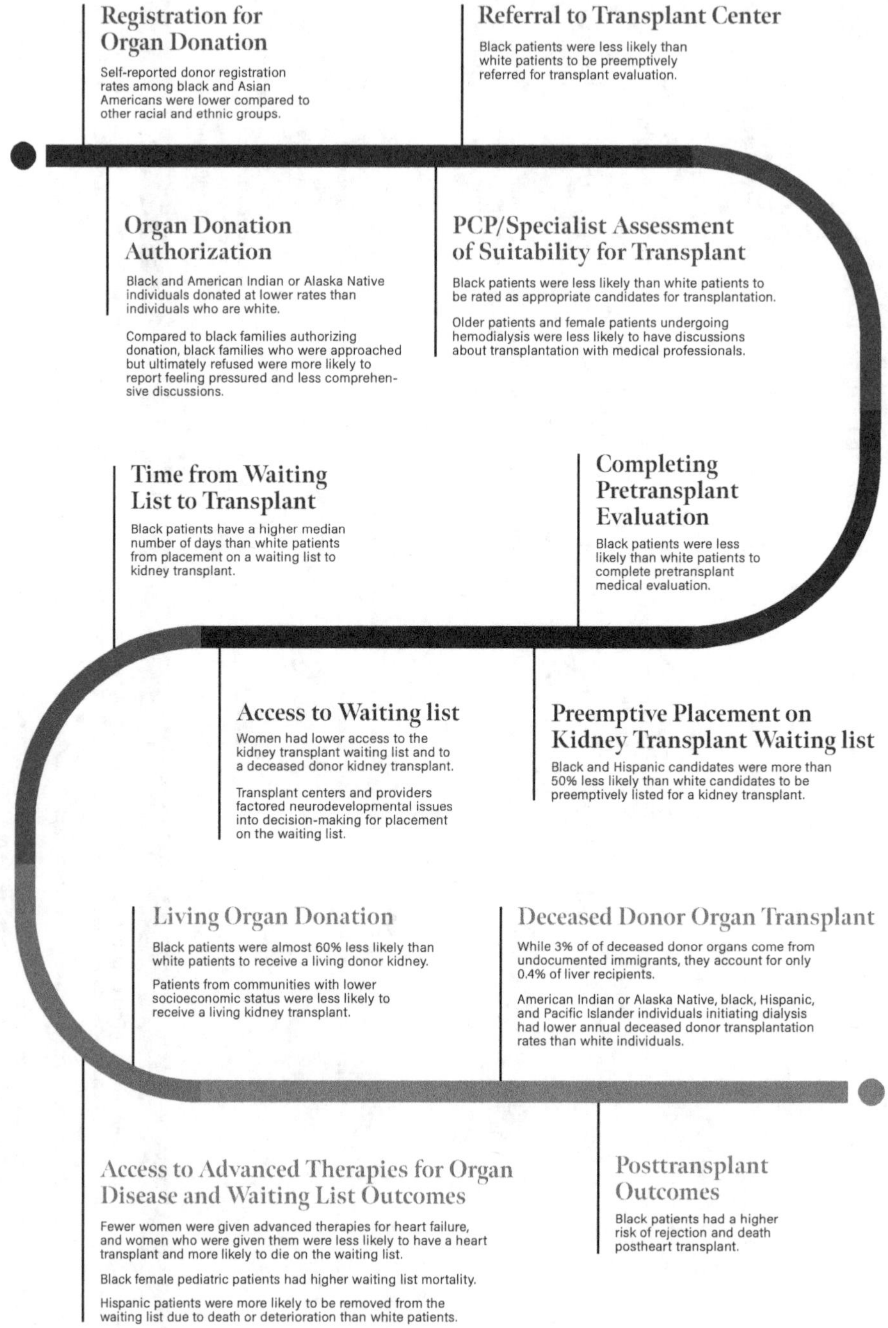

## Registration for Organ Donation

Self-reported donor registration rates among black and Asian Americans were lower compared to other racial and ethnic groups.

## Referral to Transplant Center

Black patients were less likely than white patients to be preemptively referred for transplant evaluation.

## Organ Donation Authorization

Black and American Indian or Alaska Native individuals donated at lower rates than individuals who are white.

Compared to black families authorizing donation, black families who were approached but ultimately refused were more likely to report feeling pressured and less comprehensive discussions.

## PCP/Specialist Assessment of Suitability for Transplant

Black patients were less likely than white patients to be rated as appropriate candidates for transplantation.

Older patients and female patients undergoing hemodialysis were less likely to have discussions about transplantation with medical professionals.

## Time from Waiting List to Transplant

Black patients have a higher median number of days than white patients from placement on a waiting list to kidney transplant.

## Completing Pretransplant Evaluation

Black patients were less likely than white patients to complete pretransplant medical evaluation.

## Access to Waiting list

Women had lower access to the kidney transplant waiting list and to a deceased donor kidney transplant.

Transplant centers and providers factored neurodevelopmental issues into decision-making for placement on the waiting list.

## Preemptive Placement on Kidney Transplant Waiting list

Black and Hispanic candidates were more than 50% less likely than white candidates to be preemptively listed for a kidney transplant.

## Living Organ Donation

Black patients were almost 60% less likely than white patients to receive a living donor kidney.

Patients from communities with lower socioeconomic status were less likely to receive a living kidney transplant.

## Deceased Donor Organ Transplant

While 3% of of deceased donor organs come from undocumented immigrants, they account for only 0.4% of liver recipients.

American Indian or Alaska Native, black, Hispanic, and Pacific Islander individuals initiating dialysis had lower annual deceased donor transplantation rates than white individuals.

## Access to Advanced Therapies for Organ Disease and Waiting List Outcomes

Fewer women were given advanced therapies for heart failure, and women who were given them were less likely to have a heart transplant and more likely to die on the waiting list.

Black female pediatric patients had higher waiting list mortality.

Hispanic patients were more likely to be removed from the waiting list due to death or deterioration than white patients.

## Posttransplant Outcomes

Black patients had a higher risk of rejection and death postheart transplant.

**FIGURE 4-1** Known disparities in the organ transplantation pathway.
NOTE: PCP = primary care physician.
SOURCE: See full list of references in Table 4-1.

## BOX 4-1    THE USE OF RACE AND ETHNICITY TERMS

Across medicine and health care today there remains a challenge in accurately categorizing, defining, and studying differences across populations, especially for racial and ethnic groups and the effect of these differences on health. Social science has an advanced understanding about cultural constructions of social identity. Medicine and health care services lag behind in terms of translating societal understandings into the practice of medical care as well as understanding the socioeconomic mechanisms responsible for the origins and mechanisms of many diseases and their progression (Mulligan, 2021).

Research on patient-level differences in access to transplantation commonly use the constructs of race and ethnicity to describe patients, despite the substantial methodological and conceptual limitations of using race. Although the terms race and ethnicity are commonly used together, in adherence to the U.S. government classification systems, they represent distinct cultural constructions of social identity. An ethnic group is defined in terms of shared culture. For example, those of a single ethnic group generally maintain a shared identity based on a common religion, language, nationality, ancestry, or other historical connections—that are not shared with others in their social sphere (Popejoy et al., 2020). By contrast, the construct of race is rooted in cultural, socioeconomic, political, and historical conceptions about social identity that purports a putative biological basis. There is no scientific foundation for race; however, the social function of race is racism (Yudell et al., 2020). While race is not a biological construct, it remains socially, politically, and medically ingrained in cultural beliefs about people and health (Bonham et al., 2018). Thus, it is important to understand how social, political, and medical systems may contribute to the biologic outcomes within racial and ethnic minority populations. Implicit bias continues to be a deep-rooted cultural challenge for the American health care system (Hall et al., 2015). Efforts to eradicate bias must be coupled with an ongoing investigation of how bias, discrimination, and racism contribute to the evolution of epigenetic or other biologic changes associated with disparate health outcomes (Geronimus, 2013).

It is crucial that organ donation and allocation systems understand the role that race plays in the provision of health care, classification of patients, and assignment of causality, and aim to remove the variable of race from measures used in organ allocation (Vyas et al., 2020). By contrast, using race to describe populations can help to track the effect that structural and institutional racism has on generating and perpetuating health inequities (Epstein, 2007; Center for Health Progress, 2017) in order to identify avenues for intervention and to redress inequities.

The categories *Latinx* and *Hispanic*, for example, comprise myriad cultural and ethnic groups that should be compared (e.g., Mexican Latinx share some common cultural patterns but also differ culturally from Cuban Latinx). As a result, categories are analyzed as a homogeneous group of people, despite considerable cultural variation. All groups need to be analyzed, and conceptions of racial and ethnic groups need to be better understood. For example, associated health needs exist within the categorization of racial and ethnic minority populations and studying these groups separately may help illuminate differences in outcomes.

*Conclusion 4-3: The absence of U.S. Department of Health and Human Services (HHS) requirements to collect disaggregated data by race and ethnicity, gender/sex, age, and language in organ donation and transplantation research precludes efforts to fully understand inequities in organ transplantation. Data gaps further compound challenges in provider decision making and preclude institutional priority setting for redressing inequities.*

## Geographic Disparities

In the Statement of Task, the committee was asked to consider whether deceased donor organs should be allocated to specific individuals based on need rather than groups of individuals defined by geography. Geographic disparities in organ transplantation occur for a number of reasons, including variation in OPO procedures, transplant center behavior, the number of potential organ donors and donation rates, and listing criteria. Where a potential organ transplant candidate is listed for a transplant is cited as one of the highest contributing factors associated with unintended disparities in access across multiple organ types including kidney, liver, heart, and lung (UNOS, 2021). Each organ has a specific framework for distribution among potential candidates based on various factors (e.g., medical urgency, blood type), and these policies also take into consideration cold ischemic times for various organs (e.g., heart and lung have shorter times while pancreas and kidney have longer times).[4] Because of the role geographic location plays in access to organ transplantation, there have been a number of efforts and actions to address geographic variation in transplant access, which are discussed further in Chapter 5 on equity in allocation. The committee also explores areas for improving procurement, acceptance, and use of deceased donor organs in Chapter 6.

## Individuals with Intellectual Disabilities

"So long as the decision making of medical practitioners at the evaluation stage has little to no oversight or guidance applied to it and so long as discriminatory attitudes exist, so too [will] these barriers to transplantation exist."

— Kelly Israel, Autistic Self Advocacy Network,
testimony to the committee during
July 15, 2021 public listening session

Organ transplantation for individuals with intellectual disabilities (IDs) is a controversial issue among some transplant providers, and carries varying degrees of importance in listing decisions based on the type of organ being transplanted and the severity of the disability. Prior to the 1990s, having an ID was considered by many transplant professionals as a contraindication for being listed for an organ transplant. In some cases, such as Down syndrome, there may be concerns related to immunological factors conveying potentially higher risks of infection or congenital heart disease. In other cases, reasons for contraindication include the patient potentially not understanding the procedure and assumption of a patient's lack of adherence to a strict posttransplant medication regimen required for transplant recipients. Lack of data remains a significant challenge for understanding the full breadth of disparities in access to transplantation for individuals with disabilities.

Legal protections for individuals with disabilities exist within the Americans with Disabilities Act, the Affordable Care Act (ACA), and the Rehabilitation Act. These protections specify that qualified individuals with disabilities cannot be excluded from programs receiving federal funding and that those programs should provide reasonable accommodations for individuals with disabilities.[5] However, many individuals with ID still face challenges in referral for evaluation and access to a transplant waiting list. In recent years, a number of

---

[4] *Cold ischemic time* refers to the time between when an organ is cross-clamped after being removed from the donor and when the organ is warmed with the recipient's blood.

[5] Americans with Disabilities Act of 1990 (42 U.S.C. §12182), Affordable Care Act of 2010 (42 U.S.C. §18116), Rehabilitation Act of 1973 (29 U.S.C. §794).

states have passed laws attempting to ban discrimination in organ transplantation based on an individual's ID, and other states are considering legislation. Discrimination in the context of individuals with ID is also under consideration for further action at the federal level (HHS, 2021c). Whether these laws and actions will have an effect on access remains to be seen.

## Disparities in Provider Referrals and Evaluation

Disparities in provider referral and evaluation contribute to unequal access to a waiting list for individuals with ID, and downstream, to an organ transplant. Dobbels (2014) notes that there is a lack of data on the number of individuals with ID who are found to be ineligible for transplant following an evaluation as well as the number of individuals never referred. A 2004 survey of 205 individuals and family members of those with disabilities found that about one-third of individuals for whom referral was suggested were never evaluated for an organ transplant (National Work Group on Disability and Transplantation, 2004). Provider bias may also play a role in how quality of life is assessed for individuals with ID, and ultimately, how likely they are to receive a referral for transplant or placement on the waiting list following an evaluation. For example, a systematic review by Pelleboer-Gunnink et al. (2017) found that stigmatizing attitudes regarding ID were present among mainstream health professionals.

Surveys of transplant centers and programs indicate that there is wide variability in listing decisions based on psychosocial and cognitive characteristics (Levenson and Olbrisch, 1993; Richards et al., 2009; Secunda et al., 2013; Wall et al., 2020). Because transplant programs can place varying levels of importance on cognitive characteristics and other factors, individuals with ID may experience different levels of disparities from one center to another, and transparency may be lacking for patients. During the committee's public listening session in July 2021, advocates suggested several paths forward including formalizing rules, providing individualized assessment for patients (rather than policies that consider ID as an absolute or relative contraindication for transplantation), and recognizing that some patients may need additional support in posttransplant care.

## Heart, Kidney, and Liver Transplantation and Intellectual Disabilities

Heart transplantation is one area where ID has been—and to some extent remains—controversial for providers in making decisions about listing a patient for transplant. In 2006, the International Society for Heart and Lung Transplantation (ISHLT) guidelines recommended that ID be regarded as a relative contraindication to transplantation (Mehra et al., 2006). The guidelines noted, however, the limited data on the validity of psychosocial evaluation for predicting outcomes and indicated that there may be wide variability in evaluation across centers. ISHLT updated its guidelines in 2016 and recommended that lack of adequate social support to achieve compliance could be considered a relative contraindication to heart transplant, but it recommended against heart transplant for individuals with severe cognitive-behavioral disabilities (Mehra et al., 2016). A survey by Richards et al. (2009) found that pediatric heart transplant programs tended to factor neurodevelopmental issues into the decision-making process for listing to a higher degree than kidney or liver programs with 71 percent of programs indicating that they would "always" or "usually" consider a candidate's neurodevelopmental status in their decision versus 30 percent and 33 percent for kidney and liver, respectively. Attitudes may be shifting to a small degree; of those programs considering severe ID as an absolute contraindication, 37.2 percent were heart, 44.4 percent were lung, 22.4 percent were liver, and 11.8 percent were kidney transplant programs (Wall et al., 2020). While outcomes data related to heart transplantation for individuals with ID are very limited, some studies indicate that outcomes for individuals with ID and those without ID may be similar (Samelson-Jones et al., 2012; Wightman et al., 2017).

In contrast to heart transplantation, kidney transplantation occurs more frequently in individuals with ID. This is likely attributable in part to the greater prevalence of kidney transplants in relation to other organ transplants as well as the potential for living donors. Studies have found that outcomes in this population are generally similar to patients without ID (Ohta et al., 2006; Wightman et al., 2014), though some note that long-term survival rates may be lower (Galante et al., 2010).

Data on liver transplantation in individuals with ID are limited. Wightman et al. (2016) found similar short-term graft and patient survival outcomes between pediatric patients with and without ID, but noted the need for research on long-term outcomes. A provider survey on medical and psychosocial characteristics of liver transplant recipients found that 30 percent of respondents had formal institutional policies characterizing cognitive disability as a contraindication to listing (Secunda et al., 2013). Transplant centers varied in how they viewed cognitive disability, with 42.6 percent considering moderate disability not to be a contraindication, 49.2 percent considering it a relative contraindication, and 8.2 percent considering it an absolute contraindication.

## Inequitable Access to Transplants for Undocumented Immigrants

Approximately 10.7 million undocumented immigrants live in the United States as of 2016,[6] equivalent to about 3 percent of the population (Pew Research Center, 2019). Undocumented immigrants experience disparities in gaining access to deceased donor organ transplantation. While approximately 3 percent of deceased donor organs come from undocumented immigrants, disproportionately fewer undocumented immigrants (0.4 percent) receive organ transplants (Glazier et al., 2014; Lee and Terrault, 2020). Both the National NOTA and the OPTN policy state that medical need alone should determine deceased donor organ allocation and a candidate's citizenship or residency status in the United States should not be taken into consideration (OPTN, 2021). While undocumented immigrants may be eligible to receive an organ transplant, most states do not have funding mechanisms to support necessary posttransplant care (Ackah et al., 2019). Barriers to equitable access extend well beyond funding mechanisms, raising questions about policy and ethics.

### Kidney-Specific Issues

The exact prevalence of undocumented immigrants with end-stage kidney disease (ESKD), or kidney failure, is unknown primarily because data on this population are not collected as part of the U.S. Renal Data System (Rodriguez et al., 2020). A recent estimate indicated that approximately 5,500 to 8,857 undocumented immigrants live with ESKD in the United States (Rodriguez et al., 2020). Undocumented immigrants with ESKD have been living in the United States on average for more than 5 years at the time of their diagnosis, and many continue to work despite their illness (Cervantes et al., 2017). Unlike U.S. citizens, undocumented immigrants with ESKD are not eligible for coverage of scheduled hemodi-

---

[6] An undocumented immigrant in this context refers to a person who is not a citizen of the United States, but resides in the United States (Yu and Wightman, 2021).

alysis through Medicare and are not eligible for accessing insurance through the ACA.[7] However, select state-level governments in the United States provide coverage for scheduled maintenance dialysis through Emergency Medicaid programs (Berger et al., 2020).[8] In the states that do not provide this option undocumented immigrants with ESKD must rely on emergency-only hemodialysis when their condition becomes life threatening. Emergency-only hemodialysis results in adverse health outcomes for patients, decreased quality of life, and stress on the health care system and providers (Berger et al., 2020). Recent efforts at a North Texas safety-net hospital to place undocumented immigrants with ESKD on scheduled dialysis resulted in greater survival benefit for the patients and also proved beneficial for the dialysis unit, the emergency department, and the hospital system (Berger et al., 2020).[9] Local nonprofit organizations may offer financial and placement assistance for undocumented immigrants requiring dialysis. However, these support structures are sporadic and do not cover the costs associated with kidney transplantation (cost will be discussed further in Chapter 6).

*Conclusion 4-4: Coverage of costs for scheduled dialysis for undocumented immigrants with end-stage kidney disease varies by state and results in disparities in the care available to patients. Emergency-only dialysis increases strain on hospital systems, providers, and patients.*

## DATA CHALLENGES RELATED TO ASSESSING AND ASSURING EQUITY

Assessing and promoting health equity in the organ transplantation system requires access to a wide range of timely and accurate data, including information related to the social determinants of health (Dover and Belon, 2019). Currently, the OPTN database collects the following information about patients on the transplant waiting list:

- Name
- Gender
- Race/ethnicity
- Age
- ABO blood group[10]
- Patient human leukocyte antigens (HLAs)[11]
- Patient status codes (for heart and liver)
- Number of previous transplants
- Acceptable donor characteristics[12]

---

[7] Hemodialysis is the process of cleaning the blood of individuals whose kidneys are not functioning properly. In the context of ESKD, maintenance dialysis is important for disease management and can cost thousands of dollars out of pocket if insurance coverage is unavailable.

[8] Emergency Medicaid provides temporary coverage for emergency treatment for individuals who qualify for Medicaid but are not eligible based on immigration status.

[9] Safety-net hospitals provide health care and health services to individuals who are uninsured or are insured through Medicaid.

[10] ABO blood group refers to the system by which blood type is categorized based on markers present on the surface of red blood cells (into A, B, O, or AB). The system is used to match the blood type of the donor and the recipient.

[11] HLAs are molecules present on most cells in the body that are involved in the body's immune response. HLA testing occurs prior to an organ transplant to determine whether the donor and recipient tissues match.

[12] Acceptable donor characteristics are things like body size and comorbidities.

When a patient is added to the waiting list, the transplant candidate registration form gathers information on the candidate's primary source of income, highest level of education, and employment status (OPTN, 2020). However, this pool of currently available data is not complete enough to assess the socioeconomic status of transplant candidates as there is a lack of granular information on socioeconomic and patient-centered factors, including measures of annual household income, household size, access to safe housing, job opportunities, health care access, distance to a transplant center, the patient's social networks, and neighborhood segregation. A noted gap in existing research, the influence of these social determinants of health on disparities in organ transplantation (Wesselman et al., 2021),[13] could be used to further explore the effects of waiting list time on subpopulations. Recently, the OPTN Minority Affairs Committee proposed efforts to collect additional socioeconomic information related to disparities in access to kidney transplantation, though this effort is still in progress.[14]

## Gaps in Data Present a Systems Issue

As previously noted, it is difficult to properly assess equitable referral and evaluation for organ transplantation because of a lack of national surveillance data. The U.S. Renal Data System allows for studies of these aspects related to kidney transplants, but such a nationwide data collection system does not exist for other organ transplants such as liver, heart, and lung. The absence of such data creates a systems issue—specifically around referral and admissions data. The system cannot adequately capture information on social determinants of health and may also miss capturing the medical and social needs of patients in the transplantation system. Without these data, patients may get labeled as *noncompliant*, which can lead to poorer access to transplantation and thereby poorer outcomes. In February 2021, the OPTN announced a feasibility study that would evaluate data collection related to the social determinants of health.[15] The feasibility project will look at potentially collecting aggregated third-party data to better understand how social determinants of health affect transplantation.

Gaps in data and the evidence base more broadly make it difficult for providers to make decisions, especially regarding vulnerable populations such as those with intellectual disability. As previously noted, these populations experience uneven access to referral and transplantation. To overcome some of these data gaps within the transplantation system, more patient-reported data are needed. This may include data related to education, perceived discrimination, perceived racism, distrust of the health care system, physical infrastructure and environmental factors, and access to pharmacies. Furthermore, information on the social determinants of health are needed at the time of transplant evaluation as well as follow-up data on transplant and outcomes.

In June 2021, the OPTN developed an equity dashboard with the goal of increasing transparency in access to transplantation.[16] The dashboard uses an access to transplant score

---

[13] According to the Centers for Disease Control and Prevention, the social determinants of health are "conditions in the places where people live, learn, work, and play that affect a wide range of health risks and outcomes" (CDC, 2021).

[14] For information on the Minority Affairs Committee proposal see https://optn.transplant.hrsa.gov/media/3811/202006_mac_ses_bp.pdf (accessed November 12, 2021). Public comments on the proposal raised several concerns related to implementation, including patient privacy, potential for data misuse, and the challenges in verifying socioeconomic data.

[15] For more information on the OPTN effort to collect data on the social determinants of health see https://unos.org/news/sdoh-data-collection (accessed September 12, 2021).

[16] For more information on the OPTN Equity in Access to Transplant dashboard see https://insights.unos.org/equity-in-access (accessed September 9, 2021).

derived from a Cox proportional hazards regression model measuring 15 patient characteristics such as biological (e.g., blood type, calculated panel reactive antibodies), sociocultural (e.g., ethnicity), health insurance type, and environmental (e.g., donor service area where the patient is listed). These factors are derived more broadly from the National Institute on Minority Health and Disparities Research Framework. Together, this total score is meant to convey how likely it is that a candidate on a transplant waiting list will receive a deceased donor heart, lung, kidney, or liver transplant. A major challenge to measuring equity in transplant using data collected by the OPTN—including data presented in the equity dashboard—is the lack of data regarding the referral process and steps prior to initiating evaluation. Another limitation is that the dashboard identifies a patient's gender as part of the patient characteristics collected; however, it does not separate this information from the patient's sex. Additionally, the dashboard does not identify where disparities may be occurring along the pathway to a transplant after a patient initiates a transplant evaluation because the OPTN does not have access to data on individuals starting an evaluation up to the point of placement on the waiting list (becoming a "candidate"). Consequently, little is known about where individuals are most likely to fall off the path to completing evaluation, and where disparities in falling off occur. Complicating matters in tracking the evaluation process is that transplant centers vary in the order in which tests are done in the evaluation process. Opportunities to address some of the data challenges will be discussed further in Chapter 6.

*Conclusion 4-5: It is well established that inequities arise in access to referrals, evaluation, and the waiting list for organ transplant, yet little is known where along the trajectory in that process disparities are most likely to arise, especially for vulnerable populations. There is a need to expand federal oversight to include the steps involved in identifying patients as needing a transplant before patients are added to the waiting list. Because current OPTN oversight begins only when a patient is added to the waiting list, measures and actions to advance equity throughout the system will be hampered until these earlier steps in the patients' process of gaining access to transplantation are addressed as part of the transplantation system and a source for evaluating progress in achieving equity.*

## Implicit Bias

Implicit bias, defined as "an unconscious favoritism toward or prejudice against people of a certain race, gender, or group that influences one's own actions or perceptions," has long-standing effects on health accessibility and outcomes (NASEM, 2021, p. 1). Implicit bias spans social and structural determinants of health and is often included in considerations of socioeconomic status, race/ethnicity, gender, and disability, among a host of other factors. The computer-based Implicit Association Test (IAT), first introduced in 1998, has been used to delve into the implicit biases of physicians, documenting racial and ethnic disparities in treatment and quality. The IAT can be a useful tool to help people reflect upon their implicit biases, though studies continue to assess its validity for effectively identifying implicit cognition (Meissner et al., 2019; Schimmack, 2021; Vianello and Bar-Anan, 2021). Though physicians' explicit (self-reported) attitudes regarding preferential treatment of patients based on race and attitudes regarding stereotypes about the cooperativeness of patients based on race have not been statistically significant, detection of physicians' implicit biases by the IAT show strong associations with their decisions to provide treatment (Green et al., 2007; Hall et al., 2015). Implicit attitudes may also play a role in organ donation since explicit attitudes regarding altruism toward others are likely to be subject to biases in how the donor feels they may be perceived (Joshi and Stevens, 2017). The role that implicit bias can play in patient referral will be explored further in the next section.

## STRUCTURAL BARRIERS TO EQUITY IN THE PATHWAY TO AN ORGAN TRANSPLANT

### Delays in Referral to Specialists

Delays in referrals to specialists for patients with end-stage organ failure are among the many structural barriers to equity in the pathway to an organ transplant (Anees et al., 2018; Prakash et al., 2010; Suarez et al., 2018). Delayed or late referral poses adverse consequences for patients in need of kidney, heart, liver, and lung transplants. Delayed referral is further compounded by disparities in access to primary care, which can create downstream issues in accessing necessary specialist care (Brown et al., 2016; Sabounchi et al., 2018; Tung et al., 2019).

Patient-, provider-, and system-level factors contribute to these disparities. Patient-level factors include a lack of knowledge and awareness of transplantation. In the case of kidney disease, a patient may be unaware of having kidney disease given that symptoms may not appear until advanced stages of disease. Some patients may also maintain negative attitudes and beliefs about transplantation and face socioeconomic and psychosocial challenges that preclude them from being referred or placed on the waiting list (Dageforde et al., 2015; Martin, 2014; Patzer et al., 2012; Schold et al., 2011). Provider-related factors include late referrals, which may be caused by a lack of knowledge about kidney disease and when to refer patients, and lack of bilingual or bicultural providers. In addition, evidence suggests that providers from low-wait-listing dialysis centers are unaware of the disparity in wait-listing black patients in the United States (Kim et al., 2018), and that nephrologists experience challenges building trust with ethnic minorities (Hanson et al., 2016). Similarly, providers from transplant programs may lack awareness of disparities in access to living donor transplantation at their own institution (Gordon et al., 2020). System-level factors include difficulty facilitating communication among providers across the complex health care systems for chronic care patients and the lack of culturally sensitive approaches to delivering patient education (Waterman et al., 2010).

### *Kidney*

Nearly 20 to 50 percent of chronic kidney disease patients start dialysis without a prior clinical exam by a nephrologist (Levin, 2000). A systematic literature review found that for patients with chronic kidney disease, late referral to nephrologists is associated with patient demographics, clinical factors, patient and provider attitudes, and health system characteristics. Patient demographic factors associated with late referral include older age, being a member of an ethnic or racial minority group, having less education, and being uninsured. Clinical factors include the presence of multiple comorbidities and the insensitivity of serum creatinine as a screening tool to identify patients with early-stage renal disease (Levin, 2000).[17] One study found that nondiabetic kidney disease and Charlson comorbidity index were significantly associated with late referral;[18] the authors recommended that physicians

---

[17] Serum creatinine is a laboratory measure used to assess kidney functioning. Higher levels of creatinine (a waste product) in the blood indicates impaired kidney functioning.

[18] *Charlson comorbidity index* is a method for predicting patient mortality based on a number of comorbid conditions.

pay special attention to patients with nondiabetic kidney disease and those with multiple comorbidities (Navaneethan et al., 2007). Physician and patient attitudes surrounding chronic kidney disease as a silent disease and the need for treatment influence the initiation of dialysis (Ghahramani et al., 2011, 2014; Gordon and Sehgal, 2000; Hanson et al., 2016; Levin, 2000). A study looking at nephrologist perceptions related to referring patients for kidney transplant found that the most commonly stated exclusionary factor was inadequate social support followed by the patient's limited understanding of the transplant process (Bartolomeo et al., 2019). Health system characteristics that contribute to delayed referral include lack of communication between primary care physicians and nephrologists (Navaneethan et al., 2008), as well as geographic factors (Ghahramani et al., 2014).

Late referral can contribute to increased morbidity, mortality, and resource use, as well as reduced quality of life and missed windows of opportunity for preemptive transplantation (Levin, 2000; Reese et al., 2021a). A systematic review of late referral for chronic kidney disease recommended that primary care physicians and nephrologists engage in comprehensive efforts to educate patients and physicians about the effects of delaying referral (Navaneethan et al., 2008). Patients who are referred to specialist nephrology care later in the course of renal disease when their need for dialysis is imminent tend to have poor outcomes (Levin, 2000), while a study of decline in kidney function before and after nephrology referral confirmed that early detection, specialist referral, and intervention have benefits for kidney and patient survival (Jones et al., 2006). After referral to a nephrologist, patients' decline of glomerular filtration rate slowed significantly,[19] which was also associated with better likelihood of survival. Thus, tools are needed to enhance early identification of renal insufficiency,[20] along with interventions to delay progression of renal insufficiency and prepare patients for renal replacement therapy (Levin, 2000).

## Preemptive Kidney Transplantation

Obtaining a kidney transplant before initiating maintenance dialysis is referred to as *preemptive transplantation*, and it confers longer patient survival than transplantation following dialysis initiation. However, disparities arise in preemptive referral to kidney transplantation with black patients having a 37 percent lower chance of being preemptively referred for transplant evaluation than white patients (odds ratio = 0.63 [95% confidence interval: 0.55, 0.71]) (Gander et al., 2018). Similarly, preemptive kidney transplantation occurs at significantly lower rates among patients with less than a high school education and Medicaid beneficiaries (King et al., 2019). Patients who are white, had greater health literacy, and had private health insurance have been shown to have greater access to preemptive transplantation (Grams et al., 2013; Patzer et al., 2013; Purnell and Crews, 2019; Taylor et al., 2016). Factors that affected preemptive transplantation included patient's cardiovascular disease, social deprivation, and renal units' characteristics (Kutner et al., 2012; Patzer et al., 2013). An additional challenge in preemptive kidney transplantation are the available data regarding dialysis tolerance among patients from racial and ethnic minorities, which may contribute to delays. A number of studies have shown that racial and ethnic minority dialysis patients have greater survival (Eisenstein et al., 2009; Rhee et al., 2014), though others note that there

---

[19] Glomerular filtration rate, or GFR, is a measurement of how well the kidneys filter blood. It is used to estimate how well the kidneys are functioning with lower rates indicating reduced functioning.

[20] Renal insufficiency refers to poor functioning of the kidneys; over time, this may result in the need for dialysis or transplant.

may be other contributing factors to survival advantage, such as age, that should be further studied to inform provider decision making (Johns et al., 2014; Kucirka et al., 2011).

Policy changes to the U.S. kidney allocation system have not addressed preemptive transplantation in an effort to mitigate disparities, thereby enabling such disparities to persist (Reese et al., 2021b). Researchers have suggested strategies to remediate disparities including (1) educating primary care physicians to refer patients before they reach an estimated glomerular flow rate (eGFR) of 20 or less; (2) incentivizing transplant centers to add potential candidates to the waiting list quickly; (3) implementing kidney allocation system changes (e.g., standardizing the GFR estimation to foster fairness through the use of a single standard to all patients); and (4) educating patients regarding preemptive transplantation and offering patient navigators (Reese et al., 2021b).

## Heart

A qualitative study of health care providers evaluated the association of gender and race with allocation of advanced heart failure therapies using clinical vignettes. The study found evidence of bias linked to gender and race in clinicians' decision-making process for offering advanced therapies—which was particularly evident in the case of black female patients, who tended to be judged more harshly in terms of appearance and adequacy of social support—although no association between gender and race was found in the final recommendation for allocation. However, the authors concluded that this bias could contribute to delayed allocation (Breathett et al., 2020). As one minority clinician, when presented with a patient vignette of a black female patient, observed:

> It's a shame that this lady was only diagnosed 2 years ago. I mean I get angry about that. I mean particularly being a [minority] provider, I see that many patients that are referred to me regardless of their race tend to be referred late from a heart failure standpoint. I find that my minority patients, particularly my African American patients, are referred even later....Many times it's because their symptoms were going unrecognized by the people that were taking care of them...or their symptoms weren't believed....They tell me many stories, and I'm hoping that this isn't the case for her but unfortunately if you see it enough times...it starts to dishearten you (Breathett et al., 2020, p. 7).

Delays in seeking treatment among heart failure patients (i.e., not recognizing symptoms or seeking care late into symptom onset) can compound delays in referrals to specialists, and delays in seeking treatment have been found to be significantly high (Evangelista et al., 2000). These effects could potentially be mitigated by the promotion of early symptom recognition and management among patients and families.

## Liver

Similar disparities in timely referrals have been observed among patients who need liver transplantation evaluation. Late referral to liver specialists has been identified as a major factor contributing to disproportionately low rates of liver transplantation among black individuals, despite the higher prevalence of end-stage liver disease among this racial group compared to others (Mustian et al., 2019). The same study found that black patients tend to be referred for evaluation for a transplant with more advanced disease, as evidenced by their higher median Model for End-Stage Liver Disease (MELD) score at listing. A study evaluating disparities in transplant referral patterns for alcohol-related liver disease found that gastroenterologists and transplant hepatologists were significantly more likely to refer higher-risk patients than primary care physicians (Loy et al., 2020). This suggests that there is a disparity in the referral of patients with alcohol-related liver disease based on whether the patient has access to specialty care. A retrospective evaluation of the OPTN registrants examined ethnicity and insurance-specific disparities in MELD scores at the time of waiting list registration. They found that among black patients, higher MELD scores at listing did not translate to higher waiting list mortality. However, patients with Medicare, Medicaid, or who were uninsured had significantly higher waiting list mortality than privately insured patients (Robinson et al., 2021).

## Patient Evaluation and Access to a Transplant Waiting List

Racial and ethnic groups are disproportionately less likely to be referred for transplant evaluation and to complete transplant evaluation to be placed on the transplant waiting list as compared to non-Hispanic whites (Epstein et al., 2000; Harding et al., 2017; Mucsi et al., 2017; Patzer et al., 2012; Weng et al., 2005; Wolfe et al., 1999). Specifically, black and Hispanic patients have a significantly longer time from starting dialysis to being placed on the waiting list than whites. However, effects remained only partially significant after controlling for socioeconomic status factors (i.e., Medicare insurance among patients over age 64 and zip code poverty levels) (Joshi et al., 2013). Disparities for black patients in access to the waiting list also persisted after controlling for social determinants of health (i.e., knowledge of transplantation, psychosocial factors, and cultural factors) (Ng et al., 2020). Moreover, black patients in poor neighborhoods are significantly less likely to be put on the waiting list than whites in nonpoor neighborhoods indicating that neighborhood racial composition and neighborhood poverty were related to racial disparities in access to the waiting list for black patients (Peng et al., 2018).

> *Conclusion 4-6: Based on available information, the committee does not find justifiable reasons for the demonstrable disparities between organ transplant rates for persons who would benefit from organ transplants and the burden of disease in many populations. Disproportionately fewer racial and ethnic minority patients receive organ transplants than are represented on the transplant waiting list. These inequities undermine the trust necessary for the organ transplantation system to function optimally.*

## IMPROVING QUALITY AND HEALTH EQUITY ACROSS THE ENTIRE ORGAN TRANSPLANTATION SYSTEM

### Explanation of the Proposed Framework

The committee looked at previous work on health equity as they sought to propose a framework that infuses equity, value, and transparency throughout the organ transplantation system and the points along the care pathway (Figure 4-2). The principle of health equity as a component of quality in a health care system was central. One source, *Crossing the Quality Chasm: A New Health System for the 21st Century,* described urgent changes needed in the U.S. health care delivery system to improve care for all Americans. The report established six aims for improving key dimensions in the health care system: safety, effectiveness, patient centeredness, timeliness, efficiency, and equity (IOM, 2001a). Further, the report called upon all health care constituencies to adopt these shared aims with the goal of improving the quality of care within the overall health system.

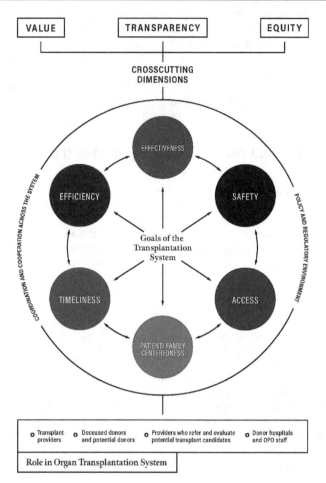

**FIGURE 4-2** A proposed framework for infusing equity, value, and transparency across the deceased donor organ transplantation system.
SOURCE: Adapted from IOM, 2010.

Equity as a crosscutting component of system performance and quality health care was further defined in *Envisioning the National Health Care Quality Report* (IOM, 2001b). The report described a two-dimensional conceptual framework in which the first dimension captures components related to quality (safety, effectiveness, patient centeredness, and timeliness) and the second dimension captures the consumer perspective on patient needs (staying healthy, improving health, living with illness or disability, coping with the end of life). Within the framework, measures of equity are meant to fit in the cells corresponding to the quality component and health care need being addressed. The *Future Directions for the National Healthcare Quality and Disparities Reports* built on the reports *Envisioning the National Health Care Quality Report* and *Crossing the Quality Chasm* to include access and efficiency as quality care components in its conceptual framework for categorizing health care quality and disparities (IOM, 2010). The framework also included care coordination and health systems infrastructure as foundational components supporting the performance measurement of the other quality components. An additional dimension was included to show the crosscutting nature of equity and value, achievable with improvements in both the quality components and foundational components.

The goal of the committee in building upon prior frameworks and developing Figure 4-2 was not to be prescriptive to the stakeholders within the organ transplantation system but rather to provide a framing for how stakeholders can discuss equity. The committee added a crosscutting dimension of transparency to highlight how the quality components can increase the overall transparency of the system in addition to equity and value. The framework may serve as a heuristic tool or decision aid to help shape future policies by promoting better access to granular data. To that end, the committee considered this framework in developing recommendations, including the dashboard of metrics (see Chapter 7). In the framework, equity is not meant to be a single activity or value; it is foundational. Given the complexity of the organ transplantation system, a framework may also serve as a means of bringing more awareness around the interconnected nature of the system to the various components and stakeholders. All stakeholders within the organ transplantation system are responsible for, and accountable to, ensuring the system is equitable.

## EVIDENCE-BASED INTERVENTIONS FOR IMPROVING HEALTH EQUITY IN THE ORGAN TRANSPLANTATION SYSTEM

A number of evidence-based interventions have been developed to reduce disparities and increase access to kidney transplantation, improve organ donation rates, and increase access to living donor kidney transplantation. These interventions include the use of patient navigators as well as a range of culturally targeted educational interventions delivered online, through mass media, or in person at transplant centers, patients' homes, or community-based venues. The appropriateness of culturally targeted efforts in organ donation authorization has been a subject of much research. As previously discussed, despite improvements in organ donation authorization rates among black and Asian individuals, some challenges remain. For example, data suggest that black families may not be approached regarding organ dona-tion requests in the same manner (or as frequently) as white families and may not view those interactions as favorably (Siminoff et al., 2003). Data from a study by Bodenheimer et al. (2012) looking at organ donation authorization in liver transplantation suggest that racial concordance between the donor and the coordinator may play a role in authorization rates and the authors highlighted the importance of adequate coordinator training to overcome barriers, though they also suggest more study is needed.

## Patient Navigators

The effect of patient navigators on reducing racial disparities in access to transplantation has been inconclusive. Patient navigators helped patients complete transplant candidate steps to be placed on the waiting list, as well as helping patients gain greater access to living donor kidney transplantation (LDKT) (Marlow et al., 2016; Sullivan et al., 2012). However, navigators did not affect the completion of transplant evaluation and did help patients to get on the waiting list, but not until after the first 500 days after starting evaluation for transplant (Basu et al., 2018).

## Culturally Targeted Interventions

Project ACTS: About Choices in Transplantation and Sharing is a culturally sensitive, family-focused intervention designed to improve readiness for organ and tissue donation among African American adults, particularly in the southeastern United States. A study evaluated the effectiveness of Project ACTS and found that the intervention was an effective tool for encouraging family discussion of deceased donation intentions among African Americans (Arriola et al., 2010). The authors concluded that OPOs, civic organizations, churches, and public health departments can use this intervention to improve organ donation intention rates among target populations. Furthermore, they concluded that intervention material could be adapted to suit the cultural needs of other populations.

A culturally tailored and linguistically congruent Hispanic Kidney Transplant Program (HKTP) at Northwestern Medicine was implemented at two other transplant programs designed to increase living donor kidney transplantation among Hispanic and Latinx patients. The HKTP comprises 16 components that redress disparities at the patient, provider, and organizational levels (Gordon et al., 2018). Through a hybrid type 2 clinical trial design, the study evaluated both the effectiveness of the HKTP intervention and the effectiveness of the intervention implementation (Gordon et al., 2021). The study found that the HKTP intervention effectively increased LDKT in Hispanic patients, compared to whites, at one intervention site that implemented the intervention with greater fidelity, in comparison to pre- and postassessments at two matched control sites. Intervention site 1 improved the Hispanic LDKT rate by 47 percent (from 20.3 percent at pre-HKTP to 29.8 percent at post-HKTP).

A study evaluated the effectiveness of interventions designed to remove barriers to living donor kidney transplantation for black patients, who receive this type of transplantation less frequently than patients of other racial groups (Rodrigue et al., 2014). Patients were randomized to one of the following three groups, in which health educators delivered interventions to (1) patients and their guests in the patient's home, (2) clusters of patients and guests in transplant centers, or (3) individual patients alone in transplant centers. The study found that patients who received house calls were more likely than those who had visits at transplant centers to have at least one donor inquiry and evaluation. Patients who received house calls had greater knowledge, fewer concerns, and greater willingness to talk about living donation 6 weeks after the intervention. The authors emphasized the importance of including the patient's social network in live donor kidney transplantation education to reduce racial disparities in live donor transplantation rates.

A mobile, customized patient education tool was developed to provide animated patient education and show individualized risk-adjusted outcomes for kidney transplant candidates following transplant. A study examined the effectiveness of this mobile, iOS-based application among a diverse group of renal transplant candidates (Axelrod et al., 2017). Most participants reported that the tool improved their knowledge and was culturally appropriate to their own race or ethnicity. Furthermore, patients scored higher on a transplant knowledge test after using the application—regardless of their health literacy level—and expressed more interest in living and deceased donor kidney transplantation.

A randomized controlled trial was conducted to test the effectiveness of a bilingual website about living kidney donation and transplantation that was culturally targeted for Hispanics and Latinos, who are disproportionately affected by kidney disease and receive disproportionately fewer LDKTs than whites (Gordon et al., 2016a,b). Compared to participants who only received routine transplant education sessions, those who were also exposed to the website had greater increases in their knowledge scores that persisted at a 3-week follow-up. These results underscore the potential benefit of supplementing transplant education using culturally tailored educational tools.

In 2010, a Spanish language mass media campaign on living organ donation attitudes and behavioral interventions was conducted among Hispanics in the southwestern United

States using an intervention community and a control community (Alvaro et al., 2010). This evaluation revealed a posttest increase in intentions related to living organ donation in the intervention group that was not observed in the control group. Moreover, those in the intervention community who were exposed to the campaign had more positive donation intentions than individuals in the same community who were not exposed to the campaign.

A religiously tailored and ethically balanced educational intervention was designed to increase living organ donation intent among Muslim Americans (Padela et al., 2020). An evaluation of this intervention found that participants in the educational intervention were more likely to donate a kidney; they were also more likely to encourage a loved one, coworker, or fellow mosque member with end-stage kidney disease to seek a living kidney donor.

## Improving Implementation of Evidence-Based Interventions

Despite the availability and effectiveness of evidence-based interventions aimed at increasing organ transplantation equity, these approaches have not been widely adopted within the organ transplantation system. For example, OPOs are responsible for discussing organ donation with a potential donor's next of kin. However, despite the importance of high-quality, positive interactions between OPO staff and the family members of a potential donor, there are no national standards for how to train OPO staff on communication skills in compassion and cultural sensitivity. One study across eight geographically distinct areas of the United States found meaningful variations in the way OPO staff communicated with family decision makers about organ donation, suggesting that "OPO staff were missing opportunities to increase the supply of available deceased donor organs...and equalize some of the regional variations in donation, conversion, and transplantation rates" (Traino et al., 2017, p. 7).

Implementation research shows that evidence-based interventions often take years to be adopted into practice; furthermore, these gaps in translation of interventions are not well understood, which can impede investment decisions for those attempting to implement interventions (Morris et al., 2011). Implementation science, which examines methods for promoting the adoption of evidence-based policies and practices in health care and public health, reveals that many factors influence the uptake of evidence-based interventions into practice. These factors pertain to the institution or organization in which an intervention is implemented, the nature of the intervention itself, and the attitudes about the intervention held by the stakeholders involved in implementing the intervention (Damschroder et al., 2009). In the context of implementing an intervention to increase Hispanics' access to transplantation and LDKT, barriers emerged including awareness of the disparity, concerns about focusing on reducing disparities for one minority group and not others in need, misperceptions about patients' payer mix, and the lack of patient disaggregated data by racial and ethnic background (Gordon et al., 2020). There is a need for more implementation science research, and implementation scientists need to be part of the effort to adopt effective interventions in the transplantation system.

> *Conclusion 4-7: Evidence-based interventions have been developed to reduce disparities and increase access to transplantation. Nonetheless, such interventions are rarely implemented into practice. Despite the availability of these interventions, dialysis centers, donor hospitals, transplant centers, OPOs, and others have not implemented the interventions to help resolve inequities in access to transplant referral, evaluation, and care.*

**Recommendation 3: Achieve equity in the U.S. organ transplantation system in the next 5 years.**

Under the direction and oversight of Congress, HHS should be held accountable for achieving equity in the transplantation system in the next 5 years. Within 1 to 2 years, HHS should identify and publish a strategy with specific proposed requirements, regulations, payment structures, and other changes for elimination of disparities. Elements of the strategy should include expanding oversight and data collection, aligning providers with the goal of equity, shared decision making with patients and public education, and elevating voices of those facing disparities.

### Expanding Oversight and Data Collection

- HHS should extend its regulatory oversight of the organ transplantation system beginning, at least, at the time a patient reaches end-stage organ failure and extending beyond 1 year posttransplant.
- HHS should update the OPTN contract to require the collection of disaggregated data by race and ethnicity, gender/sex, age, as well as language and the creation of new measures of inequity in the transplantation system.

### Aligning Providers with the Goal of Equity

- The Centers for Medicare & Medicaid Services should adopt payment policies that incentivize all providers—from primary and specialty care of patients with organ failure to referral for transplant, from care while awaiting a transplant to long-term posttransplant care—to improve equity in access to care and outcomes for patients.

### Shared Decision Making with Patients and Public Education

- HHS should develop, implement, and evaluate rigorous approaches for transplant teams to communicate routinely with (1) potential transplant recipients about their status and remaining steps in the process of transplant evaluation; (2) wait-listed candidates about organs offered to them, including information about the benefits, risks, and alternatives to accepting different types of organs to facilitate shared decision making about whether to accept the organ; and (3) wait-listed candidates about the number of organs offered and declined.
- HHS should develop, implement, and evaluate rigorous approaches for routinely educating the public about the benefits, risks, and alternatives to organ transplantation as a treatment option for end-stage organ disease or for those needing transplantation of tissue or a functional unit.
- HHS should conduct ongoing culturally targeted public education campaigns to convey the need for organ donation to save lives, to eliminate misconceptions about organ donation and transplantation, and to increase the trustworthiness of the transplantation system.

### Elevating Voices of Those Facing Disparities

- The OPTN should be required to ensure that all populations facing disparities, including persons with disabilities, are represented in the transplant policy development process.

- HHS should require and support work with OPOs to increase the diversity of their workforce to better meet the needs of donor families.

# REFERENCES

Ackah, R. L., R. R. Sigireddi, and B. V. R. Murthy. 2019. Is organ retransplantation among undocumented immigrants in the United States just? *AMA Journal of Ethics* 21(1):E17-E25.

Ahearn, P., K. L. Johansen, J. C. Tan, C. E. McCulloch, B. A. Grimes, and E. Ku. 2021. Sex disparity in deceased-donor kidney transplant access by cause of kidney disease. *Clinical Journal of the American Society of Nephrology* 16(2):241-250.

Alvaro, E. M., J. T. Siegel, W. D. Crano, and A. Dominick. 2010. A mass mediated intervention on Hispanic live kidney donation. *Journal of Health Communication* 15(4):374-387.

Anees, M., Y. Hussain, M. Ibrahim, I. Ilahi, S. Ahmad, K. I. Asif, and A. Jameel. 2018. Outcome of chronic kidney disease patients on the basis of referral to nephrologist: A one-year follow-up study. *Journal of the College of Physicians and Surgeons of Pakistan* 27(4):304-307.

Arriola, K., D. H. Robinson, N. J. Thompson, and J. P. Perryman. 2010. Project ACTS: An intervention to increase organ and tissue donation intentions among African Americans. *Health Education & Behavior* 37(2):264-274.

Axelrod, D. A., N. Dzebisashvili, M. A. Schnitzler, P. R. Salvalaggio, D. L. Segev, S. E. Gentry, J. Tuttle-Newhall, and K. L. Lentine. 2010. The interplay of socioeconomic status, distance to center, and interdonor service area travel on kidney transplant access and outcomes. *Clinical Journal of the American Society of Nephrology* 5(12):2276-2288.

Axelrod, D. A., C. S. Kynard-Amerson, D. Wojciechowski, M. Jacobs, K. L. Lentine, M. Schnitzler, J. D. Peipert, and A. D. Waterman. 2017. Cultural competency of a mobile, customized patient education tool for improving potential kidney transplant recipients' knowledge and decision-making. *Clinical Transplantation* 31(5). https://doi.org/10.1111/ctr.12944.

Bartolomeo, K., A. Tandon Gandhir, M. Lipinski, J. Romeu, and N. Ghahramani. 2019. Factors considered by nephrologists in excluding patients from kidney transplant referral. *International Journal of Organ Transplantation Medicine* 10(3):101-107.

Basu, M., L. Petgrave-Nelson, K. D. Smith, J. P. Perryman, K. Clark, S. O. Pastan, T. C. Pearson, C. P. Larsen, S. Paul, and R. E. Patzer. 2018. Transplant center patient navigator and access to transplantation among high-risk population: A randomized, controlled trial. *Clinical Journal of the American Society of Nephrology* 13(4):620-627.

Berger, J. R., H. Quinones, and M. A. Vazquez. 2020. Dialysis for undocumented immigrants: Challenges and solutions. *Kidney360* 1(6):549-552.

Bhimani, S., G. Boyle, W. Liu, S. Worley, E. Saarel, and S. Admani. 2020. Gender and racial disparities in pediatric heart transplantation in the current era: A UNOS registry analysis. *Journal of Heart and Lung Transplantation* 39(4):S461-S462.

Bodenheimer, H. C., Jr., J. M. Okun, W. Tajik, J. Obadia, N. Icitovic, P. Friedmann, E. Marquez, and M. J. Goldstein. 2012. The impact of race on organ donation authorization discussed in the context of liver transplantation. *Transactions of the American Clinical and Climatological Association* 123:64-78.

Bonham, V. L., E. D. Green, and E. J. Pérez-Stable. 2018. Examining how race, ethnicity, and ancestry data are used in biomedical research. *Journal of the American Medical Association* 320(15):1533-1534.

Boulware, L. E., and D. Mohottige. 2021. The seen and the unseen: Race and social inequities affecting kidney care. *Clinical Journal of the American Society of Nephrology* 16(5):815-817.

Boyd, R., E. Lindo, L. Weeks, and M. McLemore. 2020. On racism: A new standard for publishing on racial health inequities. *Health Affairs*. https://www.healthaffairs.org/do/10.1377/hblog20200630.939347/full (accessed December 11, 2021).

Breathett, K., E. Yee, N. Pool, M. Hebdon, J. D. Crist, R. H. Yee, S. M. Knapp, S. Solola, L. Luy, K. Herrera-Theut, L. Zabala, J. Stone, M. M. McEwen, E. Calhoun, and N. K. Sweitzer. 2020. Association of gender and race with allocation of advanced heart failure therapies. *JAMA Network Open* 3(7):e2011044.

Brown, E. J., D. Polsky, C. M. Barbu, J. W. Seymour, and D. Grande. 2016. Racial disparities in geographic access to primary care in Philadelphia. *Health Affairs* 35(8):1374-1381.

CDC (Centers for Disease Control and Prevention). 2021. *About social determinants of health.* https://www.cdc.gov/socialdeterminants/about.html (accessed September 12, 2021).

Center for Health Progress. 2017. *Race is a social construct.* https://centerforhealthprogress.org/blog/race-social-construct (accessed October 19, 2021).

Cervantes, L., S. Fischer, N. Berlinger, M. Zabalaga, C. Camacho, S. Linas, and D. Ortega. 2017. The illness experience of undocumented immigrants with end-stage renal disease. *JAMA Internal Medicine* 177(4):529-535.

Dageforde, L. A., A. Box, I. D. Feurer, and K. L. Cavanaugh. 2015. Understanding patient barriers to kidney transplant evaluation. *Transplantation* 99(7):1463-1469.

Damschroder, L. J., D. C. Aron, R. E. Keith, S. R. Kirsh, J. A. Alexander, and J. C. Lowery. 2009. Fostering implementation of health services research findings into practice: A consolidated framework for advancing implementation science. *Implementation Science* 4(50).

Darden, M., G. Parker, E. Anderson, and J. F. Buell. 2021. Persistent sex disparity in liver transplantation rates. *Surgery* 169(3):694-699.

DeFilippis, E. M., L. K. Truby, A. R. Garan, R. C. Givens, K. Takeda, H. Takayama, Y. Naka, J. H. Haythe, M. A. Farr, and V. K. Topkara. 2019. Sex-related differences in use and outcomes of left ventricular assist devices as bridge to transplantation. *Journals of the American College of Cardiology: Heart Failure* 7(3):250-257.

Dobbels, F. 2014. Intellectual disability in pediatric transplantation: Pitfalls and opportunities. *Pediatric Transplantation* 18(7):658-660.

Dover, D. C., and A. P. Belon. 2019. The health equity measurement framework: A comprehensive model to measure social inequities in health. *International Journal for Equity in Health* 18(36).

Eisenstein, E. L., J. L. Sun, K. J. Anstrom, J. A. Stafford, L. A. Szczech, L. H. Muhlbaier, and D. B. Mark. 2009. Do income level and race influence survival in patients receiving hemodialysis? *American Journal of Medicine* 122(2):170-180.

Epstein, A. M., J. Z. Ayanian, J. H. Keogh, S. J. Noonan, N. Armistead, P. D. Cleary, J. S. Weissman, J. A. David-Kasdan, D. Carlson, J. Fuller, D. Marsh, and R. M. Conti. 2000. Racial disparities in access to renal transplantation—clinically appropriate or due to underuse or overuse? *New England Journal of Medicine* 343(21):1537-1544.

Epstein, S. 2007. *Inclusion: The politics of difference in medical research.* Chicago, IL: University of Chicago Press.

Evangelista, L. S., K. Dracup, and L. V. Doering. 2000. Treatment-seeking delays in heart failure patients. *Journal of Heart and Lung Transplantation* 19(10):932-938.

Fontanarosa, P. B., and H. Bauchner. 2018. Race, ancestry, and medical research. *JAMA* 320(15):1539-1540.

Galante, N. Z., G. A. Dib, and J. O. Medina-Pestana. 2010. Severe intellectual disability does not preclude renal transplantation. *Nephrology, Dialysis, Transplantation* 25(8):2753-2757.

Gander, J. C., X. Zhang, L. Plantinga, S. Paul, M. Basu, S. O. Pastan, E. Gibney, E. Hartmann, L. Mulloy, C. Zayas, and R. E. Patzer. 2018. Racial disparities in preemptive referral for kidney transplantation in Georgia. *Clinical Transplantation* 32(9):e13380.

Geronimus, A. T. 2013. Deep integration: Letting the epigenome out of the bottle without losing sight of the structural origins of population health. *American Journal of Public Health* 103(Suppl 1):S56-563.

Ghahramani, N., Z. Y. Karparvar, M. Ghahramani, and P. Shrivastava. 2011. Nephrologists' perceptions of renal transplant as treatment of choice for end-stage renal disease, preemptive transplant, and transplanting older patients: An international survey. *Experimental and Clinical Transplantation* 9(4):223-229.

Ghahramani, N., A. Sanati-Mehrizy, and C. Wang. 2014. Perceptions of patient candidacy for kidney transplant in the United States: A qualitative study comparing rural and urban nephrologists. *Experimental and Clinical Transplantation* 12(1):9-14.

Glazier, A. K., G. M. Danovitch, and F. L. Delmonico. 2014. Organ transplantation for nonresidents of the United States: A policy for transparency. *American Journal of Transplantation* 14(8):1740-1743.

Gordon, E. J., and A. R. Sehgal. 2000. Patient-nephrologist discussions about kidney transplantation as a treatment option. *Advances in Renal Replacement Therapy* 7(2):177-183.

Gordon, E. J., J. Feinglass, P. Carney, K. Vera, M. Olivero, A. Black, K. O'Connor, J. MacLean, S. Nichols, J. Sageshima, L. Preczewski, and J. C. Caicedo. 2016a. A culturally targeted website for Hispanics/Latinos about living kidney donation and transplantation: A randomized controlled trial of increased knowledge. *Transplantation* 100(5):1149-1160.

Gordon, E. J., J. Feinglass, P. Carney, K. Vera, M. Olivero, A. Black, K. G. O'Connor, J. M. Baumgart, and J. C. Caicedo. 2016b. A website intervention to increase knowledge about living kidney donation and transplantation among Hispanic/Latino dialysis patients. *Progress in Transplantation* 26(1):82-91.

Gordon, E. J., J. Lee, R. H. Kang, J. C. Caicedo, J. L. Holl, D. P. Ladner, and M. D. Shumate. 2018. A complex culturally targeted intervention to reduce Hispanic disparities in living kidney donor transplantation: An effectiveness-implementation hybrid study protocol. *BMC Health Services Research* 18(1):368.

Gordon, E. J., E. Romo, D. Amórtegui, A. Rodas, N. Anderson, J. Uriarte, G. McNatt, J. C. Caicedo, D. P. Ladner, and M. Shumate. 2020. Implementing culturally competent transplant care and implications for reducing health disparities: A prospective qualitative study. *Health Expectations* 23(6):1450-1465.

Gordon, E. J., J. Uriarte, J. Lee, R. Kang, M. Shumate, R. Ruiz, A. Mather, D. Ladner, and J. C. Caicedo. 2021. Effectiveness of a culturally competent care intervention in reducing disparities in Hispanic live donor kidney transplantation: A hybrid trial. *American Journal of Transplantation* 22(2):474-488. https://doi.org/10.1111/ajt.16857.

Grams, M. E., B. P. Chen, J. Coresh, and D. L. Segev. 2013. Preemptive deceased donor kidney transplantation: Considerations of equity and utility. *Clinical Journal of the American Society of Nephrology* 8(4):575-582.

Green, A. R., D. R. Carney, D. J. Pallin, L. H. Ngo, K. L. Raymond, L. I. Iezzoni, and M. R. Banaji. 2007. Implicit bias among physicians and its prediction of thrombolysis decisions for black and white patients. *Journal of General Internal Medicine* 22(9):1231-1238.

Hall, W. J., M. V. Chapman, K. M. Lee, Y. M. Merino, T. W. Thomas, B. K. Payne, E. Eng, S. H. Day, and T. Coyne-Beasley. 2015. Implicit racial/ethnic bias among health care professionals and its influence on health care outcomes: A systematic review. *American Journal of Public Health* 105(12).

Hall, Y. N., A. I. Choi, P. Xu, A. M. O'Hare, and G. M. Chertow. 2011. Racial ethnic differences in rates and determinants of deceased donor kidney transplantation. *Journal of the American Society of Nephrology* 22(4):743-751.

Hanson, C. S., S. J. Chadban, J. R. Chapman, J. C. Craig, G. Wong, and A. Tong. 2016. Nephrologists' perspectives on recipient eligibility and access to living kidney donor transplantation. *Transplantation* 100(4):943-953.

Harding, J. L., A. Perez, and R. E. Patzer. 2021. Nonmedical barriers to early steps in kidney transplantation among underrepresented groups in the United States. *Current Opinion in Organ Transplantation* 26(5):501-507.

Harding, K., T. B. Mersha, P.-T. Pham, A. D. Waterman, F. J. Webb, J. A. Vassalotti, and S. B. Nicholas. 2017. Health disparities in kidney transplantation for African Americans. *American Journal of Nephrology* 46:165-175.

HHS (U.S. Department of Health and Human Services). Health Resources and Services Administration, Healthcare Systems Bureau. 2019. *2019 National Survey of Organ Donation Attitudes and Practices: Report of findings*. Rockville, MD: U.S. Department of Health and Human Services. https://www.organdonor.gov/sites/default/files/organ-donor/professional/grants-research/nsodap-organ-donation-survey-2019.pdf (accessed August 24, 2021).

HHS. 2021a. *Healthy people 2020*. https://www.healthypeople.gov/2020/about/foundation-health-measures/Disparities (accessed November 18, 2021).

HHS. 2021b. *Healthy people 2030*. https://health.gov/our-work/healthy-people/healthy-people-2030/questions-answers (accessed November 18, 2021).

HHS. 2021c. Request for Information. 45 CFR Part 84. *Discrimination on the basis of disability in critical Health and Human Services programs or activities*. https://www.hhs.gov/sites/default/files/504-rfi.pdf (accessed September 8, 2021).

IOM (Institute of Medicine). 2001a. *Crossing the quality chasm: A new health system for the 21st century*. Washington, DC: The National Academy Press.

IOM. 2001b. *Envisioning the national health care quality report*. Washington, DC: The National Academy Press.

IOM. 2010. *Future directions for the National Healthcare Quality and Disparities Reports*. Washington, DC: The National Academies Press.

Johns, T. S., M. M. Estrella, D. C. Crews, L. J. Appel, C. A. Anderson, P. L. Ephraim, C. Cook, and L. E. Boulware. 2014. Neighborhood socioeconomic status, race, and mortality in young adult dialysis patients. *Journal of the American Society of Nephrology* 25(11):2649-2657.

Jones, C., P. Roderick, S. Harris, and M. Rogerson. 2006. Decline in kidney function before and after nephrology referral and the effect on survival in moderate to advanced chronic kidney disease. *Nephrology, Dialysis, Transplantation* 21(8):2133-2143.

Joshi, M. S., and C. Stevens. 2017. Implicit attitudes to organ donor registration: Altruism and distaste. *Health Psychology and Behavioral Medicine* 5(1):14-28.

Joshi, S., J. J. Gaynor, S. Bayers, G. Guerra, A. Eldefrawy, Z. Chediak, L. Companioni, J. Sageshima, L. Chen, W. Kupin, D. Roth, A. Mattiazzi, G. W. Burke, III, and G. Ciancio. 2013. Disparities among blacks, Hispanics, and whites in time from starting dialysis to kidney transplant waitlisting. *Transplantation* 95(2):309-318.

Kernodle, A. B., W. Zhang, J. D. Motter, B. Doby, L. Liyanage, J. Garonzik-Wang, K. R. Jackson, B. J. Boyarsky, A. B. Massie, T. S. Purnell, and D. L. Segev. 2021. Examination of racial and ethnic differences in deceased organ donation ratio over time in the US. *JAMA Surgery* 156(4):e207083.

Killian, A. C., B. Shelton, P. MacLennan, M. C. McLeod, A. Carter, R. Reed, H. Qu, B. Orandi, V. Kumar, C. Sawinski, and J. E. Locke. 2021. Evaluation of community-level vulnerability and racial disparities in living donor kidney transplant. *JAMA Surgery* 156(12):1120-1129.

Kim, J. J., M. Basu, L. Plantinga, S. O. Pastan, S. Mohan, K. Smith, T. Melanson, C. Escoffery, and R. E. Patzer. 2018. Awareness of racial disparities in kidney transplantation among health care providers in dialysis facilities. *Clinical Journal of the American Society of Nephrology* 13(5):772-781.

King, K. L., S. A. Husain, Z. Jin, C. Brennan, and S. Mohan. 2019. Trends in disparities in preemptive kidney transplantation in the United States. *Clinical Journal of the American Society of Nephrology* 14(10):1500-1511.

King, L. P., L. A. Siminoff, D. M. Meyer, C. W. Yancy, W. S. Ring, T. W. Mayo, and M. H. Drazner. 2005. Health insurance and cardiac transplantation: A call for reform. *Journal of the American College of Cardiology* 45:1388–1391.

Kucirka, L. M., M. E. Grams, J. Lessler, E. C. Hall, N. James, A. B. Massie, R. A. Montgomery, and D. L. Segev. 2011. Association of race and age with survival among patients undergoing dialysis. *JAMA* 306(6):620-626.

Kutner, N. G., R. Zhang, Y. Huang, and K. L. Johansen. 2012. Impact of race on predialysis discussions and kidney transplant preemptive wait-listing. *American Journal of Nephrology* 35(4):305-311.

Lee, B. P., and N. A. Terrault. 2020. Liver transplantation in unauthorized immigrants in the United States. *Hepatology* 71(5):1802-1812.

Levenson, J. L., and M. E. Olbrisch. 1993. Psychosocial evaluation of organ transplant candidates: A comparative survey of process, criteria, and outcomes in heart, liver, and kidney transplantation. *Psychosomatics* 34(4):314-323.

Levin, A. 2000. Consequences of late referral on patient outcomes. *Nephrology Dialysis Transplantation*, 15(Suppl 3):8-13.

Loy, V. M., A. Rzepczynski, C. Joyce, S. Bello, and A. Lu. 2020. Disparity in transplant referral patterns for alcohol-related liver disease based on physician-dependent variables. *Transplantation Proceedings* 52(3):900-904.

Marlow, N. M., A. S. Kazley, K. D. Chavin, K. N. Simpson, W. Balliet, and P. K. Baliga. 2016. A patient navigator and education program for increasing potential living donors: A comparative observational study. *Clinical Transplantation* 30(5):619-627.

Martin, P. 2014. Living donor kidney transplantation: Preferences and concerns amongst patients waiting for transplantation in New Zealand. *Journal of Health Services Research & Policy* 19(3):138-144.

McEnhill, M. E., J. L. Brennan, E. Winnicki, M. M. Lee, M. Tavakol, A. M. Posselt, P. G. Stock, and A. A. Portale. 2016. Effect of immigration status on outcomes in pediatric kidney transplant recipients. *American Journal of Transplantation* 16(6):1827-1833.

Mehra, M., J. Kobashigawa, R. Starling, S. Russell, P. Uber, J. Parameshwar, P. Mohacsi, S. Augustine, K. Aaronson, and M. Barr. 2006. Listing criteria for Heart transplantation: International Society for Heart and Lung Transplantation guidelines for the care of cardiac transplant candidates—2006. *Journal of Heart and Lung Transplantation* 25(9):1024-1042.

Mehra, M. R., C. E. Canter, M. M. Hannan, M. J. Semigran, P. A. Uber, D. A. Baran, L. Danziger-Isakov, J. K. Kirklin, R. Kirk, S. S. Kushwaha, L. H. Lund, L. Potena, H. J. Ross, D. O. Taylor, E. Verschuuren, A. Zuckermann, and International Society for Heart Lung Transplantation, Infectious Diseases, Pediatric and Heart Failure and Transplantation Councils. 2016. The 2016 International Society for Heart Lung Transplantation listing criteria for heart transplantation: A 10-year update. *Journal of Heart and Lung Transplantation* 35(1):1-23.

Meissner, F., L. A. Grigutsch, N. Koranyi, F. Müller, and K. Rothermund. 2019. Predicting behavior with implicit measures: Disillusioning findings, reasonable explanations, and sophisticated solutions. *Frontiers in Psychology* 10:2483.

Morris, A. A., E. P. Kransdorf, B. L. Coleman, and M. Colvin. 2016. Racial and ethnic disparities in outcomes after heart transplantation: A systematic review of contributing factors and future directions to close the outcomes gap. *Journal of Heart and Lung Transplantation* 35(8):953-961.

Morris, Z. S., S. Wooding, and J. Grant. 2011. The answer is 17 years, what is the question: Understanding time lags in translational research. *Journal of the Royal Society of Medicine* 104(12):510-520.

Mucsi, I., A. Bansal, O. Famure, Y. Li, M. Mitchell, A. D. Waterman, M. Novak, and S. J. Kim. 2017. Ethnic background is a potential barrier to living donor kidney transplantation in Canada: A single-center retrospective cohort study. *Transplantation* 101(4):e142-e151.

Mulligan, C. J. 2021. Systemic racism can get under our skin and into our genes. *American Journal of Physical Anthropology* 175:399-405.

Mustian, M. N., B. A. Shelton, P. A. MacLennan, R. D. Reed, J. A. White, D. E. Eckhoff, J. E. Locke, R. M. Allman, and S. H. Gray. 2019. Ethnic and age disparities in outcomes among liver transplant waitlist candidates. *Transplantation* 103(7):1425-1432.

NASEM (National Academies of Sciences, Engineering, and Medicine). 2021. *The science of implicit bias: Implications for law and policy: Proceedings of a workshop–in brief.* Washington, DC: The National Academies Press. https://doi.org/10.17226/26191.

National Work Group on Disability and Transplantation. 2004. Summary report of the individual and family disability survey, March 11, 2004.

Navaneethan, S. D., S. Nigwekar, M. Sengodan, E. Anand, S. Kadam, V. Jeevanantham, M. Grieff, and W. Choudhry. 2007. Referral to nephrologists for chronic kidney disease care: Is non-diabetic kidney disease ignored? *Nephron Clinical Practice* 106(3):c113-c118.

Navaneethan, S. D., S. Aloudat, and S. Singh. 2008. A systematic review of patient and health system characteristics associated with late referral in chronic kidney disease. *BMC Nephrology* 9(3).

Ng, Y. H., V. S. Pankratz, Y. Leyva, C. G. Ford, J. R. Pleis, K. Kendall, E. Croswell, M. A. Dew, R. Shapiro, G. E. Switzer, M. L. Unruh, and L. Myaskovsky. 2020. Does racial disparity in kidney transplant waitlisting persist after accounting for social determinants of health? *Transplantation* 104(7):1445-1455.

Nissaisorakarn, P., X. Huiling, M. D. Doshi, N. Singh, K. L. Lentine, and S. E. Rosas. 2021. Eliminating racial dispari-ties in kidney transplantation. *Clinical Transplantation* 35(8):e14397.

Ohta, T., O. Motoyama, K. Takahashi, M. Hattori, S. Shishido, N. Wada, Y. Gotoh, T. Yanagihara, A. Hasegawa, and T. Sakano. 2006. Kidney transplantation in pediatric recipients with mental retardation: Clinical results of a multicenter experience in Japan. *American Journal of Kidney Diseases* 47(3):518-527.

OPTN (Organ Procurement and Transplantation Network). 2020. *Briefing to the OPTN board of directors on data collection to assess socioeconomic status and access to transplant.* https://optn.transplant.hrsa.gov/me-dia/3811/202006_mac_ses_bp.pdf (accessed September 9, 2021).

OPTN. 2021. *Policies.* https://optn.transplant.hrsa.gov/media/1200/optn_policies.pdf (accessed September 9, 2021).

Padela, A. I., R. Duivenbode, M. R. Saunders, M. Quinn, and E. Koh. 2020. The impact of religiously tailored and ethically balanced education on intention for living organ donation among Muslim Americans. *Clinical Transplantation* 34(12):e14111.

Patzer, R. E., J. P. Perryman, J. D. Schrager, S. Pastan, S. Amaral, J. A. Gazmararian, M. Klein, N. Kutner, and W. M. McClellan. 2012. The role of race and poverty on steps to kidney transplantation in the southeastern United States. *American Journal of Transplantation* 12(2):358-368.

Patzer, R. E., B. A. Sayed, N. Kutner, W. M. McClellan, and S. Amaral. 2013. Racial and ethnic differences in pediatric access to preemptive kidney transplantation in the United States. *American Journal of Transplantation* 13(7):1769-1781.

Pelleboer-Gunnink, H. A., W. Van Oorsouw, J. Van Weeghel, and P. Embregts. 2017. Mainstream health profes-sionals' stigmatising attitudes towards people with intellectual disabilities: A systematic review. *Journal of Intellectual Disability Research* 61(5):411-434.

Peng, R. B., H. Lee, Z. T. Ke, and M. R. Saunders. 2018. Racial disparities in kidney transplant waitlist appearance in Chicago: Is it race or place? *Clinical Transplantation* 32(5):e13195.

Pew Research Center. 2019. *U.S. unauthorized immigrant population estimates by state, 2016.* https://www.pew research.org/hispanic/interactives/u-s-unauthorized-immigrants-by-state (accessed September 2, 2021).

Popejoy, A. B., K. R. Crooks, S. M. Fullerton, L. A. Hindorff, G. W. Hooker, B. A. Koenig, N. Pino, E. M. Ramos, D. I. Ritter, H. Wand, M. W. Wright, M. Yudell, J. Y. Zou, S. E. Plon, C. D. Bustamante, and K. E. Ormond, Clinical Genome Resource (ClinGen) Ancestry and Diversity Working Group. 2020. Clinical genetics lacks standard definitions and protocols for the collection and use of diversity measures. *American Journal of Hu-man Genetics* 107(1):72-82.

Prakash, S., R. A. Rodriguez, P. C. Austin, R. Saskin, A. Fernandez, L. M. Moist, and A. M. O'Hare. 2010. Racial composition of residential areas associates with access to Pre-ESRD nephrology care. *Journal of the American Society of Nephrology* 21(7):1192-1199.

Purnell, T. S., and D. C. Crews. 2019. Persistent disparities in preemptive kidney transplantation. *Clinical Journal of the American Society of Nephrology* 14(10):1430-1431.

Reese, P. P., O. Aubert, M. Naesens, E. Huang, V. Potluri, D. Kuypers, A. Bouquegneau, G. Divard, M. Raynaud, Y. Bouatou, A. Vo, D. Glotz, C. Legendre, C. Lefaucheur, S. Jordan, J. P. Empana, X. Jouven, and A. Loupy. 2021a. Assessment of the utility of kidney histology as a basis for discarding organs in the United States: A comparison of international transplant practices and outcomes. *Journal of the American Society of Nephrol-ogy* 32(2):397-409.

Reese, P. P., S. Mohan, K. L. King, W. W. Williams, V. S. Potluri, M. N. Harhay, and N. D. Eneanya. 2021b. Racial disparities in preemptive waitlisting and deceased donor kidney transplantation: Ethics and solutions. *American Journal of Transplantation* 21(3):958-967.

Rhee, C. M., P. Lertdumrongluk, E. Streja, J. Park, H. Moradi, W. L. Lau, K. C. Norris, A. R. Nissenson, A. N. Amin, C. P. Kovesdy, and K. Kalantar-Zadeh. 2014. Impact of age, race and ethnicity on dialysis patient survival and kidney transplantation disparities. *American Journal of Nephrology* 39(3):183-194.

Richards, C. T., L. M. Crawley, and D. Magnus. 2009. Use of neurodevelopmental delay in pediatric solid organ transplant listing decisions: Inconsistencies in standards across major pediatric transplant centers. *Pediatric Transplantation* 13(7):843-850.

Robinson, A., G. Hirode, and R. J. Wong. 2021. Ethnicity and insurance-specific disparities in the model for end-stage liver disease score at time of liver transplant waitlist registration and its impact on mortality. *Journal of Clinical and Experimental Hepatology* 11(2):188-194.

Rodrigue, J. R., M. J. Paek, O. Egbuna, A. D. Waterman, J. D. Schold, M. Pavlakis, and D. A. Mandelbrot. 2014. Making house calls increases living donor inquiries and evaluations for blacks on the kidney transplant waiting list. *Transplantation* 98(9):979-986.

Rodriguez, R., L. Cervantes, and R. Raghavan. 2020. Estimating the prevalence of undocumented immigrants with end-stage renal disease in the United States. *Clinical Nephrology* 93(1):108-112.

Sabounchi, N., N. Sharareh, F. Irshaidat, and S. Atav. 2018. Spatial dynamics of access to primary care for the Medicaid population. *Health Systems* 9(1):64-75.

Salter, M., M. A. McAdams-Demarco, A. Law, R. J. Kamil, L. A. Meoni, B. G. Jaar, S. M. Sozio, W. H. L. Kao, R. S. Parekh, and D. L. Segev. 2014. Age and sex disparities in discussions about kidney transplantation in adults undergoing dialysis. *Journal of the American Geriatrics Society* 62(5):843-849.

Samelson-Jones, E., D. M. Mancini, and P. A. Shapiro. 2012. Cardiac transplantation in adult patients with mental retardation: Do outcomes support consensus guidelines? *Psychosomatics* 53(2):133-138.

Schimmack, U. 2021. The Implicit Association Test: A method in search of a construct. *Perspectives on Psychological Science* 16(2):396-414.

Schold, J. D., J. A. Gregg, J. S. Harman, A. G. Hall, P. R. Patton, and H. U. Meier-Kriesche. 2011. Barriers to evaluation and wait listing for kidney transplantation. *Clinical Journal of the American Society of Nephrology* 6(7):1760-1767.

Secunda, K., E. J. Gordon, M. W. Sohn, L. A. Shinkunas, L. C. Kaldjian, M. D. Voigt, and J. Levitsky. 2013. National survey of provider opinions on controversial characteristics of liver transplant candidates. *Liver Transplantation* 19(4):395-403.

Siminoff, L. A., R. H. Lawrence, and R. M. Arnold. 2003. Comparison of black and white families' experiences and perceptions regarding organ donation requests. *Critical Care Medicine* 31(1):146-151.

Siminoff, L. A., G. P. Alolod, H. M. Gardiner, R. D. Hasz, P. A. Mulvania, and M. Wilson-Genderson. 2020. A comparison of the content and quality of organ donation discussions with African American families who authorize and refuse donation. *Journal of Racial and Ethnic Health Disparities* 8:485-493.

Suarez, J., J. B. Cohen, V. Potluri, W. Yang, D. E. Kaplan, M. Serper, S. P. Shah, and P. P. Reese. 2018. Racial disparities in nephrology consultation and disease progression among veterans with CKD: An observational cohort study. *Journal of the American Society of Nephrology* 29(10):2563-2573.

Sullivan, C., J. B. Leon, S. S. Sayre, M. Marbury, M. Ivers, J. A. Pencak, K. A. Bodziak, D. E. Hricik, E. J. Morrison, J. M. Albert, S. D. Navaneethan, C. M. Reyes, and A. R. Sehgal. 2012. Impact of navigators on completion of steps in the kidney transplant process: A randomized, controlled trial. *Clinical Journal of the American Society of Nephrology* 7(10):1639-1645.

Taylor, D. M., J. A. Bradley, C. Bradley, H. Draper, R. Johnson, W. Metcalfe, G. Oniscu, M. Robb, C. Tomson, C. Watson, R. Ravanan, P. Roderick, and ATTOM Investigators. 2016. Limited health literacy in advanced kidney disease. *Kidney International* 90(3):685-695.

Thuluvath, P. J., W. Amjad, and T. Zhang. 2020. Liver transplant waitlist removal, transplantation rates and post-transplant survival in Hispanics. *PLoS ONE* 15(12):e0244744

Traino, H. M., A. J. Molisani, and L. A. Siminoff. 2017. Regional differences in communication process and outcomes of requests for solid organ donation. *American Journal of Transplantation* 17(6):1620-1627.

Tung, E. L., D. A. Hampton, M. Kolak, S. O. Rogers, J. P. Yang, and M. E. Peek. 2019. Race/ethnicity and geographic access to urban trauma care. *JAMA Network Open* 2(3).

UNOS (United Network for Organ Sharing). 2021. *Equity in access to transplant.* https://insights.unos.org/equity-in-access (accessed August 10, 2021).

USRDS (United States Renal Data System). 2020. *Annual data report: Epidemiology of kidney disease in the United States.* Bethesda, MD: National Institute of Diabetes and Digestive and Kidney Diseases.

Vianello, M., and Y. Bar-Anan. 2021. Can the Implicit Association Test measure automatic judgment? The validation continues. *Perspectives on Psychological Science* 16(2):415-421.

Vyas, D. A., L. G. Eisenstein, and D. S. Jones. 2020. Hidden in plain sight—reconsidering the use of race correction in clinical algorithms. *New England Journal of Medicine* 383(9):874-882.

Wall, A., G. H. Lee, J. Maldonado, and D. Magnus. 2020. Genetic disease and intellectual disability as contraindications to transplant listing in the United States: A survey of heart, kidney, liver, and lung transplant programs. *Pediatric Transplantation* 24(7):e13837.

Waterman, A. D., J. R. Rodrigue, T. S. Purnell, K. Ladin, and L. E. Boulware. 2010. Addressing racial and ethnic disparities in live donor kidney transplantation: Priorities for research and intervention. *Seminars in Nephrology* 30(1):90-98.

Waterman, A. D., J. D. Peipert, S. S. Hyland, M. S. McCabe, E. A. Schenk, and J. Liu. 2013. Modifiable patient characteristics and racial disparities in evaluation completion and living donor transplant. *Clinical Journal of the American Society of Nephrology* 8(6):995-1002.

Weng, F. L., M. M. Joffe, H. I. Feldman, and K. C. Mange. 2005. Rates of completion of the medical evaluation for renal transplantation. *American Journal of Kidney Diseases* 46(4):734-745.

Wesselman, H., C. G. Ford, Y. Leyva, X. Li, C. H. Chang, M. A. Dew, K. Kendall, E. Croswell, J. R. Pleis, Y. H. Ng, M. L. Unruh, R. Shapiro, and L. Myaskovsky. 2021. Social determinants of health and race disparities in kidney transplant. *Clinical Journal of the American Society of Nephrology* 16(2):262-274.

Wightman, A., B. Young, M. Bradford, A. Dick, P. Healey, R. McDonald, and J. Smith. 2014. Prevalence and outcomes of renal transplantation in children with intellectual disability. *Pediatric Transplantation* 18(7):714-719.

Wightman, A., E. Hsu, Q. Zhao, and J. Smith. 2016. Prevalence and outcomes of liver transplantation in children with intellectual disability. *Journal of Pediatric Gastroenterology and Nutrition* 62(6):808-812.

Wightman, A., H. L. Bartlett, Q. Zhao, and J. M. Smith. 2017. Prevalence and outcomes of heart transplantation in children with intellectual disability. *Pediatric Transplantation* 21(2). https://doi.org/10.1111/petr.12839.

Wolfe, R. A., V. B. Ashby, E. L. Milford, A. O. Ojo, R. E. Ettenger, L. Y. Agodoa, P. J. Held, and F. K. Port. 1999. Comparison of mortality in all patients on dialysis, patients on dialysis awaiting transplantation, and recipients of a first cadaveric transplant. *New England Journal of Medicine* 341(23):1725-1730.

Yu, E., and A. Wightman. 2021. Pediatric kidney transplant in undocumented immigrants: An American perspective. *Pediatric Transplant* 25(1):e13788.

Yudell, M., D. Roberts, R. DeSalle, S. Tishkoff, 70 signatories. 2020. NIH must confront the use of race in science. *Science* 369(6509):1313-1314.

# 5

# Saving More Lives and Enhancing Equity with Deceased Donor Organ Allocation Policies

llocation systems—that is, how patients are prioritized on the waiting list and organs are rated for transplant—differ by organ type. The U.S. Department of Health and Human Services (HHS) Final Rule directs the Organ Procurement and Transplantation Network (OPTN) to design organ allocation policies "to achieve the best use of donated organs.[1] Specifically, the OPTN must rank candidates from "most to least medically urgent" while "taking into account...that life-sustaining technology allows alternative approaches." However, allocation systems differ by organ. Heart, liver, and lung allocation comply with the OPTN regulation and have allocation systems designed specifically on candidate urgency. Donated livers are allocated based on the transplant candidate's likelihood of dying while on the wait list. Lung allocation is similar, but takes into account a transplant candidate's likelihood of dying within a year after the transplant (Friedewald et al., 2013). Heart allocation relies on treatment choices as a proxy for medical urgency rather than by calculations coming from a scoring system. The kidney allocation system (KAS) ranks candidates primarily by waiting time.

According to the United Network for Organ Sharing (UNOS),[2] several logistical and medical factors must be taken into account before a donated organ can be allocated to a patient. First, an organ needs to match the candidate; waiting list candidates who are incompatible (i.e., because of blood type, organ size, or other medical issues) are removed from consideration for that particular donated organ. Next, the order of eligible candidates is decided using what UNOS calls a *match run*, which is a rank-order list of candidates for a particular organ. The computed match run is unique for every organ and every donor. The match run also takes into consideration factors that affect the likely success of a transplant, including geographical factors such as transplant hospital locations or organ-specific time constraints that may limit the distance an organ is able to travel and still be viable for transplant (Table 5-1) and organ size (i.e., a pediatric-sized organ is best for a pediatric patient). Matching criteria do

---

[1] 42 C.F.R. §121.8 e-CFR: Title 42: Public Health.
[2] For more specific information, see https://unos.org/transplant/how-we-match-organs (accessed October 21, 2021).

**TABLE 5-1** Structural Factors and Key Disparities in Organ Allocation

| Organ | Before the Waiting List and Offer Process | Factors Considered in Allocation[a] | Key Disparities |
|---|---|---|---|
| Kidney | A candidate must undergo evaluation by the transplant team, and given blood tests, diagnostics tests, and a mental health evaluation. The transplant team will review medical history to determine eligibility for transplant, then the candidate is added to the UNOS waiting list.[b]<br><br>Average wait time: 3–5 years[c] | Proceeds through the Kidney Allocation System, which includes estimated 1-year posttransplant survival (EPTS), distance from donor hospital, pediatric status, waiting time, prior living donor, donor/recipient immune system incompatibility (CPRA)[d,e]<br><br>Max organ preservation time: 24–36 hours | Black patients, patients with diabetes, patients with prior solid organ transplantations<br><br>Driven largely by inequitable access to donors, disparities in wait time vary widely across geographic location |
| Heart | A candidate must be referred by their physician, then be evaluated by the transplant team. The transplant team reviews their medical history to determine eligibility for transplant. A candidate who smokes must also cease smoking and be nicotine free for several months before they are allowed on the waiting list.<br><br>Candidates are rank ordered for transplant by the treatments they need, and assigned 1 of 6 total adult status levels. Candidates with higher medical urgency (i.e., adult status 1) are prioritized for transplantation. Status levels are based primarily on use and complexity of treatments and devices needed (advanced support therapies), with some consideration of medications and additional heart conditions.<br><br>Average wait time: 7–10 months | Medical need; distance from donor hospital[f]<br><br>Max organ preservation time: 4–6 hours | |
| Lung | A candidate must first be evaluated by a transplant team then given blood tests, diagnostics tests, and a mental health evaluation.<br><br>Similar to heart transplant, the transplant team also reviews the patient's medical history to determine eligibility for transplant. A candidate who smokes must also cease smoking and be nicotine free for several months before being allowed on the waiting list.[g]<br><br>Once a candidate is deemed eligible, they are added to the UNOS waiting list.<br><br>Average wait time: a few months to many years depending on lung disease diagnosis | Lung allocation system, which includes medical urgency and survival benefit; waiting time; distance from donor hospital[h]<br><br>Max organ preservation time: 4–6 hours | |
| Liver | Candidates must be evaluated by the transplant team, and will be given blood tests, imaging, and physical exams to determine the origin and severity of their liver disease, if any other diseases are affecting them, and estimate their likelihood to survive transplant.<br><br>Those not eligible for transplant are candidates with a severe infection, current alcohol or drug abuse, serious heart or lung diseases, or cancer (outside the liver). | Model of End-Stage Liver Disease or Pediatric End-Stage Liver Disease score; medical need; distance from donor hospital[j]<br><br>Max organ preservation time: 8–12 hours | Adult patients of small size<br><br>Pediatric patients of color, due to less frequent application for exception points; pediatric patients older than 1 year but less than 2 years old; and potentially pediatric patients aged 12–17[k] |

| Organ | Process | Allocation criteria | |
|---|---|---|---|
| | Once a candidate is deemed eligible, they are added to the UNOS waiting list.[i]<br><br>Average waiting time: less than 30 days to more than 5 years | | |
| Intestine | A candidate must undergo evaluation by the transplant team.<br><br>Candidates are then assigned a status for transplant—1, 2, or inactive. Status 1 candidates are prioritized for transplant. Status-level assignments are based on medical criteria.[j] | Time on the waiting list, abnormal liver function, limited access points for intravenous feeding tubes, or presence of other medical indications warranting urgent transplant; blood type identical to or compatible with donor; geographic distance from transplant hospital (priority for within 500 NM, then sharing is national).[a] | |
| VCA | A candidate must undergo evaluation by the transplant team.<br><br>Candidates are registered on the waiting list by VCA type.[m] | Time on the waiting list, blood type compatibility with donor, and geographic distance from the transplant hospital (priority for within 500 NM, then sharing is national). | |
| Pancreas | Candidates must undergo evaluation by the transplant team, and testing to determine their CPRA value. Only candidates diagnosed with diabetes, pancreatic exocrine insufficiency, or that require a pancreas as part of a multiorgan transplant for technical reasons are permitted to enter the waiting list.[n] | Time on the waiting list, CPRA, distance from the transplant hospital (priority for within 250 NM, then 2,500 NM, then sharing is national). | |
| Multiorgan | Candidates are evaluated by the transplant team according to the policies governing the types of organ transplants they need. | Multiorgan transplant specific policies for heart–lung, liver–kidney, and kidney–pancreas transplants; time on the waiting list, distance from the transplant hospital, and needed medical support without transplant, in line with single-organ transplant policies. | Kidney-alone transplant candidates[o] |

NOTE: NM = nautical miles; CPRA = calculated panel reactive antibody; VCA = vascularized composite allotransplantation; UNOS = United Network for Organ Sharing.

SOURCES:
a https://unos.org/transplant/how-we-match-organs.
b https://www.hopkinsmedicine.org/health/treatment-tests-and-therapies/kidney-transplant.
c https://www.kidney.org/atoz/content/transplant-waitlist.
d https://www.srtr.org/transplant-centers/university-of-wisconsin-hospital-and-clinics-wiuw/?organ=kidney&recipientType=adult&donorType=.
e https://www.srtr.org/transplant-centers/university-of-chicago-medical-center-iluc/?organ=kidney&recipientType=adult&donorType=.
f https://www.upmc.com/services/transplant/heart/process/waiting-list.
g https://www.hopkinsmedicine.org/health/treatment-tests-and-therapies/lung-transplant.
h https://my.clevelandclinic.org/health/articles/9971-lung-transplant-finding-an-organ-donor.
i https://www.niddk.nih.gov/health-information/liver-disease/liver-transplant/preparing-transplant.
j Singal and Kamath, 2003.
k Hsu et al., 2003.
l UNOS. 2021a.
m https://optn.transplant.hrsa.gov/media/4211/bp_202012_programming-vca-allocation-in-unet.pdf.
n OPTN, n.d.-b.
o Reese et al. 2021.

not consider income, celebrity status, or insurance status in determining allocation priority. The committee is mindful that its charge is to consider all types of solid organ transplants. While each of these organs is considered in this chapter, the majority of this text focuses on kidneys since the vast majority of candidates on any waiting list for any organs are waiting for a kidney transplant.

## DISPARITIES EXACERBATED BY ALLOCATION SCORING SYSTEMS

As described in previous chapters, factors contributing to disparity in the waiting list for transplantation include gaps in access to health care, uneven referral rates to specialist providers, and differing education efforts on treatment options and preparation for end-stage disease. These upstream factors are inextricable from the end result of the organ transplantation system and therefore crucial to highlight again.

Chapter 4 of this report discusses disparities in detail as they relate to many aspects of the organ transplantation system. Only a few key inequities are summarized here as fundamental underlying problems plaguing current allocation policies.

### Implications of Current Policies Regarding Measurement of Organ Function and Recipient Suitability in Allocation Decisions[3]

Black organ donors receive a higher Kidney Donor Profile Index (KDPI) score because of the inclusion of *race/ethnicity* as a term in KDPI calculation (see Table 5-6). Few patients with diabetes or who have had a previous solid organ transplant will meet the current criteria for priority kidney allocation. In addition, because of the known high prevalence of diabetes among black and Hispanic patients, these groups may be less likely to gain the advantages of priority allocation when longevity matching[4] patients with a 20 percent estimated post-transplant survival (EPTS) to donated organs with a 20 percent KDPI (Delgado et al., 2021; Freedman et al., 2016; Julian et al., 2017).

Changes to allocation with the new kidney allocation system in 2014 improved allocation by introducing sharing of donor organs at local, regional, and national levels for patients with high calculated panel reactive antibody (CPRA) scores. However, some disparities still exist. Black candidates with a CPRA of 80 percent or more continue to have lower access to transplantation compared with white candidates, whereas Hispanic candidates have similar access as white candidates with the changes. Patients who live in rural areas continue to have lower probability of finding a donor organ, especially if they do not get priority nationally (Kulkarni et al., 2019; Stewart et al., 2018).

There are regional differences in longevity matching, such that areas that do not have very many candidates with a low EPTS may not be able to optimize organs donated with a low KDPI, thus donated kidneys calculated to be least medically complex may go to candidates with a lower estimated survival posttransplant (Husain et al., 2019; Schold et al., 2014). As discussed in the section later in this chapter on survival benefit, it is not clear that this is a disparity with respect to the organ transplantation system overall, but it may affect patient outcomes on an individual or regional level. Waiting list mortality for liver transplant

---

[3] Much of this section is excerpted or slightly modified from papers commissioned by the committee for this study (Ku, 2021; Lai, 2021). Commissioned papers are in the study's public access file and are available upon request from the National Academies' Public Access Records Office (paro@nas.edu).

[4] Longevity matching refers to better matching the life span of an organ with the life span of the recipient.

candidates is comparable between patients of different race and ethnic backgrounds, likely driven by the objective measurements used in calculating the Model for End-Stage Liver Disease (MELD) scores.

Women waiting for liver transplants are much more likely to die while on the waiting list than men, likely caused by creatinine measures underestimating kidney function in women that is further exacerbated by serum sodium level calculations (Locke et al., 2020). However, sex differences also play a crucial role in liver diseases, their evolution and outcome, and in liver transplantation in terms of graft survival, metabolic levels, and quality of life after liver transplantation (Rodriquez-Castro et al., 2014). Disparities in access to liver transplants are exacerbated by considerations of body and organ size as well as differences in the etiology of underlying liver disease in addition to the previously mentioned limitations of the MELD score, especially regarding creatinine levels (Axelrod and Pomfret, 2008). Exception points granted to patients diagnosed with hepatocellular carcinoma are also more likely to be given to men, given the disease prevalence. Updated guidance to granting exception points for these patients may address this but has yet to be studied.

Exception points for Pediatric End-Stage Liver Disease (PELD) calculations are frequently requested and granted. However, patients identifying as nonwhite request exception points at lower rates. A National Liver Review Board, introduced in 2019, aims to standardize exception points, but the effects of this board on racial and ethnic disparities is still unknown.

There may also be age-based disparities in PELD calculations. Children older than 1 year but less than 2 years of age have a higher risk of dying while on the waiting list. In addition, children aged 12–17 years are prioritized for transplant using MELD, but MELD was based on blood values in adults and has not been verified for its accuracy in adolescents.

Kidney-alone transplant candidates may be disadvantaged by multiorgan allocation policies, where the "next sequential" candidate who would have received a donated kidney had it not gone to a multiorgan transplant recipient tended to be younger, more highly sensitized, and more likely to identify with a minority group (Westphal et al., 2021).

## CURRENT ALLOCATION POLICIES AND SCORING SYSTEMS

Within the context of the structural factors and key disparities described in Table 5-1, each organ has varying policies and procedures governing transplantation. Some of the historical context around these policies is described in Chapter 3. The current policies and procedures working to govern allocation, including relevant factors for prewaiting list, waiting list, and postwaiting list, are described in this section.

### Waiting List Management

Organ transplant waiting list management has become increasingly complex across all organ types but especially in the kidney population. Large transplant programs report upward of 1,000 or more kidney patients on their waiting list, underscoring the importance of assessing individual patients for transplant readiness, communication of waiting list status, and patient education. Husain et al. (2018) reported that nearly one in five kidneys is offered as a primary offer to a deceased patient on the waiting list, contributing to less efficiency in the process of organ offers, and perhaps contributing to organ nonuse.

In late 2011, regulatory changes led to the Social Security Administration (SSA) not including protected state death records in the Death Master File used by the OPTN, among others, to verify patient status. Although changes affected access to the SSA, dialysis units and transplant centers are obligated to report all kidney patient deaths to the U.S. Renal Data System in almost real time. Though death data ultimately are reported via a different mechanism, offers to deceased candidates highlight the lack of patient engagement around organ offers being declined on their behalf by transplant centers (Husain et al., 2018; see Figure 5-1). With national death data available to update the waiting list in a timely fashion, it is perplexing why the OPTN and/or transplant centers choose not to update the waiting list with this information. Understanding that 20 percent of kidney offers are to deceased individuals on the transplant waiting list is a situation that undermines public trust in the organ transplantation system. Updating patient data can improve the organ offer process, and make it possible for the right organ to get to the right recipient in a timely manner. A real opportunity exists for better data management of waiting list candidates by transplant centers and the OPTN.

In 2016, the OPTN implemented the 3-year Collaborative Improvement and Innovation Network (COIIN), a study designed to improve the use of kidneys with a KDPI score of greater than 50 percent (Wey et al., 2020). Although COIIN did not have an effect on kidney use, waiting list management was a key focus area of the intervention guide and included referring patients for transplant evaluation, evaluating and selecting candidates for listing, and reevaluating wait-listed candidates. A visual analytics tool that displays information related to the active and inactive status of kidney patients on transplant center waiting lists was launched by UNOS in early 2020 and is available to all kidney transplant programs on its data analytics portal (OPTN, 2021b).

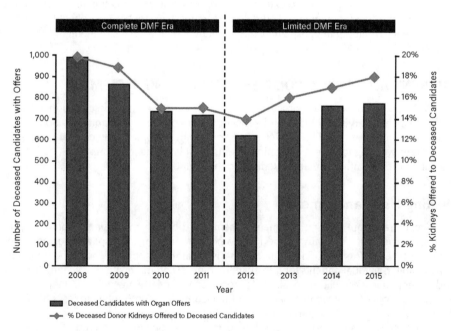

**FIGURE 5-1** Number of deceased candidates with offers by year.
NOTE: DMF = Death Master File.
SOURCE: Husain et al., 2018.

## Overview of Efforts to Address Geographic Disparities

Certain organ allocation and distribution policies have been highly debated among the transplantation community over the years. As a recent example, there was a change in 2018 to the adult heart allocation system that was made to improve stratification of waiting list candidates and provide broader access to the most medically urgent cases. Waiting list stratification changed from a three-tiered to six-tiered system. There were concerns that the changes would encourage a different approach to the care of critically ill heart failure patients, and early data suggest that may be the case (Cogswell et al., 2020). Following this change, which went into effect in October 2018, the number of heart transplants increased from 2,954 to 3,032, though this was most likely not related to the change. However, 78 percent of transplants after the change were from the most medically urgent categories (status 1, 2, and 3) versus 68 percent in status 1a (the most urgent before the change) (Goff et al., 2020). In addition, the median distance between the donor and transplant hospital increased from 83 to 216 nautical miles. Six-month posttransplant survival did not change significantly (93.6 percent vs. 92.8 percent). Use of extra corporeal membrane oxygenation was also statistically significantly higher than before the allocation change (1.93 percent vs. 1.06 percent; $P < .001$). More intra-aortic balloon pumps were also implanted following the change (8.84 percent vs. 3.86 percent; $P < .001$). It is too early to determine the overall effect of the change, but the challenges point to the complexities in making sweeping changes to the allocation system. One cohort study comparing heart transplant rates before and after the 2018 allocation change found significant variation in heart transplantation rates among centers in the same geographic region and those sharing the same organ procurement organization (OPO)—the largest variation being 27 percent for two transplant centers with the same OPO (Tran et al., 2022). Centers with higher transplant volumes and a greater proportion of candidates with intra-aortic balloon pump had higher transplant rates (Tran et al., 2022).

The evolution of liver allocation and distribution policies is another example of changes that have occurred. It was first developed in 1987 using a points-based system and relied on defined distribution units. Within this system, there was concern that candidates with the highest medical need could be bypassed for candidates with a lower medical need if the individual with the highest need were outside of the service area of the OPO that procured the liver. The OPTN Final Rule in 1998 sought to address some of these geographic disparities in deceased donor organ allocation. Specifically, the Final Rule directs that organ allocation policies not be based on a transplant candidate's place of residence or listing except to the extent required by other requirements of the Final Rule and that allocation should achieve equitable allocation among patients, including through the distribution of organs over as "broad a geographic area as feasible" under the other allocation policies.[5] The ensuing controversy prompted Congress to request a study from the Institute of Medicine (IOM) to ascertain the effects of the Final Rule; the IOM committee later issued a report recommending broader sharing of livers (IOM, 1999).

Implementation of the MELD system of allocation in 2002 was intended to better address medical urgency in liver transplantation. A number of distribution efforts related to expanded allocation followed, including the Share 15 policy in 2005, which sought to improve access for candidates with the highest need by making liver offers to those with a MELD score of 15 or higher at the regional level prior to the local level. The Share 35 policy in 2013 further extended regional and national sharing to candidates with MELD scores over 35 before local candidates with scores under 35. Massie et al. (2015) found that nonuse rates and waiting

---

[5] OPTN Final Rule, 42 C.F.R. §121.8.

list mortality both decreased following implementation. However, regional variation in transplant outcomes following implementation of this policy was also noted (Halazun et al., 2016). In 2018, liver distribution policy moved away from the donation service area to acuity circles based on 150, 250, and 500 nautical miles from a donor hospital.[6] While implementation was delayed because of legal action, the policy went into effect in February 2020.

In an effort to address geographic disparities more broadly, the OPTN created an ad hoc committee in 2017 focused on the geographic distribution of organs. The committee recommended, and the OPTN board of directors subsequently adopted in 2018, a continuous distribution framework as the best option for future distribution policies and directed its organ-specific committees to move in this direction. Whether these changes to allocation policies will result in the desired corrections to geographic disparities in access to transplant remains to be seen; however, as with any new policy changes, it will be important to monitor implementation efforts for unintended consequences.

## Continuous Distribution

Continuous distribution is a framework for allocating and distributing deceased donor organs developed by the OPTN. The framework aims to eliminate fixed geographic boundaries currently used to separate groups of candidates based on distance between donor hospital and transplant hospital. Prior deceased donor organ distribution frameworks have considered patient characteristics in a defined sequence, whereas continuous distribution will create a composite score that considers multiple patient and donor attributes all at once with an overall score that includes medical urgency, posttransplant survival, candidate biology, patient access (such as pediatric or prior living donor), and placement efficiency, defined as efficient use of resources to match, transport, and transplant a donated organ (OPTN, n.d.-a).

The OPTN gives the following illustration on its website to describe some of the differences under a continuous distribution framework (Figure 5-2). Under current classification systems, one factor alone (e.g., distance from donor hospital) can determine the order in which hypothetical transplantation candidates A, B, C, and D receive an organ offer. Taking distance from the donor hospital as the example, candidate C would receive an organ offer first, followed by A, B, and finally D.

Taking this same example in a continuous distribution framework instead, depending on the weight and value of attributes selected by the organ-specific committee and transplant community, candidate B may be the first to receive an organ offer owing to their combination of medical urgency, survival probability, and distance to the donor hospital. Under this hypothetical framework, candidate A would receive the next offer, followed by C and then D.

> *Conclusion 5-1: Assigning a relatively large weight to the placement efficiency factor (based on potential recipients' proximity to the donor hospital) in the continuous distribution policy would violate the Final Rule and defeat the goals of the policy, which the OPTN adopted to ensure that organs are allocated fairly and efficiently among patients nationally.*

Organ-specific committees, with input from transplant communities, are identifying and confirming relevant attributes for candidates on the waiting list; prioritizing the attri-

---

[6] For more information on allocation based on acuity circles, see https://optn.transplant.hrsa.gov/governance/key-initiatives/liver (accessed August 10, 2021).

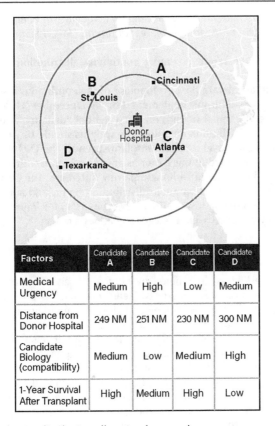

| Factors | Candidate A | Candidate B | Candidate C | Candidate D |
|---|---|---|---|---|
| Medical Urgency | Medium | High | Low | Medium |
| Distance from Donor Hospital | 249 NM | 251 NM | 230 NM | 300 NM |
| Candidate Biology (compatibility) | Medium | Low | Medium | High |
| 1-Year Survival After Transplant | High | Medium | High | Low |

**FIGURE 5-2** Continuous distribution allocation framework.
NOTE: NM = nautical mile.
SOURCE: OPTN, n.d.-a.

butes and assigning waiting list point values to them; developing, modeling, and analyzing the proposed frameworks; seeking formal public comment on the proposals; incorporating changes proposed in the public comment period as appropriate; and then seeking approval from the OPTN board of directors before implementing the new frameworks (see Chapter 2 for a further description of the OPTN policy-making process).

The continuous distribution for lung transplantation is the furthest along in the process, with the board of directors reviewing it in December 2021 and anticipated implementation in 2023. The kidney and pancreas policy completed its public comment phase at the end of September 2021,[7] and it will go to the board of directors in 2022 for review. Continuous distribution policy development for liver and intestine will begin next, anticipated in 2022, followed by heart and vascularized composite allotransplantation (VCA), anticipated in 2023.

*Conclusion 5-2: The OPTN is developing the continuous distribution formulas for each organ type consecutively, which pushes full system implementation of the*

---

[7] To read the public comments on this policy, see https://optn.transplant.hrsa.gov/governance/public-comment/update-on-continuous-distribution-of-kidneys-and-pancreata (accessed November 5, 2021).

*policy additional years into the future and delays achieving an equitable, transparent, and efficient system of organ transplantation in the United States.*

**Recommendation 4: Accelerate finalizing continuous distribution allocation frameworks for all organs.**

The OPTN should accelerate the development of the continuous distribution framework for all organ types with full implementation by December 31, 2024. The OPTN should set organ-specific upper bounds on the weight of "distance to the donor hospital" in the continuous distribution equation. The weights should be proportional to the effect of increased organ travel on posttransplant survival. The OPTN should regularly reevaluate the weight assigned to this factor as advances in normothermic preservation permit travel time to be extended without impairing outcomes. The OPTN should annually evaluate the effects of the continuous distribution policy and adjust the equations for organs that are not moving toward the goals set by HHS for improved equity, organ use, and patient outcomes, as well as steady or reduced costs.

## Heart Allocation

Heart allocation in adults is determined by clinical observations and medical information, rather than a series of laboratory tests. Heart allocation is prioritized by medical urgency, with the highest priority for transplantation given to candidates who are sickest and using mechanical circulatory support devices for circulation and breathing (Table 5-2). This policy went into effect in 2018, adding additional stratification levels to the previous heart medical urgency statuses for a total of six categories (see Chapter 2). In addition to directing donated hearts to the most medically urgent candidates, the 2018 policy change altered the geographic distribution priorities for transplantation. Following the change, significant increases in regional and national distribution of donated hearts was observed coupled with a higher percentage of transplants going to candidates with a higher urgency status.[8] This policy change also appears to have driven a change in strategies for managing patients on the waiting list, such as increased use of extracorporeal membrane oxygenation and temporary use of a ventricular assist device. For example, one study found that the use of temporary percutaneous endovascular mechanical circulatory support was an efficient, safe, and effective intervention for tier 2 candidates until a heart transplant could be received (Clerkin et al., 2022), potentially indicating a change in the heart transplant community's practices of caring for patients prior to transplantation (Silvestry and Rogers, 2022). Another study compared the use of short-term mechanical circulatory support—an intervention as a bridge to transplant—before and after the 2018 heart allocation changes and found the use of this circulatory support increased and continued to expand following the allocation policy changes (Cascino et al., 2021). However, the increased use of short-term mechanical circulatory support was not consistent across transplant centers. While the allocation change may have had the intended effect of increasing access to transplantation for patients using this mechanical support, there could be variations in equitable access to heart transplantation due to the variations in transplant center behavior (Cascino et al., 2021).

In January 2020, the use of zones for heart and lung distribution was replaced with nautical mile (NM) fixed distance circles from the donor hospital. This change to using nautical

---

[8] For more detailed information, see https://optn.transplant.hrsa.gov/media/3701/data_report_thoracic_committee_heart_subcommittee_20200227_rpt1_revised_508_compliant.pdf (accessed October 20, 2021).

**TABLE 5-2** Heart Allocation System

| Allocation System | Factors and Variables |
|---|---|
| Heart (adult) | Using advanced support therapies, such as implanted medical devices to assist with circulation or breathing<br>Required stay in hospital<br>Experiencing complications from infection or blood clotting<br>Using other support for circulation or breathing<br>Using heart function-stimulating medication<br>Experiencing difficult to control, life-threatening condition<br>Needing one or more other organ transplants |

SOURCE: https://transplantliving.org/organ-facts/heart/heart-faq (accessed October 21, 2021).

miles for thoracic organ distribution was the first step toward a full continuous distribution policy.

## Liver Allocation

Liver allocation in adults is determined by either three or four laboratory blood tests (Table 5-3) to calculate a MELD score. The MELD-based liver allocation system improves on the prior allocation system based on Child-Turcotte-Pugh classification and wait time, with advantages in objectivity, simplicity, and use of easily acquired standardized components (see Chapter 3). Similar to MELD, the PELD score is calculated to allocate livers to children aged 12 and younger using similar blood tests plus age and relative growth pattern (Table 5-3) (Lai, 2021).

## Lung Allocation

Lung allocation is determined by the lung allocation score (LAS) (UNOS, 2021). The LAS is calculated from a number of factors, from clinical data or laboratory tests, and from daily-living factors like age or how easy it is to perform everyday tasks (Table 5-4). The LAS reflects the seriousness of each candidate's medical status before transplant, as well as the

**TABLE 5-3** Measurements of Organ Function and Recipient Suitability Typically Considered in Liver Allocation Decisions

| Allocation Scoring System | Factors and Variables |
|---|---|
| Model for End-Stage Liver Disease (MELD) Liver (adult) | Serum creatinine<br>Bilirubin<br>International Normalized Ratio (INR) for prothrombin time<br>Serum sodium |
| Pediatric End-Stage Liver Disease (PELD) Liver (pediatric) | Albumin<br>Serum bilirubin<br>INR for prothrombin time<br>Growth failure (based on gender, height, and weight)<br>Age at listing |

SOURCE: https://optn.transplant.hrsa.gov/data/allocation-calculators/about-meld-and-peld (accessed January 14, 2022).

**TABLE 5-4** Measurements of Organ Function and Recipient Suitability Typically Considered in Lung Allocation Decisions

| Algorithm | Factors and Variable |
|---|---|
| Lung Allocation Score (LAS) | Age at offer |
| | Bilirubin |
| | Bilirubin increase of at least 50% |
| | Body mass index |
| | Cardiac index prior to any exercise |
| | Central venous pressure |
| | Continuous mechanical ventilation, if candidate is hospitalized |
| | Serum creatinine |
| | Diabetes |
| | Diagnosis of lung ailment |
| | Predicted forced vital capacity |
| | Functional status |
| | Oxygen need to maintain saturation at rest |
| | $pCO_2$ |
| | $pCO_2$ increase of at least 15% |
| | Resting pulmonary artery systolic pressure |
| | 6-minute walk distance (with oxygen if needed) |

SOURCE: UNOS, 2021.

likelihood of a successful transplant. It also estimates how long a patient will survive following transplant relative to other patients on the waiting list (UNOS, 2021). Lung will be the first organ fully transitioned to continuous distribution allocation, beginning in early 2023.[9]

## Intestine and VCA Allocation

Intestine and VCA transplants make up relatively small percentages of total annual transplants in the United States. The OPTN policies regulating allocation of these types of transplants are concordantly less complex than they are for many other types of transplants. Allocation for these types of transplants is primarily based on necessary medical support without transplant, clinical judgment or diagnoses, geographic distance from transplant hospitals, and length of time spent on the waiting list.

## Additional Policies for Multiorgan Transplant Allocation

The OPTN currently has formal policies regarding allocation to heart–lung, liver–kidney, and kidney–pancreas multiorgan transplant candidates. For heart transplant candidates that also need a lung transplant, the heart is matched first and the lungs come from the same deceased donor. If a lung transplant candidate also needs a heart transplant, the lungs are matched first but the donated heart is first offered to transplant candidates in "allocation classifications 1 through 12." In June 2021, the OPTN clarified policies surrounding multiorgan allocation to resolve issues with variation in OPO interpretations as to the prioritization of organ offers for the second required organ (kidney or liver), if available, from the same donor to a potential transplant recipient. The updated policy also increased the allocation prioritization for heart and lung multiorgan candidates from 250 to 500 nautical miles, to better align with thoracic allocation policies (OPTN, 2021a,b).

---

[9] https://unos.org/news/new-lung-allocation-policy-approved (accessed January 14, 2022).

## Kidney Allocation

### *Estimating Kidney Function for Entering the Waiting List*

For a patient to be registered on the kidney transplant waiting list, they must either be on dialysis or have an estimated glomerular filtration rate (eGFR) that falls below 20 mL/min; eGFR is determined by serum creatinine, age, gender, and race. Serum creatinine levels in the body vary. In an attempt to account for this variability, eGFR has included race in its calculations. However, as discussed in Chapter 4 of this report, race is not defined by biology but is rather a social construct. Inclusion of race in eGFR has led to disparities in medical practice. For the same serum creatinine, a black patient will be wait-listed later than a patient of any other race or ethnicity, given the adjustment factor that is applied in the Chronic Kidney Disease Epidemiology Collaboration equation inflates the estimated kidney function of black individuals by approximately 16 percent (Ku et al., 2021; Zelnick et al., 2021).

### *Race and eGFR*

The committee acknowledges that the use of race in eGFR is and has been part of a larger debate about the continued use of race-based medicine in health care (AABA, 2021; American Society of Human Genetics, 2020).[10] Using race in clinical equations generally, and in transplant clinical equations specifically, poses urgent ethical and scientific challenges. Because the concept of race has no scientific basis, retaining race as a variable in clinical equations is unethical and can reinforce and perpetuate structural racism (Emanuel et al., 2000). Chapters 4 and 5 have explored inequities among racial and ethnic groups throughout the process of organ transplantation, from end-stage organ failure to posttransplant outcomes. As stakeholders in the organ transplantation system move toward a more equitable system that better addresses the needs of minority and underserved populations who have experienced limited access to transplantation and worse transplant outcomes, reevaluating the use of race in eGFR and other clinical equations (e.g., KDPI) is warranted. Indeed, many organizations and groups have been working toward this end, including a National Kidney Foundation/American Society of Nephrology (NKF/ASN) taskforce, the OPTN and Health Resources and Services Administration (HRSA), as well as research supported by the National Institute of Diabetes and Digestive and Kidney Diseases of the National Institutes of Health (NIDDK) (OPTN Minority Affairs and Kidney Transplantation Committees, 2021).

The NKF/ASN taskforce recently examined alternatives to race-based estimations of kidney functions and evaluated the effects of including race in eGFR estimations. After a careful deliberative process, the taskforce concluded that revising the current eGFR calculations to remove race was an immediate first step that could reduce disparity, as well as yielding other medical benefits. For all individuals at high risk of developing chronic kidney disease, the task force recommended widespread use of a new measure that incorporates a blood test for

---

[10] In defining *race-based medicine*, the American Academy of Family Physicians (AAFP) states that "Race is a social construct that is used to group people based on physical characteristics, behavioral patterns, and geographic location. Racial categories are broad, poorly defined, vary by country, and change over time. People who are assigned to the same racial category do not necessarily share the same genetic ancestry; therefore, there are no underlying genetic or biological factors that unite people within the same racial category. By using race as a biological marker for disease states or as a variable in medical diagnosis and treatment, the true health status of a patient may not be accurately assessed, which can lead to racial health disparities. AAFP opposes the use of race as a proxy for biology or genetics in clinical evaluation and management and in research. AAFP encourages clinicians and researchers to investigate alternative indicators to race to stratify medical risk factors for disease states." https://www.aafp.org/about/policies/all/racebased-medicine.html (accessed November 15, 2021).

cystatin C along with serum creatinine in the calculation; this would improve the accuracy of estimation over either individual measure without adversely affecting any populations (Delgado et al., 2021). A study funded by the NIDDK based on the Chronic Renal Insufficiency Cohort (CRIC) registry similarly recommended use of cystatin C in calculating eGFR based on analyses of the CRIC data under several conditions (Hsu et al., 2021).

*Conclusion 5-3: Use of race in eGFR estimations is one factor leading to systematic underestimation of kidney disease severity in black individuals. This results in health inequities in that black patients have to wait longer for transplants, are sicker than other patients when they get a transplant, and disproportionately die of kidney disease.*

## Race and KDPI

Given current scientific evidence and the recent advice to remove race from eGFR (Delgado et al., 2021), it is appropriate for the scientific community to continue efforts to develop and refine clinical equations so they do not include race as a variable. Some on the committee wanted to recommend the immediate removal of race from KDPI and other clinical equations because race is a social construct, lacks a biological basis, is not scientifically founded, and perpetuates racialized medicine (Ioannidis et al., 2021). Thus, as an unscientific variable, continuing to use race would be unethical (Emanuel et al., 2000). For these reasons, some on the committee argued race should neither be used in medical practice nor used as a biological proxy and that this committee should recommend the immediate removal of race from KDPI. Others on the committee were hesitant to recommend complete removal of race in these equations because of having insufficient information on the unintended consequences of doing so. Some committee members also felt that the issue was not a particular focus of this committee's charge and would be better assessed by a properly constituted group of subject matter experts with specific instructions for considering the use of race in KDPI and other clinical equations. Based on the available information the committee believes that to achieve a more equitable organ transplantation system race should be eliminated from any equation or measurement used to determine access to the waiting list or eventual transplant (e.g., KDPI), understanding that doing so might have unintended consequences. The potentiality of such consequences needs to be considered by a group of experts knowledgeable in the multiple dimensions of this matter. The HHS should expeditiously convene such an expert group.

While the organ transplantation system moves toward a vision of non-race-based measures in assessing kidney function, some have suggested that

- Changing practice guidelines will require significant education efforts within health systems and consideration of the increased number of patients that may be classified with chronic kidney disease (Ahmed et al., 2021). The authors suggest further study to better define whether differences in creatinine-based eGFR are based on social or ancestry factors and advocate for increased transparency with patients if race-adjusted eGFR is used.
- There will be many short- and long-term consequences that should be addressed, including access to clinical trials (Delgado et al., 2021), antibiotic dosing (Eneanya et al., 2019), patients being classified with advanced stage kidney disease, and implications for health insurance (Ahmed et al., 2021).
- There may also be a number of benefits including increasing referral rates to specialists, reducing disparities in access to a transplant waiting list, and the potential for better management of chronic kidney disease (Powe, 2020).

- New equations should be developed using scientifically validated variables such as height and weight, while more research should be done to ascertain the potential benefits and harms of eliminating race in eGFR calculations (Eneanya et al., 2019).
- Use a stepped approach that incorporates patient voices and moves toward an evidence-based solution in the long term (Powe, 2020). Variability across institutions may create more confusion and unreliable trends.

As highlighted in Chapter 4, black patients experience disproportionate rates of kidney disease compared to white patients yet have less access to specialist care. While black populations make up approximately 13 percent of the U.S. population, adjusted prevalence of end-stage kidney disease was 3.4 times higher than white individuals in 2018 (USRDS, 2020). Black patients with chronic renal insufficiency also progressed through end-stage renal disease at five times the rate of whites with chronic renal insufficiency, which suggests that a refinement of the NKF chronic kidney disease (CKD) classification for stages of CKD may be warranted given the differences in progression among black and white patients (Hsu et al., 2003). Important strategies for slowing CKD progression include hypertension management and albuminuria management. Early referral to nephrologists is associated with improved CKD patient outcomes, but there are known disparities by race in referral (Gander et al., 2018).

*Conclusion 5-4: Non-race-based ways of measuring organ function are greatly needed and deserve prioritization by federal agencies to set the standards for what is scientifically and ethically acceptable in determining patient prioritization for the transplant waiting list and eventual transplantation.*

*Conclusion 5-5: Using race in surveillance approaches for measuring outcomes across populations is useful for identifying the existence and persistence of disparities. However, researchers need to provide the rationale for how and why race is used in any such analysis.*

## Predialysis Wait Time

In the current allocation system, a transplant candidate's access to transplantation before beginning dialysis (predialysis) is determined by the time of registration on the waiting list. The U.S. kidney allocation system currently gives priority "waiting time" points for years on dialysis but simultaneously allows unlimited predialysis "waiting time" points to accumulate. This substantially advantages white, educated individuals with private insurance who are able to gain timely access to transplant referral and join the waiting list before beginning dialysis (King et al., 2019; Reese et al., 2021). Black and Hispanic patients are approximately four times less likely to receive a preemptive transplant (Figure 5-3). Furthermore, candidates with longer dialysis time are at a higher risk of death without a transplant (Aufhauser et al., 2018); therefore, transplanting individuals already on dialysis saves more lives than preemptive transplants.

Prior to implementation of the KAS in 2014, transplantation candidates preemptively entered on the waiting list with a qualifying eGFR accrued waiting time from their listing date onward, while candidates wait-listed after starting maintenance dialysis accrued waiting time from their listing date onward.

One of the goals of the KAS was to improve equity in organ allocation for candidates who were wait-listed after spending years undergoing dialysis. In the current policy, candidates wait-listed after the onset of maintenance dialysis accrue a priority point for each year of prelisting dialysis. However, candidates wait-listed before dialysis onset (preemptive wait-listing) continue to receive a point for each year waiting after reaching the qualifying eGFR of 20 (Harhay et al., 2018).

The revisions to the kidney allocation system also prioritized deceased donor kidney transplantation for candidates with long dialysis durations. Early studies have shown that the KAS has been successful in closing the gap in transplant rates between wait-listed white and minorities. Preemptive transplants have not experienced the same closing of the gap (Figure 5-3). In 2019, 11 percent of all adult deceased donor kidney transplants nationwide were preemptive. White patients received 65 percent, and black patients received only 17 percent of those preemptive kidneys, though the waiting list was made up of 38 percent white and 31 percent black patients (Reese et al., 2021). Also in 2019, 48 percent of wait-listed white patients, but only 22 percent of wait-listed black patients, began to accrue waiting time priority before dialysis (Reese et al., 2021).

A first-come, first-served approach that allows transplant priority to accrue for patients prior to the point of dialysis initiation is not in line with equity (Reese et al., 2021). Patients who already have advantage with both residual kidney function and greater ability to navigate the health system (primarily white, educated, privately insured) get greater access.

It is also the case that black patients with elevated creatinine will have a higher eGFR (thereby making them ineligible for wait-listing) but nonetheless may need kidney transplantation sooner than similar white patients because of rapid disease progression.

Another consideration for preemptive transplant is long-term management of patients who have already received a kidney transplant. It is common for transplant recipients to experience failure of their donated kidney; on average, more than half of transplant recipients experience loss of their donated kidney within 10 years. Emotional effects of this loss notwithstanding, there are also many medical decisions to make to best manage disease including a decision about whether or not to enroll on the waiting list for a new transplant. Repeat transplant patients are enrolled on the waiting list at lower rates than would be expected given their and their clinicians' familiarity with the system. There were about

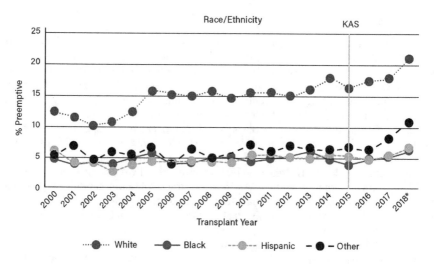

**FIGURE 5-3** Percentage of preemptive transplants grouped by racial or ethnic groups.
SOURCE: King et al., 2019.

4,000 patients in 2019 or just under 11 percent of the total waiting list (Davis and Mohan, 2021).

Many countries require that a patient must be on dialysis in order to be added to the waiting list (although different policies may apply to children or multiorgan transplant candidates).[11] The criteria to start dialysis for end-stage kidney disease is regulated tightly by the Centers for Medicare & Medicaid Services (CMS) in the United States. It is possible that removing predialysis wait time from the kidney allocation system could reduce structural racism in kidney allocation and save more lives. It would be important that any policy change not ban preemptive deceased donor kidney transplants, but rather represent that these transplants may confer less benefit than transplanting patients with significant dialysis time. For example, preemptive deceased donor transplants could still occur if the candidate had a high enough priority based on the other components in the kidney allocation system. It would also be important that any policy change have no direct effect on candidate listing for planned living donor transplantation by inadvertently disincentivizing or limiting this type of transplantation.

A recommendation to remove waiting time was made in the 1999 Institute of Medicine report *Organ Procurement and Transplantation for Liver Allocation* under Recommendation 2 and read: "Discontinue use of waiting time as an allocation criterion for patients in statuses 2B and 3." This recommendation was instrumental in the transition to a MELD-based liver allocation system. Similarly, removing preemptive waiting list time as a factor in kidney allocation policies could (1) improve access for patients on dialysis by making available deceased donor kidneys that were previously going to individuals who had not yet started dialysis; (2) improve equity in access to a transplant for individuals previously disadvantaged; (3) increase living donation as patients previously advantaged by preemptive access to deceased donor kidneys would seek living donation if they wish to receive a preemptive transplant; and (4) align with the intention of some other countries without completely limiting access to the waiting list to only those who have started dialysis as some other countries do. *It is important to note that the committee's recommendation is not to categorically eliminate preemptive transplants with deceased donor kidneys. These preemptive transplants would still be possible if the candidate has accrued a sufficiently high allocation priority via other mechanisms in the kidney allocation system (i.e., high CPRA, proximity to the donor, prior living donor points).* It is also important to note that children do not typically tolerate lengthy time on dialysis very well (de Galasso et al., 2020; Verghese, 2017), so a policy change may need to exempt pediatric patients.

Ultimately, national efforts to advance early recognition of kidney disease are needed such that individuals needing a transplant are able to access the waiting list in an equitable manner. All transplant candidates—minorities, individuals without private health insurance, and those with limited access to the health care system—deserve access to transplantation based on their medical need. While this longer-term goal (see Recommendation 1) is advanced, the elimination of predialysis waiting time points is an immediate policy lever to increase equity and efficiency in the transplantation system.

*Conclusion 5-6: Although the new kidney allocation system may be narrowing transplant rates between white and ethnic minority populations, a large disadvantage remains in access to preemptive transplants, in large part because of the accumulation of waiting time points for predialysis wait time.*

---

[11] Canada, Germany, Australia, and Korea require individuals to be on dialysis before being added to the waiting list. The UK, France, and other European countries (excluding Germany) allow preemptive wait-listing.

*Conclusion 5-7: The use of a single tool, eGFR, measured at one point in time to determine kidney function and an individual's eligibility for the waiting list, is inadequate and does not appropriately account for the rapidity with which a patient's condition is likely to decline and have an urgent need for transplantation.*

*Conclusion 5-8: Transplant centers can also select one of three eGFR measures to determine kidney function; this can greatly affect an individual's access to the waiting list and thereby increase the accident of geography.*

**Recommendation 5: Eliminate predialysis waiting time points from the kidney allocation system.**

**To reduce racial and ethnic disparities in the application of kidney transplant allocation policies, the OPTN should discontinue the use of predialysis waiting time credit, or points, in the current kidney allocation system, leaving only the date that the patient began regularly administered dialysis as an end-stage renal disease patient as the basis for an individual to accumulate points based on wait time. While this committee is *not* recommending that access to the deceased donor kidney waiting list be limited to only those who have started dialysis, the committee is recommending that predialysis waiting time should be discontinued as a basis for accumulating waiting time points. This change would ultimately save more lives in a fairer and more equitable manner by eliminating the current preferential access to deceased donor kidneys for individuals able to gain timely access to referral for transplant and the transplant waiting list. Considerations may be necessary for pediatric transplant candidates, multiorgan transplant candidates, prior transplant recipients, and those currently listed with predialysis waiting time. The OPTN should closely monitor any unintended consequences of removing predialysis waiting time points. To avoid manipulating the system by earlier dialysis initiation, the OPTN policy should include penalties for providers who engage in the premature initiation of dialysis.**

## Wait-Listing and the Kidney Allocation System

In general, the Scientific Registry of Transplant Recipients (SRTR) holds that when considering the distribution of a scarce resource such as donated kidneys, the methods must be derived from and based upon sound ethical principles, including the two key principles of utility and equity (Table 5-5). As previously mentioned, the KAS was implemented in 2014 by the OPTN to address high rates of procured organ nonuse and variability in access to organ transplantation. The KAS also attempts to match the amount of time donated kidneys are expected to function with estimated transplant recipient length of life, in some cases. For instance, kidneys with the longest expected function are allocated to the individuals with the longest expected lifetime—after initial allocation to multiorgan recipients and children—via metrics of EPTS and the KDPI (Table 5-6). The majority of the kidneys are still allocated primarily by length of time on the waiting list. The KAS also assigns additional priority to highly sensitized transplant candidates to give them access to the national donor pool via the CPRA metric (Table 5-6). In 2019, additional changes to the policy were approved to allow kidney distribution based on geographical distance between donor and recipient, as opposed to the previous policy where match sequencing relied on donation service area and the OPTN region.

Within its first year, the KAS reduced age mismatch between donated organs and transplant recipients, and increased transplant access for previously disadvantaged patients, such

**TABLE 5-5** Guiding Principles Considered in the Redesigned Kidney Allocation System

| Proposed Goals of the Kidney Allocation System (KAS) | Ethical Principle Addressed |
|---|---|
| More accurately estimate graft and recipient longevity to maximize the potential survival of every transplanted kidney and to provide acceptable levels of access for candidates on the waiting list. | Utility/Equity |
| Promote posttransplant kidney function for candidates with the longest estimated posttransplant survival who are also the most likely to require additional transplants because of early age of ESRD onset. | Utility |
| Minimize loss of potential functioning years of deceased donor kidney grafts through improved matching. | Utility |
| Improve the efficiency of the offering system and organ use through the introduction of a new scale for kidney quality, the Kidney Donor Profile Index. | Utility |
| Reduce differences in transplant access for populations described in the National Organ Transplant Act (e.g., candidates from racial/ethnic minority group, pediatric candidates, and sensitized candidates). | Equity |

SOURCE: https://www.srtr.org/media/1072/friedewald_the_kidney_allocation_system_surg_clin_n_am_2013.pdf (accessed January 20, 2022).

**TABLE 5-6** Measurements of Organ Function and Recipient Suitability Typically Considered in Kidney Allocation Decisions

| Algorithm | Factors and Variables |
|---|---|
| Calculated panel reactive antibody (CPRA) | Calculates unacceptable human leukocyte antigens to measure a transplant candidate's sensitization level and likelihood of the presence or intensity of acute or antibody-mediated rejection. Transplant programs define unacceptable antigens for each transplant candidate, and there is variation in the definition among different transplant centers. |
| Estimated posttransplant survival (EPTS) | EPTS factors include (1) candidate time on dialysis, (2) diabetes diagnosis, (3) prior solid organ transplantation, and (4) age. |
| Kidney Donor Profile Index (KDPI) | Age<br>History of diabetes<br>Height<br>Cause of death<br>Weight<br>Serum creatinine<br>Race or ethnicity<br>Hepatitis C virus (HCV) status, from serological or NAT testing<br>History of hypertension<br>Donation after circulatory death (DCD) status |

SOURCES: https://optn.transplant.hrsa.gov/learn/professional-education/kidney-allocation-system (accessed January 15, 2022); https://optn.transplant.hrsa.gov/resources/allocation-calculators (accessed January 15, 2022); Cecka, 2010.

as highly sensitized candidates or those who had been on dialysis for long periods (Wang et al., 2017). However, despite these accomplishments, rates of kidney nonuse were not reduced. Because there are many more transplant candidates than there are donated organs, the KAS and its underlying principles prioritize allocating kidneys to younger and healthier candidates (Table 5-5).

## EPTS and KDPI[12]

The EPTS score is assigned to all adult candidates on the kidney waiting list as part of the KAS. Its intent is to match high-quality organs to candidate recipients with the best estimated survival following transplant, and it is calculated relative to all candidates on the waiting list (Chopra and Sureshkumar, 2015).

The EPTS is used with the KDPI to introduce the concept of longevity matching into the new allocation system. Only candidates with EPTS scores of 20 percent or less will receive increased priority for offers for kidneys with KDPI scores of 20 percent or less, meaning that in the context of these two calculations, the 20 percent of highest-quality donated kidneys are prioritized to candidates with the longest estimated survival after transplantation. For the remaining 80 percent of kidney allocations, EPTS is not used at all. Independent assessment of how EPTS performs judged it to be a "moderately good tool for discriminating posttransplant survival of adult kidney-only transplant recipients" by testing the algorithm on Australia and New Zealand's combined dialysis and transplant registry (Clayton et al., 2014). Allocation proceeds by geography and local candidates—even those with an EPTS score exceeding 20 percent—appear on the match list before candidates listed outside the donor service area.

The KDPI score estimates the risk of graft failure, and it is intended to help assess the suitability of donated kidneys for particular patients as well as with longevity matching. KDPI is a scoring system based on 10 donor factors as a screening tool for donor quality and has been shown to be generally predictive of both short- and long-term graft survival, and though it may have other shortcomings it has the advantage of creating a sliding scale of assessment rather than a distinct decision, as with the standard criteria donor/extended criteria donor designations it replaced.

This longevity matching in allocation has two effects: (1) younger and healthier patients on the waiting list are prioritized to receive the kidneys that are expected to survive the longest posttransplant, and (2) medically urgent candidates receive kidneys with lower estimated survival posttransplant, which potentially worsens the patient's long-term outcomes.

Other countries do not use KDPI as a consideration in their allocation decisions. For example, Alexandre Loupy and colleagues estimated that the U.S. rate of nonuse for procured organs is nearly double the rate in France (Aubert et al., 2019). France tends to use donated kidneys with higher KDPI, largely driven by use of organs from older donors, and transplanted patients still realize significant survival benefit.

*Conclusion 5-9: The United States is alone in constructing its allocation policies around a single measure of kidney quality (KDPI), which reduces the number of deceased donor transplants without improving average outcome. This results in fewer total transplants than would occur if these patients had access to donated kidneys that are expected to produce better results. The committee concludes that constructing U.S. allocation policies around KDPI is an inappropriate focal point that does not exist in other countries and may lead to perverse regulatory incentives for U.S. transplant centers to be overly selective and risk averse in the kidneys they choose to transplant. As a result, many opportunities are missed to provide transplantation to a greater number of individuals on the waiting list.*

---

[12] Much of this section is excerpted or slightly modified from a paper commissioned by the committee for this study (Ku, 2021). Commissioned papers are in the study's public access file and are available upon request from the National Academies' Public Access Records Office (paro@nas.edu).

## SURVIVAL BENEFIT OF TRANSPLANTATION

The survival benefit of transplantation is the counterfactual difference between a patient's estimated survival with transplantation and without transplantation. Traditionally, the benefit of transplantation has been restricted to posttransplant survival, typically 1-year posttransplant survival. This is a measure of graft survival, and maximizing 1-year graft survival leads to the selection of the healthiest candidates and most viable organs. By contrast, survival benefit measures additional lives saved by comparing the expected waiting list survival to the expected posttransplant survival for a given patient and organ dyad, in a given transplant center. Maximizing survival benefit may lead to the selection of the most medically urgent[13] candidates that still have high likelihood of posttransplant survival.

The survival benefit of deceased donor organ transplantation has been quantified in lung (Vock et al., 2017), heart (Parker et al., 2019; Singh et al., 2014), liver (Luo et al., 2018), and kidney (Merion et al., 2005; Pérez-Sáez et al., 2016; Wolfe et al., 1999). The current kidney transplantation system conveys a significant overall 5-year survival benefit of 31.6 percent (50.8 percent survival associated with remaining on the waiting list versus 82.4 percent associated with transplantation). Nevertheless, survival benefit varies widely from 24 to 39 percent owing to variation in candidate characteristics. Similarly, survival benefit varies widely across transplant centers, from 20 to 48 percent for a median KDPI kidney (KDPI = 43 percent) (Parker et al., 2021).

During the course of the committee's work, the idea of survival benefit was introduced and seemed promising as a way to reduce inequities in the organ transplantation system. However, the committee—being acutely aware and mindful of the extent of the organ transplantation system's complexity—understands that any change of this magnitude could introduce both intended and unintended effects. The committee is also aware that the policy revision process is a laborious one that involves input from many stakeholders and thoughtful debate. There was disagreement between some on the committee about the degree to which statistical modeling should play a role in changing allocation. Nevertheless, a substantial amount of modeling and further work and testing would need to be done to verify the committee's impression that this could be a step forward—rather than a rehashing of similar discussions that took place prior to implementation of the KAS in 2014—and also to identify potential unintended consequences that could undermine the intended change.

Further evaluation of survival benefit through simulation and further studies should be undertaken expeditiously. Given the magnitude of potential benefit to patients and possibility to reduce inequity, sufficient evidence should be accrued within the next 3 years to determine whether further incorporating a survival benefit metric into allocation decisions for all organs—but especially kidneys—could be made by that time.

*Conclusion 5-10: If transplant centers are ranked based on 1-year survival of transplant recipients, any measure of organ quality will result in organ nonuse based on*

---

[13] According to OPTN policy, a new definition of the *medically urgent* classification within all kidney allocation categories "creates priority for candidates at imminent risk of death due to an inability, or anticipated inability, to accept dialysis treatment for renal failure" (OPTN, 2020a). While the committee recognizes this as the OPTN definition for *medically urgent classification* for kidney transplant patients, the committee defines *medical urgency* in this report differently than the OPTN (Parker et al., 2021). This committee's definition of *medical urgency* is "risk of death without receiving an organ transplant." The committee recognizes that patients in renal failure without any viable dialysis access are certainly the candidates in the most dire need of transplantation. However, the kidney allocation system does not yet clearly allocate organs to the candidates with highest risk of dying without transplantation. Therefore, in order to align kidney allocation with the other organs, throughout the remainder of the report the term *medical urgency* refers to the "risk of death without receiving an organ transplant" and not the exhaustion of dialysis access options.

138     REALIZING THE PROMISE OF EQUITY IN THE ORGAN TRANSPLANTATION SYSTEM

the assumption that they will lower a center's ranking and increase costs. A ranking system is needed that is based on saving lives, not 1-year graft survival, and a reimbursement system is needed that acknowledges the importance of reimbursing transplant centers for the increased costs associated with transplanting lifesaving medically complex organs.

## Constructing a Good Survival Benefit Estimator

Survival benefit is not a new concept (Massie et al., 2014). Prior to implementing the KAS, the OPTN and the transplant community considered survival benefit as a basis for kidney organ allocation, but they rejected the idea when the calculation proposed was found to favor younger and healthier candidates in contrast to the HHS Final Rule. However, there may be other ways to estimate survival benefit that are less likely to favor younger, healthier candidates and that could improve the efficiency of kidney allocation. First, by focusing on a finite time interval, it is possible that more medically urgent candidates with high waiting list mortality will derive increased benefit from a transplant relative to remaining on the list than young healthy candidates whose waiting list mortality is more similar to their posttransplant survival. Second, survival benefit is not constant over time; rather, it varies significantly from the short term to the long term, and any improved model would reflect this variation. Third, there is variability in survival benefit among transplant centers (Parker et al., 2019, 2021). A good survival benefit estimator would include adjustment to estimated survival benefit for a given candidate that is specific to the transplant center at which that person is listed. Fourth, a good survival benefit estimator should include detailed candidate characteristics (e.g., age, diabetes, dialysis time, prior transplantation) and donor characteristics (e.g., KDPI or an improved estimator of quality of the donor organ) and allow them to interact in producing a survival benefit estimate. The more detailed the measured characteristics, the better the estimator. A limitation of the current KAS is that many important characteristics of the candidate and donor are not routinely collected (e.g., cardiac risk).

Conclusion 5-11: Better estimators of survival benefit, focusing on saving more lives, are available and would benefit from being reviewed by the SRTR via simulation to determine their operating characteristics relative to the current KAS allocation system.

Conclusion 5-12: The concept of survival benefit, the difference between estimated waiting list and posttransplant survival over a fixed interval of time, focuses on saving more lives relative to the current metric of 1-year graft survival. The use of survival benefit has the potential to improve allocation, center rankings, and share decision making between transplant candidates and transplant teams. The application of a survival benefit is particularly relevant to kidney allocation, where allocation is based largely on histocompatibility and waiting time regardless of medical urgency.

## Racial Disparities

As discussed in Chapter 4, disparities research often focuses on differences in care for black and white patients, and other ethnic and racial groups receive less research focus. Racial disparities between black and white patients are discussed here with the understanding that additional research on the effects of allocation changes in other ethnic and racial groups is needed.

Prior to the implementation of the KAS in 2014, dialysis time prior to wait-listing was ignored by the allocation system. In fact, structural racism in health care often prevents black patients from accessing transplant centers for listing in the first place (Gander et al., 2018; Joshi et al., 2013; Peng et al., 2018). Racial disparities in dialysis time at transplant persisted between 2010 and 2020 despite the implementation of the KAS in 2014. In 2013, the median dialysis time at transplant for a white recipient was 2.6 years compared to 4.5 years for black recipients. In 2019, the median dialysis time at transplant for a white recipient was 2.5 years compared to 4.8 years for black recipients (Joshi et al., 2013). The KAS did reduce the race gap in transplant rate (Melanson et al., 2017), likely because of a backlog in minority candidates with very long dialysis times who finally got credit for the years they suffered waiting. The racial disparity in rates of preemptive transplants has continued to increase since the implementation of the KAS. In 2020, the rate was 20 percent for whites and only 7 percent for black patients, a disparity that has only worsened since implementation of the KAS in 2014 (Patzer et al., 2009).

Survival benefit increases with increasing dialysis time. Therefore, minorities who enter the waiting list with almost twice the dialysis time could have a higher likelihood of receiving a kidney offer if allocation is based on survival benefit rather than 1-year posttransplant survival, for which their rates are lower and lead to increased racial disparity because of existing allocation algorithms.

*Conclusion 5-13: Black candidates enter the kidney transplant waiting list with double the length of dialysis time than white candidates and as a consequence have increased medical urgency as evidenced by their increased risk of mortality without transplantation. Under the current allocation system, which focuses on 1-year post-transplant survival and waiting list time, the disparity will persist. There is need to understand whether a shift in allocation policy to survival benefit would prioritize those populations currently disadvantaged because of their increased waiting list mortality.*

# Longevity Matching[14]

In the KAS, candidates with low scores on the high EPTS measure are given priority for the top 20 percent KDPI kidneys. The KAS was designed in this manner to better match the life span of an organ with the life span of the recipient (i.e., longevity matching). While this policy may extend total graft survival, it may also lower the total number of lives saved by the KAS because healthier transplant candidates receive the higher-quality kidneys. Overall, the top 20 percent EPTS candidates have much lower estimated survival benefit than the top 20 percent most medically urgent candidates. Transplanting the median patient without diabetes after the median amount of dialysis time (3.8 years of dialysis) was associated with 5-year survival benefit of 32 percent compared to only 19 percent for preemptively transplanting the same patient (i.e., dialysis time of 0, see Figure 5-4). This translates to more than 1 life saved for every 10 transplants performed in dialysis recipients compared to preemptive transplant recipients. Figure 5-4 illustrates the survival benefit of transplantation for a 55-year-old recipient without diabetes—transplanted after 3.8 years of dialysis and 848 days of waiting list time—compared to preemptively transplanting the same patient after 433 days of waiting

---

[14] Much of this section is excerpted or slightly modified from a paper commissioned by the committee for this study (Parker et al., 2021). Commissioned papers are in the study's public access file and are available upon request from the National Academies' Public Access Records Office (paro@nas.edu).

list time. The preemptive transplant recipient has higher 5-year posttransplant survival (93 percent vs. 88 percent), but transplantation is significantly less urgent than the recipient on dialysis (survival without transplant 73 percent vs. 56 percent). In combination, this means the patient on dialysis experiences a much greater benefit from transplantation (32 percent) compared to the preemptive recipient (19 percent). This raises important questions regarding the effectiveness of longevity matching.

Furthermore, the top 20 percent most urgent candidates experience a greater benefit from lower KDPI kidneys than the top 20 percent EPTS candidates. For both a 15 percent and 85 percent KDPI kidney, allocation to the top 20 percent most medically urgent candidates produces large increases in survival benefit relative to the longevity matching (top 20 percent EPTS recipients). The difference in 5-year survival benefit between receiving a 15 percent versus an 85 percent KDPI kidney is near zero for the top 20 percent EPTS recipients, but 7 percent greater for the 15 percent KDPI kidney relative to the 85 percent KDPI kidney for the top 20 percent most medically urgent recipients. These data suggest that longevity match-ing—at least through 5 years posttransplant—is having the opposite of its intended effect. Relative to receiving a high KDPI kidney, lower KDPI kidneys produce greater survival benefit for sicker recipients than they do for the younger and healthier EPTS recipients.

Finally, with respect to the use of KDPI in general, there was a small but statistically significant decrease in posttransplant survival with higher KDPI kidneys. For every 10 percent increase in KDPI, 5-year survival benefit decreased by 1 percent. However, kidneys with a KDPI greater than 85 percent were associated with a 5-year survival benefit of 28 percent, which is still an appreciable benefit of transplantation relative to remaining on the waiting list. In 2019, there were 1,356 transplants performed using donor kidneys with a KDPI of 85 percent or more. If these transplants had not been performed, an estimated 377 candidates would have died within 5 years.

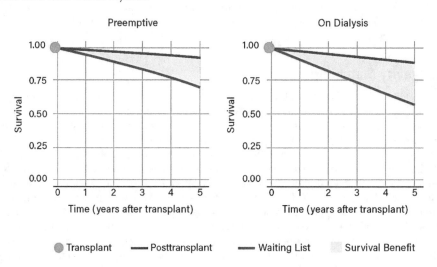

**FIGURE 5-4** Five-year survival benefit for the median recipient on dialysis compared to a preemptive transplant.
NOTE: Survival benefit of transplantation for a 55-year-old recipient without diabetes transplanted after 3.8 years of dialysis and 848 days of waiting list time (survival benefit = 32%) compared to preemp-tively transplanting the same patient after 433 days of waiting time (survival benefit = 19%).
SOURCE: Parker et al., 2021.

*Conclusion 5-14: The current kidney allocation system includes longevity matching of the highest-quality kidneys (top 20 percent KDPI kidneys) with the healthiest candidates on the transplant waiting list. This policy gives priority for the highest-quality kidneys to younger and healthier patients on the waiting list who are estimated to have the longest survival posttransplantation. While this policy increases overall graft survival, it may save fewer lives than allocating these high-quality kidneys to the most urgent candidates.*

## Survival Benefit as a Potential Tool for Organ Allocation

In addition to facilitating greater acknowledgement and incorporation of patient preferences in accepting or declining organ offers, survival benefit could potentially be used to inform changes to allocation policy more broadly. CMS and the OPTN regulate transplant program performance primarily through 1-year posttransplant patient and graft survival (Parker et al., 2019; Singh et al., 2014). Focusing on posttransplant survival does not account for health lost while waiting for transplant—which is particularly important for medically urgent candidates who are at higher risk of death or deterioration and who tend to lose health more rapidly—and reduces the efficiency of deceased donor kidney allocation. This regulatory pressure creates an incentive to prioritize the healthiest candidates. This regulation also promotes excess selectivity of donors, leading transplant programs to not use one in five procured deceased donor kidneys recovered for transplantation owing to an incorrect perception of low quality. In contrast, allocation based on survival benefit could prioritize medically urgent patients with decreased waiting list survival. Such an allocation system would actively counter the disparities in access to transplantation that lead to minority candidates entering the waiting list with greater medical urgency.

**Recommendation 6: Study opportunities to improve equity and use of organs in allocation systems.**

**HHS should require the OPTN to study the effect of changing the kidney allocation system to include a measure of survival benefit and dialysis waiting time as a method of improving access to transplant for all patients without unintended consequences for patients with disabilities, socioeconomically disadvantaged populations, and racially diverse patients. Additional endpoints for study should include patient-centered and patient-identified metrics as well as waiting list mortality, organ nonuse rates, and overall survival from the time of entry onto the waiting list.**

**Recommendation 7: Increase equity in organ allocation algorithms.**

**HHS should quickly resolve areas of inequity in current organ allocation algorithms. The committee identified numerous aspects of the current organ allocation algorithms that require revision, further study, or immediate implementation. The committee recommends that HHS do the following:**

- Require the OPTN to update its prediction models (e.g., KDPI, EPTS, and MELD) using the most recent data no less frequently than every 5 years. During this time, the models themselves should be reconsidered by adding or removing predictors that will either improve predictive accuracy or increase equity (e.g., adding serum sodium to the MELD score, replacing race with scientifically valid biologic predictors in the KDPI). Statistical aspects of the prediction models themselves should also be reviewed to ensure that the best performance possible is achieved and that they are properly validated using data not used to derive the prediction models.

- Modify the MELD scoring system for liver allocation and prioritization or establish an alternative overall prioritization scheme to include a modifier based on body size or muscle mass to overcome the demonstrated disparities observed for patients of smaller size.
- Immediately implement the recommendations of the National Kidney Foundation and American Society of Nephrology joint task force to use the revised equation, which eliminates race, in calculating eGFR for all individuals and to use the revised equation for high-risk individuals that incorporates a blood test for cystatin C along with serum creatinine.
- Require the OPTN to ensure that all laboratories in the transplantation system become capable of conducting validated cystatin C tests within 12 months.
- Resolve the use of race in KDPI and other clinical equations. Within 12 months HHS should make a decision on the continued use of race in KDPI and how best to eliminate race from KDPI and other clinical equations used in organ allocation and access.
- Continue to gather data on factors that may result in disparities in access to, and outcomes of, organ transplantation (e.g., socioeconomic status, place of residence, access to health care, race and ethnicity, presence in patient or family of stressors caused by racism) and use such data to determine whether faster progression to end-stage kidney disease is experienced by patients with any particular factor or combination of factors, and if so whether this evidence should be used to establish a new threshold for listing on the transplant list and for allocation of an organ for transplantation.

## MODELING ALLOCATION POLICY CHANGES

The current process for modeling allocation policy begins when the OPTN notices a problem with waiting lists, such as the case study in geographic disparities in liver allocation (Mulligan, 2021). The OPTN takes into account factors such as organ transportation time limits, geographic boundaries of service areas, organ donation rates, transplantation rates, when in their disease patients enter the waiting list, and variation in how likely a patient is to die or be removed from the waiting list for being too sick. The OPTN determines the most pressing underlying problem and requests models of how different policy changes might affect those numbers from the SRTR. The OPTN agrees on practical parameters to restrict the modeling to solutions that are feasible, such as a minimum number of districts in a sharing area to make sure donated livers were not traveling for longer than transportation time limit. With a few options for changing policy, the OPTN conducts community forums to gather feedback on those potential changes from patients, transplant centers, OPOs, and other stakeholders in the transplantation community. IT then iterates the proposed changes with this feedback to update the models and present a "concept document" and a recommendation for proposed changes to the OPTN board of directors.

The SRTR builds and updates simulated allocation models (SAMs) to model alternative organ allocation policies and predicted outcomes for patients on the waiting lists for each organ type. The models also predict patient outcomes following transplant. Currently, the SRTR maintains SAMs for liver, heart and lung together or separately as thoracic organs, and kidney and pancreas. The SAMs "use a variety of allocation rules to determine how organs would be allocated to potential recipients under each rule considered" (SRTR, 2019). The models include and try to predict variation for factors in organ allocation such as individual accept/reject decisions or estimating life expectancy with or without receiving a transplant. SRTR is developing new simulation software, the Organ Allocation Simulator, that uses more modern coding language, cross-platform compatibility, and built-in parameters for error checking that will make the simulator more accurate and easier to use. As of October 2021, the Organ Allocation Simulator was not yet officially launched or accessible.

The data used to build all of these simulations come from the OPTN database of historical data of patients on the related waiting list over the past year, donated organs that became available in the same time frame, and characteristic organ offer acceptance practices (Snyder, 2021). The OPTN database collects only information on a patient's name, gender, race/ethnicity (as 1 variable), age, ABO blood group, human leukocyte antigen, status codes, number of previous transplants, and acceptable donor characteristics. No information is collected regarding socioeconomic or patient-centered factors such as health care access, distance to a transplant center, perceived discrimination or trust (see Chapter 4), candidate cardiac risk factors, or information from donors including secondary diseases or conditions other than cause of death.

Other limitations of the current modeling system pertain to behavior change, as reported by Snyder (2021). The simulators do not capture behavior change in response to new allocation policies, nor do they predict behavior change when it comes to accept/reject decisions in the context of the policy change being modeled because of its basis in historical data. For example, in the case of modeling changing geographic boundaries in allocation, the existing models do not account for how the characteristics of eligible donors may change for a given transplant candidate in a revised geographic area. Moreover, the available data do not adequately capture instances when an offered organ is declined in the match run system. Lastly, Snyder highlighted a need for the simulations to model and account for predicted changes in behavior following a policy change, saying,

> I often hear from the expert in the field that we know how behavior might change in response to this [new] policy. Can the simulator actually implement that change? We'd like to…develop modules so that the user of the simulator—[SRTR] or any independent researcher—could actually implement those behavior changes as suggested and show the [OPTN] committee how that might work.

The data on which some allocation algorithms are based are not frequently updated. For example, the current KDPI model is derived from deceased donor kidney transplants from 1995 to 2005 (OPTN, 2020b), likely rendering its predictions for transplants in 2021 biased. Even when it is clear an update is necessary, there are multiple-year delays. For example, including sodium significantly improved the accuracy of MELD (Kim et al., 2008). However, MELD was not updated to include this variable until 2016.

*Conclusion 5-15: The process and output of modeling allocation policy changes would be improved by*

- *Addressing current gaps in OPTN data collection, including socioeconomic and patient-centered factors, transplant candidate cardiac risk factors, information about organ donors regarding secondary diseases or conditions, and meaningful justifications for when a donated organ is declined by a transplant team;*
- *Accounting and allowing for more predictive models that include effects from anticipated behavior changes following allocation policy implementation;*

- *Including metrics and analyses of the cost and any other associated economic implications of proposed allocation changes; and*
- *Running randomized controlled trials of major allocation policy changes when possible.*

*Conclusion 5-16: Equitable and efficient organ allocation in the United States relies on the performance of several multivariable prediction models, such as the KDPI, EPTS, and the MELD. The OPTN infrequently updates these scores, despite their critical role in rank-ordering candidates and donors.*

## INFORMATION TECHNOLOGY INFRASTRUCTURE OPPORTUNITIES

UNOS, a nonprofit, private voluntary organization, holds the subcontract for the OPTN and has been the sole administrator of the OPTN since the initial contract was awarded by HRSA in 1986 (see Chapter 2). The OPTN is responsible for matching donated organs with potential recipients at the national level. The specific contract ensures that

- the national organ waiting list is maintained,
- the information technology (IT) system operates to match organs with patients,
- system performance is monitored and based on transplant data gathered, and
- organ allocation policies are developed (Proctor, 2019).

Since 1986 there have been open opportunities for other organizations or entities to bid on the OPTN contract. However, the contractual needs of the IT system and the complex infrastructure needed to support the organ donation and transplantation system were significant barriers to some potential bidders. For example, some have argued that the short timeline for response, unreachable requirements for organizational experience for an entity other than UNOS, and overall uncertainty about the transition period for key software systems discouraged innovative approaches to the OPTN and competitive bids outside of UNOS (Gentry and Segev, 2019). In 2020, the Senate Finance Committee questioned UNOS's presumed ownership of its IT, given funding with taxpayer dollars, and the perception of an incumbency advantage (U.S. Senate Committee on Finance, 2020). In 2021, the House of Representatives Appropriations Committee expressed encouragement for HHS to promote competition for the OPTN contract.[15]

The perceived risks and challenges to accomplishing the mission of the OPTN contract include

- time considerations (delays in implementing the Final Rule resulted in unforeseen time constraints that would make this contract challenging),
- financial considerations, and
- an unstable legal and regulatory environment (RAND, 1999).

In 2019, under an executive order from the president calling for improvements for those with end-stage kidney failure, HHS issued a request for information (RFI) regarding the OPTN IT infrastructure (HHS, 2019). The RFI established that it was in search of "ideas and

---

[15] *Departments of Labor, Health and Human Services, and Education, and Related Agencies Appropriations Bill, 2022.* 117th Cong., 1st sess. See pages 63-64 at https://docs.house.gov/meetings/AP/AP00/20210715/113908/HMKP-117-AP00-20210715-SD003.pdf (accessed February 4, 2022).

information about how to improve the national information technology system for matching transplantable organs and managing detailed, confidential medical data on transplant patients and organ donors" (HHS, 2019). In announcing HHS's RFI on the OPTN technology, then-HHS Secretary Alex Azar said: "The Health Resources and Services Administration will issue a Request for Information about more effective ways in which modern IT systems may be able to manage allocating organs and handling patient and donor data on a national scale. We especially want to hear from entities that are capable of developing a system that is more effective than the one we have today" (HHS, 2019). Additionally, in 2020, an external analysis of UNOS's technology, endorsed by all five past, bipartisan HHS Chief Technology Officers, concluded that "[UNOS] maintains an antiquated technology and limited technical acumen" (Bloom Works, 2020).

Many years ago, organ donation used to be managed by one man with one voice mail box (Crichton, 2021). In the early 1980s, Don Denny relied on messages left on his voice mail box to coordinate organ donations and matches. Nearly 2,700 transplants were conducted this way over a 4.5-year period (Crichton, 2021). By 1986, shortly after UNOS became incorporated, information technology was beginning to evolve which led to more computerized systems to deal with organ matching. In 2012, a large improvement came in UNOS' adoption of a mobile application called TransNet, which allowed OPOs to "electronically package and label organs" reducing errors in handwriting and data entry mistakes (Crichton, 2021).

## Committee Considerations

The committee considered the limited available evidence on the performance of the OPTN IT infrastructure as well as anecdotal end-user experiences, but gaps remain in the committee's understanding of any specific enhancements to the IT system that have been made in recent years and generally how well the IT system is supporting the achievement of an equitable, efficient system of organ transplantation. If the IT system is unable to support the goals of the organ transplantation system then change is needed. The committee is aware that previously the OPTN contract was changed to separate out the data analysis function—a role currently implemented successfully through a HRSA contract for the SRTR.

Committee members recognize that potential changes and restructuring of the OPTN IT functions creates risk. The greatest risks are that the government contracts for a new, separate IT infrastructure to perform the organ allocation and other OPTN IT functions currently performed by UNOS, and the new system does not work or does not work properly. Healthcare.gov is a recent example in a long line of similar examples where government contracting for large IT systems resulted in initial failures that took time to overcome. The current organ transplantation IT system performs key functions every hour, and enables the matching of available organs with wait-listed candidates, using complex algorithms associated with transplant allocation for all organ types. The committee recognizes that great care must be taken to ensure the continued, effective lifesaving operations of any system used to perform the IT functions.

Committee members discussed several ways to manage the risks associated with procuring the IT functionality necessary to perform the basic and sophisticated operations of a system such as the OPTN. One of them was to operate the current UNOS IT infrastructure in parallel with the new IT infrastructure over a prescribed period of time in order to ensure that a fallback capability remains available as the new IT infrastructure comes online. It may be necessary to clarify that the National Organ Transplant Act (NOTA) authority would permit the temporary operations of dual systems as part of potential transitions. Another way to mitigate risk is by contracting for agile system development where key basic IT functions are made operational in a new system; once the first several functions are operational, then additional functions are systematically developed and added over time. This approach ensures that the eventual complete system is functional from day 1 of its full operational status and not subject to catastrophic system development failure. While agile development is an effective way to prevent catastrophic failures associated with new, large IT systems, in the case of the OPTN, the existing IT infrastructure would most likely need to function alongside the agile development of the new one, which would involve funding considerations and potential statutory issues as well.

It may also be necessary for the government to use contracting mechanisms to create a stepped approach to ensuring government ownership and control of the existing IT functionality operated by UNOS. This becomes even more important if the government were to award a new contract to a non-UNOS organization to potentially operate the UNOS system as a backup during the development of a new and improved IT infrastructure.

The committee recognizes that competitive government contracting for IT systems is complex, and there are likely additional or other ways of mitigating risks beyond or instead of those outlined here.

> *Conclusion 5-17: While a significant amount of data are currently collected about various aspects of the transplantation system, few metrics are well defined, have consistent definitions, or aim to capture the patient experience. Opportunities exist to improve the types of data collected about the transplantation system to prioritize standardized, meaningful, patient-centered data to inform the development of performance measures for OPOs and transplant centers.*

> *Conclusion 5-18: Significant improvements could be needed in the IT infrastructure underpinning the organ transplantation system to improve the efficiency and equity of organ allocation and make the system more user friendly.*

**Recommendation 8: Modernize the information technology infrastructure and data collection for deceased donor organ procurement, allocation, distribution, and transplantation.**

**HHS should ensure that the OPTN uses a state-of-the-art information technology infrastructure that optimizes the use of new and evolving technologies to support the needs and future directions of the organ transplantation system. Toward this end, HHS should do the following:**

- Within the next 1 to 2 years, evaluate how well the current IT system meets the needs of the transplantation system by collecting and analyzing data from IT end users (e.g., OPOs and transplant teams) and other stakeholders.
- Using the user needs assessment and input from external IT experts, identify needed improvements in the current IT system used by the OPTN that would make it more efficient, equitable, and user friendly.
- Assess the pros and cons of various contracting approaches to mitigate and prevent the risks of system failures if substantial changes in IT contracting are pursued.

**Based on the evaluation of the current IT system, HHS should consider pursuing one of the following three noted courses of action:**

- Immediately separate the IT infrastructure components from the remainder of the OPTN contract and institute a new competitive process for an IT services contractor. or
- Incorporate the identified improvements in the next OPTN contract bidding process in 2023. This could include smart approaches to mitigate potential system failure risks, separating the IT infrastructure components from the OPTN contract to address necessary improvements, and keeping the contract intact but with updated expectations for the winning contractor. or
- Pursue an alternative approach that would achieve the same desired outcome.

**If HHS determines that separating the IT infrastructure from the current OPTN contract requires a change in the NOTA, then HHS should work with Congress to revise NOTA accordingly.**

# REFERENCES

AABA (American Association of Biological Anthropologists). 2021. *AABA statement on race & racism.* https://physanth.org/about/position-statements/aapa-statement-race-and-racism-2019 (accessed December 31, 2021).

Ahmed, S., C. T. Nutt, N. D. Eneanya, P. P. Reese, K. Sivashanker, M. Morse, T. Sequist, and M. L. Mendu. 2021. Examining the potential impact of race multiplier utilization in estimated glomerular filtration rate calculation on African-American care outcomes. *Journal of General Internal Medicine* 36(2):464-471.

American Society of Human Genetics. 2020. *American Society of Human Genetics statement regarding concepts of "good genes" and human genetics.* https://www.ashg.org/publications-news/ashg-news/statement-regarding-good-genes-human-genetics (accessed December 31, 2021).

Aubert, O., P. P. Reese, B. Audry, Y. Bouatou, M. Raynaud, D. Viglietti, C. Legendre, D. Glotz, J. P. Empana, X. Jouven, C. Lefaucheur, C. Jacquelinet, and A. Loupy. 2019. Disparities in acceptance of deceased donor kidneys between the United States and France and estimated effects of increased US acceptance. *JAMA Internal Medicine* 179(10):1365-1374.

Aufhauser, D. D., A. W. Peng, D. R. Murken, S. J. Concors, P. L. Abt, D. Sawinski, R. D. Bloom, P. P. Reese, and M. H. Levine. 2018. *Clinical Transplantation* 32(6):e13260.

Axelrod, D. A., and E. A. Pomfret. 2008. Race and sex disparities in liver transplantation: Progress toward achieving equal access? *JAMA* 300:2425-2426.

Bloom Works. 2020. *Bloom Works: The costly effects of an outdated organ donation system: Technology recommendations.* https://bloomworks.digital/organdonationreform/Technology (accessed February 2, 2022).

Cascino, T. M., J. Stehlik, W. S. Cherikh, Y. Cheng, T. M. F. Watt, A. A. Brescia, M. P. Thompson, J. S. McCullough, M. Zhang, S. Shore, J. R. Golbus, F. D. Pagani, D. S. Likosky, and K. D. Aaronson. 2021. A challenge to equity in transplantation: Increased center-level variation in short-term mechanical circulatory support use in the context of the updated U.S. heart transplant allocation policy. *Journal of Heart and Lung Transplantation* 41(1):95-103.

Cecka, J. M. 2010. Calculated PRA (CPRA): The new measure of sensitization for transplant candidates. *American Journal of Transplantation* 10(1):26-29.

Chopra, B., and K. K. Sureshkumar. 2015. Changing organ allocation policy for kidney transplantation in the United States. *World Journal of Transplantation* 5(2):38-43.

Clayton, P. A., S. P. McDonald, J. J. Snyder, N. Salkowski, and S. J. Chadban. 2014. External validation of the estimated posttransplant survival score for allocation of deceased donor kidneys in the United States. *American Journal of Transplantation* 14(8):1922-1926.

Clerkin, K. J., O. Salako, J. A. Fried, J. M. Griffin, J. Raikhelkar, R. Jain, S. Restaino, P. C. Colombo, K. Takeda, M. A. Farr, G. Sayer, N. Uriel, and V. K. Topkara. 2022. Impact of temporary percutaneous mechanical circulatory support before transplantation in the 2018 heart allocation system. *JACC: Heart Failure* 10(1):12-23.

Cogswell, R., R. John, J. D. Estep, S. Duval, R. J. Tedford, F. D. Pagani, C. M. Martin, and M. R. Mehra. 2020. An early investigation of outcomes with the new 2018 donor heart allocation system in the United States. *Journal of Heart and Lung Transplantation* 39(1):1-4.

Crichton, D. 2021. *How technology is transforming organ procurement.* https://techcrunch.com/2021/09/22/how-technology-is-transforming-organ-procurement/?guccounter=1 (accessed November 1, 2021).

Davis, S., and S. Mohan. 2021. Managing patients with failing kidney allograft. *Clinical Journal of the American Society of Nephrology* 17(3):444-451. https://doi.org/10.2215/cjn.14620920.

de Galasso, L., S. Picca, and I. Guzzo. 2020. Dialysis modalities for the management of pediatric acute kidney injury. *Pediatric Nephrology (Berlin, Germany)* 35(5):753-765.

Delgado, C., M. Baweja, N. R. Burrows, D. C. Crews, N. D. Eneanya, C. A. Gadegbeku, L. A. Inker, M. L. Mendu, W. G. Miller, M. M. Moxey-Mims, G. V. Roberts, W. L. St. Peter, C. Warfield, and N. R. Powe. 2021. Reassessing the inclusion of race in diagnosing kidney diseases: An interim report from the NKF-ASN task force. *Journal of the American Society of Nephrology* 32(6):1305-1317.

Emanuel, E. J., D. Wendler, and C. Grady. 2000. What makes clinical research ethical? *JAMA* 283:2701-2711.

Eneanya, N. D., W. Yang, and P. P. Reese. 2019. Reconsidering the consequences of using race to estimate kidney function. *JAMA* 322(2):113-114.

Freedman, B. I., S. O. Pastan, A. K. Israni, D. Schladt, B. A. Julian, M. D. Gautreaux, V. Hauptfeld, R. A. Bray, H. M. Gebel, A. D. Kirk, R. S. Gaston, J. Rogers, A. C. Farney, G. Orlando, R. J. Stratta, S. Mohan, L. Ma, C. D. Langefeld, D. W. Bowden, P. J. Hicks, and J. Divers. 2016. APOL1 Genotype and kidney transplantation outcomes from deceased African American donors. *Transplantation* 100(1):194-202.

Friedewald, J. J., C. J. Samana, B. L. Kasiske, A. K. Israni, D. Stewart, W. Cherikh, and R. N. Formica. 2013. The kidney allocation system. *Surgical Clinics of North America* 93(6):1395-1406.

Gander, J. C., X. Zhang, L. Plantinga, S. Paul, M. Basu, S. O. Pastan, E. Gibney, E. Hartmann, L. Mulloy, C. Zayas, and R. E. Patzer. 2018. Racial disparities in preemptive referral for kidney transplantation in Georgia. *Clinical Transplantation* 32(9):e13380.

Gentry, S. E., and D. L. Segev. 2019. Restructuring the OPTN contract to achieve policy coherence and infrastructure excellence. *American Journal of Transplantation* 19(6):1622-1627.

Goff, R. R., K. Uccellini, K. Lindblad, S. Hall, R. Davies, M. Farr, S. Silvestry, and J. G. Rogers. 2020. A change of heart: Preliminary results of the United States 2018 adult heart allocation revision. *American Journal of Transplantation* 20(10):2781-2790.

Halazun, K. J., A. K. Mathur, A. A. Rana, A. B. Massie, S. Mohan, R. E. Patzer, J. P. Wedd, B. Samstein, R. M. Subramanian, B. D. Campos, and S. J. Knechtle. 2016. One size does not fit all—Regional variation in the impact of the share 35 liver allocation policy. *American Journal of Transplantation* 16(1):137-142.

Harhay, M. N., M. O. Harhay, K. Ranganna, S. M. Boyle, L. L. Mizrahi, S. Guy, G. E. Malat, G. Xiao, D. J. Reich, and R. E. Patzer. 2018. Association of the kidney allocation system with dialysis exposure before deceased donor kidney transplantation by preemptive wait-listing status. *Clinical Transplantation* 32(10):e13386.

HHS (U.S. Department of Health and Human Services). 2019. *Modern National Resource Allocation System: Request for Information.* https://sam.gov/opp/69bd972384b8480283bd2599fc8805a9/view;%20 (accessed October 19, 2021).

Hsu, C.-Y., F. Lin, E. Vittinghoff, and M. G. Shlipak. 2003. Racial differences in the progression from chronic renal insufficiency to end-stage renal disease in the United States. *Journal of the American Society of Nephrology* 14(11):2902-2907.

Hsu, C.-Y., W. Yang, R. V. Parikh, A. H. Anderson, T. K. Chen, D. L. Cohen, J. He, M. J. Mohanty, J. P. Lash, K. T. Mills, A. N. Muiru, A. Parsa, M. R. Saunders, T. Shafi, R. R. Townsend, S. S. Waikar, J. Wang, M. Wolf, T. C. Tan, H. I. Feldman, and A. S. Go. 2021. Race, genetic ancestry, and estimating kidney function in CKD. *New England Journal of Medicine* 385(19):1750-1760.

Husain, S. A., F. S. Winterhalter, and S. Mohan. 2018. Kidney transplant offers to deceased candidates. *American Journal of Transplantation* 18(11):2836-2837.

Husain, S. A., K. L. King, G. K. Dube, D. Tsapepas, D. J. Cohen, L. E. Ratner, and S. Mohan. 2019. Regional disparities in transplantation with deceased donor kidneys with Kidney Donor Profile Index less than 20% among candidates with top 20% estimated post transplant survival. *Progress in Transplantation (Aliso Viejo, California)*, 29(4):354-360.

Ioannidis, J. P., N. R. Powe, and C. Yancy. 2021. Recalibrating the use of race in medical research. *JAMA* 325(7):623.

IOM (Institute of Medicine). 1999. *Organ procurement and transplantation: Assessing current policies and the potential impact.* Washington, DC: National Academy Press.

Joshi, S., J. J. Gaynor, S. Bayers, G. Guerra, A. Eldefrawy, Z. Chediak, L. Companioni, J. Sageshima, L. Chen, W. Kupin, D. Roth, A. Mattiazzi, G. W. Burke III, and G. Ciancio. 2013. Disparities among blacks, Hispanics, and whites in time from starting dialysis to kidney transplant waitlisting. *Transplantation* 95(2):309-318.

Julian, B. A., R. S. Gaston, W. M. Brown, A. Reeves-Daniel, A. K. Israni, D. P. Schladt, S. O. Pastan, S. Mohan, B. I. Freedman, and J. Divers. 2017. Effect of replacing race with apolipoprotein L1 genotype in calculation of kidney donor risk index. *American Journal of Transplantation* 17(6):1540-1548.

Kim, W. R., S. W. Biggins, W. K. Kremers, R. H. Wiesner, P. S. Kamath, J. T. Benson, E. Edwards, and T. M. Therneau. 2008. Hyponatremia and mortality among patients on the liver-transplant waiting list. *New England Journal of Medicine* 359(10):1018-1026.

King, K. L., S. A. Husain, Z. Jin, C. Brennan, and S. Mohan. 2019. Trends in disparities in preemptive kidney transplantation in the United States. *Clinical Journal of the American Society of Nephrology* 14(10):1500-1511.

Ku, E. 2021 (unpublished). *Review of algorithms used in kidney allocation—Issues of fairness, equity, and system variation*. Paper commissioned by the Committee on a Fairer and More Equitable, Cost-Effective, and Transparent System of Donor Organ Procurement, Allocation, and Distribution, National Academies of Sciences, Engineering, and Medicine, Washington, DC.

Ku, E., C. E. McCulloch, D. B. Adey, L. Li, and K. L. Johansen. 2021. Racial disparities in eligibility for preemptive waitlisting for kidney transplantation and modification of EGFR thresholds to equalize waitlist time. *Journal of the American Society of Nephrology* 32(3):677-685.

Kulkarni, S., K. Ladin, D. Haakinson, E. Greene, L. Li, and Y. Deng. 2019. Association of racial disparities with access to kidney transplant after the implementation of the New Kidney Allocation System. *JAMA Surgery* 154(7):618.

Lai, J. C. 2021 (unpublished). *Review of algorithms in liver allocation*. Paper commissioned by the Committee on a Fairer and More Equitable, Cost-Effective, and Transparent System of Donor Organ Procurement, Allocation, and Distribution, National Academies of Sciences, Engineering, and Medicine, Washington, DC.

Locke, J. E., B. A. Shelton, K. M. Olthoff, E. A. Pomfret, K. A. Forde, D. Sawinski, M. Gray, and N. L. Ascher. 2020. Quantifying sex-based disparities in liver allocation. *JAMA Surgery* 155(7).

Luo, X., J. Leanza, A. B. Massie, J. M. Garonzik-Wang, C. E. Haugen, S. E. Gentry, S. E. Ottmann, and D. L. Segev. 2018. MELD as a metric for survival benefit of liver transplantation. *American Journal of Transplantation* 18(5):1231-1237.

Massie, A. B., X. Luo, E. K. Chow, J. L. Alejo, N. M. Desai, and D. L. Segev. 2014. Survival benefit of primary deceased donor transplantation with high-KDPI kidneys. *American Journal of Transplantation* 14(10):2310-2316.

Massie, A. B., E. K. Chow E, C. E. Wickliffe, X. Luo, S. E. Gentry, D. C. Mulligan, and D. L. Segev. 2015. Early changes in liver distribution following implementation of Share 35. *American Journal of Transplantation* 15:659-667.

Melanson, T. A., J. M. Hockenberry, L. Plantinga, M. Basu, S. Pastan, S. Mohan, D. H. Howard, and R. E. Patzer. 2017. New kidney allocation system associated with increased rates of transplants among black and hispanic patients. *Health Affairs (Project Hope)* 36(6):1078-1085.

Merion, R. M., V. B. Ashby, R. A. Wolfe, D. A. Distant, T. E. Hulbert-Shearon, R. A. Metzger, A. O. Ojo, and F. K. Port, F. 2005. Deceased-donor characteristics and the survival benefit of kidney transplantation. *JAMA* 294(21):2726-2733.

Mulligan, D. 2021. *The role of modeling in proposed organ allocation policy changes*. Presentation at the February 4-5, 2021 public workshop of the Committee on a Fairer and More Equitable, Cost-Effective, and Transparent System of Donor Organ Procurement, Allocation, and Distribution, National Academies of Sciences, Engineering, and Medicine Virtual Meeting, Washington, DC. https://www.nationalacademies.org/event/02-04-2021/a-fairer-and-more-equitable-cost-effective-and-transparent-system-of-donor-organ-procurement-allocation-and-distribution-a-virtual-workshop (accessed January 26, 2022).

OPTN (Organ Procurement and Transplantation Network). 2020a. *Briefing to the OPTN Board of Directors on addressing medically urgent candidates in the new kidney allocation system*. https://optn.transplant.hrsa.gov/media/3813/202006_kidney_medical_urgency_bp.pdf (accessed February 3, 2022).

OPTN. 2020b. *A guide to calculating and interpreting the Kidney Donor Profile Index (KDPI)*. https://optn.transplant.hrsa.gov/media/1512/guide_to_calculating_interpreting_kdpi.pdf (accessed January 2, 2022).

OPTN. 2021a. *Clarify multi-organ allocation policy*. https://optn.transplant.hrsa.gov/governance/public-comment/clarify-multi-organ-allocation-policy (accessed December 31, 2021).

OPTN. 2021b. *OPTN metrics: Waitlist details*. https://insights.unos.org/OPTN-metrics (accessed December 13, 2021).

OPTN. n.d.-a. *Continuous distribution*. https://optn.transplant.hrsa.gov/policies-bylaws/a-closer-look/continuous-distribution (accessed December 13, 2021).

OPTN. n.d.-b https://optn.transplant.hrsa.gov/professionals/by-topic/guidance/kidney-pancreas-allocation-system-frequently-asked-questions/= (accessed January 27, 2022).

OPTN Minority Affairs and Kidney Transplantation Committees. 2021. *Reassess inclusion of race in estimated glomerular filtration rate (eGFR) calculation*. https://optn.transplant.hrsa.gov/media/pdrel25h/20210819_ki_mac_-egfr_meeting_summary.pdf (accessed January 2, 2022).

Parker, W. F., A. S. Anderson, R. D. Gibbons, E. R. Garrity, L. F. Ross, E. S. Huang, and M. M. Churpek. 2019. Association of transplant center with survival benefit among adults undergoing heart transplant in the United States. *JAMA* 322(18):1789.

Parker, W. F., Y. Becker, and R. D. Gibbons. 2021 (unpublished). *Saving more lives with deceased donor kidney transplantation*. Paper commissioned by the Committee on a Fairer and More Equitable, Cost-Effective, and Transparent System of Donor Organ Procurement, Allocation, and Distribution, National Academies of Sciences, Engineering, and Medicine, Washington, DC.

Patzer, R. E., S. Amaral, H. Wasse, N. Volkova, D. Kleinbaum, and W. M. McClellan. 2009. Neighborhood poverty and racial disparities in kidney transplant waitlisting. *Journal of the American Society of Nephrology* 20(6):1333-1340.

Peng, R. B., H. Lee, Z. T. Ke, and M. R. Saunders. 2018. Racial disparities in kidney transplant waitlist appearance in Chicago: Is it race or place? *Clinical Transplantation* 32(5):e13195.

Pérez-Sáez, M. J., E. Arcos, J. Comas, M. Crespo, J. Lloveras, and J. Pascual. 2016. Survival benefit from kidney transplantation using kidneys from deceased donors aged ≥75 years: A time-dependent analysis. *American Journal of Transplantation* 16(9):2724-2733.

Powe, N. R. 2020. Black kidney function matters: Use or misuse of race. *JAMA* 324(8):737-738.

Proctor, G. 2019. *HRSA Healthy Grants Workshop. HRSA examined: The Healthcare Systems Bureau.* https://www.hrsa.gov/sites/default/files/hrsa/grants/manage/technicalassistance/hsb-2019.pdf (accessed October 18, 2021).

RAND informs government it will not bid on contracts to administer OPTN, SRTR. 1999. The Free Library. https://www.thefreelibrary.com/RAND+informs+government+it+will+not+bid+on+contracts+to+administer...-a058091072 (accessed December 16, 2021).

Reese, P. P., S. Mohan, K. L. King, W. W. Williams, V. S. Potluri, M. N. Harhay, and N. D. Eneanya. 2021. Racial disparities in preemptive waitlisting and deceased donor kidney transplantation: Ethics and solutions. *American Journal of Transplantation* 21(3):958-967.

Rodríguez-Castro, K. I., E. De Martin, M. Gambato, S. Lazzaro, E. Villa, and P. Burra. 2014. Female gender in the setting of liver transplantation. *World Journal of Transplantation* 4(4):229-242.

Schold, J. D., L. D. Buccini, P. P. Reese, E. D. Poggio, and D. A. Goldfarb. 2014. Effect of dialysis initiation for preemptively listed candidates in the revised kidney allocation policy. *American Journal of Transplantation* 14(12):2855-2860.

Silvestry, S. C., and J. G. Rogers. 2022. Rinse, wash, repeat: The evolution of the UNOS heart transplant allocation system. *JACC: Heart Failure* 10(1):24-26.

Singal, A. K., and P. S. Kamath. 2013. Model for end-stage liver disease. *Journal of Clinical and Experimental Hepatology* 3(1):50-60.

Singh, T. P., C. E. Milliren, C. S. Almond, and D. Graham. 2014. Survival benefit from transplantation in patients listed for heart transplantation in the United States. *Journal of the American College of Cardiology* 63(12):1169-1178.

Snyder, J. 2021. *Simulated allocation models: Strengths, limitations, and data availability.* Presentation at the February 4-5, 2021 public workshop of the Committee on a Fairer and More Equitable, Cost-Effective, and Transparent System of Donor Organ Procurement, Allocation, and Distribution, National Academies of Sciences, Engineering, and Medicine Virtual Meeting, Washington, DC. https://www.nationalacademies.org/event/02-04-2021/a-fairer-and-more-equitable-cost-effective-and-transparent-system-of-donor-organ-procurement-allocation-and-distribution-a-virtual-workshop (accessed January 26, 2022).

SRTR (Scientific Registry of Transplant Recipients). 2019. *Simulated allocation models.* https://www.srtr.org/requesting-srtr-data/simulated-allocation-models (accessed January 1, 2022).

Stewart, D. E., A. R. Wilk, A. E. Toll, A. M. Harper, R. R. Lehman, A. M. Robinson, S. A. Noreen, E. B. Edwards, and D. K. Klassen. 2018. Measuring and monitoring equity in access to deceased donor kidney transplantation. *American Journal of Transplantation* 18(8):1924-1935.

Tran, Z. T., R. Hernandez, J. Madrigal, S. T. Kim, A. Verma, D. G. Rabkin, and P. Benharash. 2022. Center-level variation in transplant rates following the heart allocation policy change. *JAMA Cardiology.* https://doi.org/10.1001/jamacardio.2021.5370.

UNOS. 2021. *Lung calculation.* https://unos.org/wp-content/uploads/unos/Lung_Calculation.pdf (accessed December 16, 2021).

USRDS (United States Renal Data System). 2020. *Annual data report: Epidemiology of kidney disease in the United States.* Bethesda, MD: National Institute of Diabetes and Digestive and Kidney Diseases.

U.S. Senate Committee on Finance. 2020. *FinalSIGNED - Grassley Wyden to HHS 23Oct2002.* https://www.finance.senate.gov/imo/media/doc/FinalSIGNED%20-%20Grassley%20Wyden%20to%20HHS%20 23Oct2020.pdf (accessed February 4, 2022).

Verghese, P. S. 2017. Pediatric kidney transplantation: A historical review. *Pediatric Research* 81(1-2):259-264.

Vock, D. M., M. T. Durheim, W. M. Tsuang, C. A. Finlen-Copeland, A. A. Tsiatis, M. Davidian, M. L. Neely, D. J. Lederer, and S. M. Palmer. 2017. Survival benefit of lung transplantation in the modern era of lung allocation. *Annals of the American Thoracic Society* 14(2):172-181.

Wang, C. J., J. B Wetmore, and A. K. Israni. 2017. Old versus new: Progress in reaching the goals of the new kidney allocation system. *Human Immunology* 78(1):9-15.

Westphal, S. G., E. D. Langewisch, A. M. Robinson, A. R. Wilk, J. J. Dong, T. J. Plumb, R. Mullane, S. Merani, A. L. Hoffman, A. Maskin, and C. D. Miles. 2021. The impact of multi-organ transplant allocation priority on waitlisted kidney transplant candidates. *American Journal of Transplantation* 21(6):2161-2174.

Wey, A., J. Foutz, S. K. Gustafson, R. J. Carrico, K. Sisaithong, H. Tosoc-Haskell, M. McBride, D. Klassen, N. Salkowski, B. L. Kasiske, A. K. Israni, and J. J. Snyder. 2020. The collaborative innovation and improvement network (COIIN): Effect on donor yield, waitlist mortality, transplant rates, and offer acceptance. *American Journal of Transplantation* 20(4):1076-1086.

Wolfe, R. A., V. B. Ashby, E. L. Milford, A. O. Ojo, R. E. Ettenger, L. Y. C. Agodoa, P. J. Held, and F. K. Port. 1999. Comparison of mortality in all patients on dialysis, patients on dialysis awaiting transplantation, and recipients of a first cadaveric transplant. *New England Journal of Medicine* 341(23):1725-1730.

Zelnick, L. R., N. Leca, B. Young, and N. Bansal. 2021. Association of the estimated glomerular filtration rate with vs without a coefficient for race with time to eligibility for Kidney Transplant. *JAMA Network Open* 4(1).

# 6

# Improving Procurement, Acceptance, and Use of Deceased Donor Organs

"Our vision of the transplant ecosystem is patient centered, designed to improve organ failure and patient survival by doing four things: Improving organ availability, maximizing use, achieving high-quality outcomes, and fostering innovation."
—A. Osama Gaber, President, American Society of Transplant Surgeons,
Houston Methodist Department of Surgery, testimony to the committee
during July 15, 2021 public listening session

The U.S. organ transplantation system is dependent on many factors, as discussed in this chapter, but most importantly, it depends on the generosity of individuals and their families who, at the time of death, make the decision to donate organs to someone they have never met. The success of this system is founded on and maintained by the public's trust in that system—both trust in the end-of-life decision-making process and trust in the process of providing transplants to patients who need them. In the context of evolving organ allocation and distribution policies and new organ procurement organization (OPO) regulations, there are notable tensions in the donation and transplant community that have resulted in the task of this report. After analyzing the performance of the organ transplantation and donation system—and OPOs and transplant centers in particular—and reviewing the scientific literature and publicly available data, the committee found that the current organ transplantation system, similar to other systems, is *perfectly designed to achieve the results it gets* (Berwick, 1996; IOM, 2006). That is, the results of the organ transplantation system, in terms of procuring, allocating, distributing, and transplanting organs into waiting recipients, are precisely the results permitted by the features of the system. The current deficiencies in the organ transplantation system present opportunities for improvement. Data on the performance of system components (e.g., OPOs and transplant centers) reveals significant shortfalls in the degree to which the potential transplant recipient is at the center of the decision-making process, but there are effective ways to address these shortfalls.

This chapter analyzes the performance data of OPOs and transplant centers with a focus on opportunities to standardize and bring innovations and best practices to OPOs and transplant centers nationwide. Inadequacies in OPO and transplant center performance are currently detracting from getting the best organ for, and to, the right recipient in the most efficient and equitable manner. This chapter discusses the sources and types of data in the organ transplantation system and opportunities for standardization to improve understanding of system performance; the committee analyzed this evidence through a systems perspective and the underlying principle that putting the patient at the center of system improvements is always best.

There are two key areas with high variability in performance and therefore great room for improvement that are a major focus of this chapter: (1) OPO pursuit and procurement of donation after circulatory determination of death (DCDD) donors,[1] and (2) transplant centers accepting and using more of the deceased donor organs offered to individuals on the waiting list. The committee's identification of these two key areas was influenced by these striking statistics on performance: (1) An over five-fold variation exists across the nation's OPOs in terms of recovery of DCDD donors, and (2) the 2019 transplant center rates at which organs were recovered for transplant but not transplanted (i.e., the nonuse rate)[2] ranged from 20 percent for kidneys, 10 percent for livers, 6.5 percent for lungs, to 0.85 percent for hearts (Israni et al., 2021; SRTR, 2021) That is, one in five deceased donor kidneys are procured but not used (Israni et al., 2021; SRTR, 2021). Furthermore, there are organs offered and declined before they are ever procured, so the number of potentially transplantable organs that are not used for transplant may be even higher. To increase efficiency, the organ transplantation system must prioritize the use of already available organs, while simultaneously expanding the donor pool in all ways possible, especially including procurement and use of more DCDD donors to meet the needs of those on the transplant waiting list.

In all systems, including the organ transplantation system, variations exist for any number of reasons and are not, in and of themselves, an indicator of poor performance (NQF, 2021). However, meaningful performance comparisons are only possible, and variations explained, when standardized measures are used. Although an abundance of data has been collected on the organ transplantation system, the committee found that large, core segments of data are not standardized. For instance, while all 57 OPOs collect a variety of data related to the processes of organ donation in their geographic area, standardization of those data is lacking. Also, as discussed in Chapter 4, there are no national standards for how to train OPO staff on communication skills in compassion and cultural sensitivity, despite evidence suggesting that OPO staff were missing opportunities to increase the supply of available deceased donor organs and equalize regional variations in donation and transplantation rates (Traino et al., 2017).

This lack of standardization limits efforts in identifying causes of system variation. Despite the knowledge and sharing of many best practices for OPOs and transplant centers, underperformance and a lack of systemwide adherence will become further entrenched without the implementation of reliable process and outcome measures. All stakeholders benefit when variations are readily discernible, promoting both continuous improvement initiatives and the transfer of best practices among donor hospitals, OPOs, and transplant centers (Lynch et al., 2021).

## INCREASING DECEASED ORGAN DONATION AND PROCUREMENT

As transplantation has become a treatment modality for end-stage organ failure of all types, the gap has continued to widen between the national waiting list and the number of available deceased organ donors. The National Academies have been called on in the past

---

[1] *Donation after circulatory death* (DCD) is the most well-known term, but the committee uses the more precise term *donation after circulatory determination of death* (DCDD). Historically, this was also known as *non–heart-beating cadaveric donation*.

[2] This report uses the term *nonuse rate*; this is equivalent to the more commonly used *discard rate*.

to provide advice on ways to increase deceased organ donation in the United States (see Appendix B). National efforts in the years since the National Organ Transplant Act (NOTA)—and especially since the Organ Donation and Transplant Breakthrough Collaborative was initiated in 2003—have resulted in the widespread sharing of proven practices among all 57 OPOs (Shafer et al., 2008) and hundreds of the nation's largest trauma centers where most donors originate. These efforts, and others, have resulted in a steady growth in the rate of deceased organ donation: the total number of deceased donors increased annually between 2010 and 2020 from 7,943 to 12,588 donors, and organ donation from deceased donors grew 39 percent between 2015 and 2020 (OPTN, 2021a). In 2020, the United States led the world in the deceased organ donor rate with 38.03 donors per million population (IRODaT, 2021). However, this committee did not conduct an analysis of differential death rates across countries or of the ways that differences in the cause of death could impact international comparisons. Relative to other high-income countries, the United States has disproportionately high numbers of drug overdose deaths (Ho, 2019), gun deaths (Grinshteyn and Hemenway, 2019), suicides (The Commonwealth Fund, 2020), and fatal car accidents (WHO, 2018). These differences, which may contribute to more potential donors per million population in the United States compared with other countries, deserve further research.

## OPO REGULATORY FRAMEWORK AND PERFORMANCE METRICS

As described earlier in this report, OPOs have the responsibility for identifying potential organ donors, receiving authorization for deceased donor donation, providing support to donor families, clinically managing organ donors, allocating and procuring organs, and confirming that organs reach the transplant hospital (CMS, 2020a). In addition, OPOs provide professional and public education on organ donation. Therefore, organ donation is most closely linked to OPO performance, but the use of organs by transplant centers creates an interconnectedness between OPO and transplant center behaviors. For instance, the willingness of transplant centers to accept different types of organs has often driven OPO practices of pursuing medically complex, older, or DCDD donors. If a transplant center has been unwilling to accept and use organs from medically complex donors, then the OPO has been unlikely to pursue procuring these types of donors (Yu et al., 2020). With the advent of broader distribution of organs to transplant candidates, and as evidenced by increases in DCDD donation, many OPOs have proven to be more willing to pursue these donors and transplant centers are more willing to use the organs.

The formal system and structure of OPOs as regulated nonprofit monopolies was created under NOTA with regulatory authority assigned to the Centers for Medicare & Medicaid Services (CMS). CMS conducts surveys of OPOs every 4 years and evaluates whether they meet CMS conditions for coverage for recertification. There are currently 57 OPOs, each assigned to their own donation service area (DSA). Although an OPO has never been decertified, decertification would require the OPO's geographic area—its DSA—to be opened to competition from other OPOs qualified to compete. On a monthly basis, the Scientific Registry of Transplant Recipients (SRTR) receives data collected from OPOs by the United Network for Organ Sharing (UNOS), contracted to act as the Organ Procurement and Transplantation Network (OPTN). The OPO data include the number of deaths reported by hospitals within their DSAs, the number of those deaths meeting standardized definitions of "eligible" or "imminent" deaths,[3] the frequency with which deceased individuals become donors, and the

---

[3] The definitions "eligible" and "imminent" are still in OPTN policies, but have been removed in the new OPO regulations.

number of organs that are successfully placed for transplant (SRTR, 2022a). Program-specific data for all OPOs are available on the SRTR website.

OPO performance measures are widely recognized as insufficient, largely because each OPO self-reports their outcomes in a nonstandardized way, making valid comparisons of OPO performance nearly impossible. For years, some within and beyond the OPO community requested defined, standardized performance regulations. In November 2020, CMS issued a long-awaited Final Rule that updates the conditions for coverage to evaluate OPOs on the outcomes of new measures of the donation rates and transplantation rates (CMS, 2020a). OPO performance on the new outcome measures will be publicly released each year, and OPOs will face increased competition under the new measures. At the end of each 4-year recertification cycle, DSAs for Tier 2 and Tier 3 OPOs will be opened for competition; the new CMS measures will be implemented in August 2022, and full application and enforcement will begin in 2026 (CMS, 2020a) (see Box 6-1 for key provisions).

This committee's charge includes consideration of the following:

> "self-reported donation metrics (e.g., "eligible deaths") and the impact on estimates of the true donor supply....and the development of a new, standardized, objective, and verifiable donation metric to permit the transplant community to evaluate DSAs and OPOs and establish best practices" (see Chapter 1).

The revisions to the CMS Final Rule were a matter of much debate by stakeholders in the organ transplantation system. One area of particular relevance to this report is the reliance on death certificate data for the donation rate measure. In theory, death certificate data could be considered independent of bias, as it is not self-reported by OPOs, and able to provide a larger picture of the number of potential deceased donors. However, death certificates do not require the listing of secondary diagnoses, which may include medical conditions that would preclude deceased donation, such as cancer or an infectious disease like COVID-19. Without these secondary diagnoses, a deceased person who would never be medically acceptable for donation could be inadvertently counted in the donation rate denominator, negatively affecting the OPO's performance metrics under the proposed donation rate metric. Additionally, the reliability and accuracy of death certificate data is a challenge. The percent of death certificates inaccurately or incompletely reporting cause of death or having other significant errors ranges from 25 to 50 percent (Gill and DeJoseph, 2020; McGivern et al., 2017; POGO, 2021; Pritt et al., 2005; Wexelman et al., 2013). Also, death certificate data often do not become available until 1 to 2 years after the death occurred, a problem when considering the need to evaluate OPO performance in a timely manner. Notwithstanding these concerns, some authors indicate that irregularities in death certificate data would not impact the reporting of eligible donor deaths since stroke, trauma, and drug overdose deaths constitute a large portion of organ donors, and these conditions are rarely miscategorized on death certificates (Karp and Segal, 2021).

An alternative source of data suggested during the CMS comment period as a more accurate source of data for calculating donor potential is ventilated death data from hospitals' electronic health records (EHRs). These hospital data refer to whether the patient died on a ventilator, a medical requirement for organ donation to occur. This is a key data point which is not specified on death certificates (UNOS, 2020). Advocates for this metric suggest that in the future these hospital-level patient data could come from individual patient EHRs upon referral of the donor to the OPO. However, some authors, including a former U.S. chief data scientist, have noted that ventilated death definitions are not standardized and there is currently no reporting mechanism or automated system to capture the relevant information,

| BOX 6-1 | KEY PROVISIONS OF THE REVISED ORGAN PROCUREMENT ORGANIZATION (OPO) CONDITIONS FOR COVERAGE FINAL RULE |
| --- | --- |

- *Donation rate measure*: CMS is changing the OPO donation rate measure to the number of organ donors in the OPO's DSA as a percentage of inpatient deaths among patients 75 years old or younger with a primary cause of death that is consistent with organ donation. Death that is consistent with organ donation means all deaths from the state death certificates with the primary cause of death listed as the ICD–10–CM codes I20–I25 (ischemic heart disease) and I60–I69 (cerebrovascular disease), as well as V–1–Y89 (external causes of death), such as blunt trauma, gunshot wounds, drug overdose, suicide, drowning, and asphyxiation. A key change from the previous outcome measures is that a donor is now defined as a deceased individual from whom at least one vascularized organ (heart, liver, lung, kidney, pancreas, or intestine) is transplanted, not just procured for transplant, or an individual from whom a pancreas is procured and is used for research or islet cell transplantation.
- *Transplantation rate measure:* CMS is changing the OPO transplantation rate measure to the number of transplanted organs from an OPO's DSA as a percentage of inpatient deaths among patients 75 years old or younger with a primary cause of death that is consistent with organ donation.
- *Performance benchmark:* The performance rates that OPOs will be encouraged to meet for the donation and transplantation rates will be established by the lowest rates of the top 25 percent of OPOs from the previous 12-month period, a ranking that will be publicly available. OPOs with performance rates that are below the top 25 percent will be required to take action to improve their rates through a quality assurance and performance improvement program.
- *12-month review periods:* CMS will review OPO performance every 12 months throughout the 4-year recertification cycle to ensure fewer viable organs are wasted and more timely transplants occur. If an OPO ultimately does not improve enough to meet the outcome measures before the end of the recertification cycle, the OPO may be decertified and lose its DSA.
- *Performance tiers:* At the end of each recertification cycle, each OPO will be assigned a tier ranking based on its performance for both the donation rate and transplantation rate measures and its performance on the recertification survey. The highest-performing OPOs that are ranked in the top 25 percent will be assigned to Tier 1 and automatically recertified for another 4 years. Tier 2 OPOs are the next-highest-performing OPOs, where performance on both measures exceeds the median but does not reach Tier 1. Tier 2 OPOs will not automatically be recertified and will have to compete to retain their DSAs. Tier 3 OPOs are the lowest-performing OPOs that have one or both measures below the median. Tier 3 OPOs will be decertified and will not be able to compete for any other open DSA.
- *Increased competition:* CMS will ensure that OPO DSAs are awarded to the highest-performing OPOs. At the end of each 4-year recertification cycle, DSAs for Tier 2 and Tier 3 OPOs will be opened for competition. Only Tier 1 and Tier 2 OPOs will be able to compete for DSAs. Tier 2 OPOs will need to successfully compete for their DSA or another open DSA in order to be recertified for another 4 years. All the DSAs for Tier 3 OPOs will be replaced by a better-performing OPO, and DSAs for Tier 2 OPOs could be replaced by a higher-performing OPO.
- *Transparent OPO performance*: The new outcome measures improve on the prior measures by using objective, transparent, and reliable data, rather than OPO self-reported data, to establish the donor potential in the OPO's DSA. CMS will publish OPO performance on the outcome measures annually.

SOURCE: CMS, 2020a.

thereby requiring manual review of patient medical records using complex definitions and patient-specific details. Among other problems, the authors suggest this complexity in using ventilated death definitions leaves the data vulnerable to manipulation and inaccuracy (Karp et al., 2020).

During consideration of the new OPO performance metrics, CMS reported that commenters raised concerns about the burden on donor hospitals if data on ventilated deaths were required for reporting. CMS agreed that requiring these additional reporting requirements or combining disparate data sources to estimate donor potential via ventilated deaths "could not be obtained by reasonable efforts" but would continue to be evaluated as new data sources become available (CMS, 2020b). In December 2021, CMS also issued a request for information regarding, among other parts of the organ donation process, input on data collection of patient-level data, underscoring the urgency in making accurate assessments of organ donor potential and suggesting there is room for ongoing clarity and improvement in current regulations (CMS, 2021).

In the end, the committee agreed that no single metric—whether based on death certificates or ventilated deaths data—would be adequate to fully understand and assess the performance of the interconnected parts of the organ transplantation system. Rather, performance measures in multiple domains are needed to assess the performance of donor hospitals, OPOs, and transplant centers in achieving overall system performance goals (see Recommendation 12 in Chapter 7 for greater discussion of the metrics that could populate a standardized dashboard of performance metrics). As organ donation, procurement, and transplantation practices evolve, performance metrics will need to evolve accordingly. For example, if donor care units are adopted by all OPOs in the United States, as recommended in this report (see Recommendation 11 later in this chapter), this would constitute a significant change in procurement practices that may warrant reconsideration of the performance measures used to assess OPO functionality given the new standard of practice. The committee believes that the organ transplantation system's consideration of these issues should be informed by the experience of organizations such as the National Quality Forum that have demonstrated specific expertise in evaluating performance metrics across complex systems.

Box 6-2 provides the committee's rationale for an integrated and holistic approach to the measurement and assessment of OPO performance.

*Conclusion 6-1: The CMS OPO performance metrics taking effect in 2022 will provide standardization and allow for more meaningful reporting on system performance. However, timely, verifiable, and currently available data—ideally hospital patient-level data—would provide the most accurate assessment of deceased donor potential.*

## KEY AREA FOR IMPROVEMENT FOR OPOS: DONATION AFTER CIRCULATORY DETERMINATION OF DEATH

While there are many factors related to increasing the organ supply, the more than five-fold variation of DCDD donors by OPOs across the country provides a striking example that significant improvements are possible and needed in this area. The committee reviewed levels of achievement by the highest performers in the system to provide valuable insight into the possibilities within the existing statutory, regulatory, and clinical practice-based elements of the transplantation system to increase deceased organ donation.

| | COMMITTEE'S RATIONALE FOR METRICS TO EVALUATE |
|---|---|
| **BOX 6-2** | **ORGAN PROCUREMENT ORGANIZATION (OPO)** **PERFORMANCE** |

The committee affirms the need for

- A reliable, accurate, and timely donation rate, or how often do eligible deceased individuals become donors, as a key measure of OPO performance;
- This measure should not be self-reported; and
- Donation rate measurement should be standardized across OPOs.

The committee calls for

- The donation rate as one measure in a dashboard of metrics (see Chapter 7) to assess OPO performance, which include additional measurement elements to address disparities, referrals responded to, and others;
- The use of a consensus-based process to arrive at the donation rate measure;
- Patient-level data that use a measure denominator that is accurate and granular enough to contain essential information about referrals of ventilated deaths, medical suitability of donors, and other key information;
- A measure denominator that is electronically reported and does not have lag periods of 1–2 years; and
- A measure that will be defensible in court, if challenged.

## Historical Perspective

Early transplant programs obtained organs either from healthy, living, related donors or from deceased donors who were declared dead by cardiopulmonary criteria. A determination of death by neurological criteria, although a legal option in the sense that state laws allowed clinicians to make determinations of death according to their own practice and custom, was not generally accepted historically as clinicians were reluctant to pronounce death in a patient who had continued heart function. These deceased donors provided kidneys most frequently, although there were some successful attempts to transplant other solid organs (IOM, 1997). In 1981, the National Conference of Commissioners on Uniform State Laws, the entity that promulgates many uniform laws, published the Uniform Determination of Death Act that was adopted very quickly by almost all 50 states. As more donors were being declared dead by neurological criteria, the number of donors declared by circulatory criteria decreased significantly, and virtually all DCDD donation in the United States came to a standstill.

In response to a 1997 request from the U.S. Department of Health and Human Services (HHS), the Institute of Medicine (IOM) studied ways to increase the availability of organs while ensuring the ethically and medically sound treatment of donor patients before and after death. The IOM study concluded that organ recovery after circulatory death provided an opportunity to increase the availability of organs to individuals on the waiting list (IOM, 1997). The release of the IOM report correlated with subsequent increases in DCDD, with OPOs and transplant centers developing protocols and supporting infrastructure to expand the practice of DCDD in the continuum of quality end-of-life care. A national focus in the pursuit of DCDD donation developed during the 2003 Health Resources and Services Administration-sponsored Organ Donation Breakthrough Collaborative, when a national benchmark of 10 percent of deceased donors being recovered through DCDD was established.[4] While DCDD donors have increased overall, the adoption of DCDD protocols has been uneven across the United States and OPOs exhibit significant variation in their pursuit of and success with DCDD.

Some variation in procurement of DCDD organs could be related to challenges in determining death, particularly for the donation of hearts after cardiac death (Veatch, 2008). There is also consideration of variability in "hands-off" rules—that is, the time for which the decedent's condition is considered irreversible. The committee did not conduct an in-depth analysis of these issues, but notes that under current regulatory and ethical regimes, there exists an opportunity to continue and support the upward trend of DCDD organ procurement and transplantation.

## Current State of DCDD Donation and Transplantation

Since DCDD donation has been tracked by the OPTN, the consistent pursuit of DCDD donors and use by transplant centers began to systematically increase in 2004, precipitated by the Organ Donation and Transplantation Breakthrough Collaborative (Figure 6-1).

Despite these overall increases in DCDD procurement, today there is five-fold variation in the recovery of DCDD organs across the system. To analyze the variability in DCDD performance across OPOs, it is important to understand the variability in use of DCDD organs by transplant centers and the interconnected nature of OPO and transplant center behaviors and performance. Figure 6-2 shows the growth in the use of DCDD organs by transplant centers.

---

[4] A version of the program continues today as the Donation and Transplantation Community of Practice, managed by the alliance. See https://www.organdonationalliance.org/about (accessed December 23, 2021).

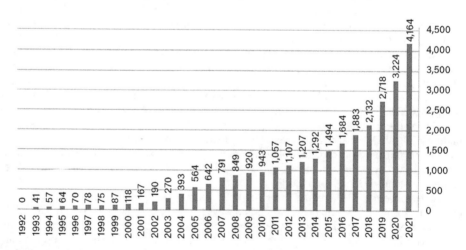

**FIGURE 6-1** DCDD donors recovered in the United States: 1992–2021.
NOTE: DCDD donors $n$ = 28,281; All DCDD + non-DCDD donors $n$ = 250,461; DCDD donor percentage = 11.3%.
SOURCE: Based on OPTN data as of January 10, 2022. https://optn.transplant.hrsa.gov/data/view-data-reports/national-data (accessed January 10, 2022).

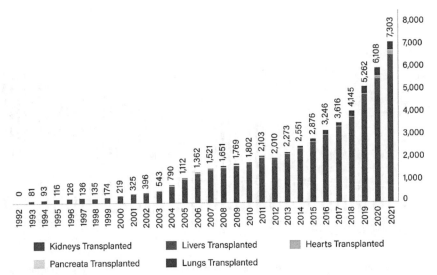

**FIGURE 6-2** DCDD organs transplanted in the United States by donor type: 1992–2021.
NOTE: Total DCDD transplants since 1992 = 53,844; total kidneys transplanted = 43,029; total livers transplanted = 7,856; total hearts transplanted = 327; total pancreata transplanted = 569; total lungs transplanted = 2,063.
SOURCE: Based on OPTN data as of January 10, 2022. https://optn.transplant.hrsa.gov/data/view-data-reports/national-data (accessed January 10, 2022).

Figure 6-3 shows the considerable variation in the proportion of DCDD donors procured at each of the 57 OPOs in 2021,[5] from a low of 11 percent to a high of 53 percent of all deceased donors within the OPO.

The committee's analysis of SRTR data for 226 out of the 240 transplant centers that had complete data from 2019 to 2021 revealed significant variation in the likelihood of transplant with a DCDD kidney across U.S. transplant centers. A small but statistically significant increasing trend was observed in use of DCDD transplants (odds ratio = 1.16, 95% confidence interval = 1.13, 1.18, $P < .0001$); the overall observed percentages were 16.2 percent in 2019, 17.4 percent in 2020, and 19.9 percent in 2021.[6]

The likelihood that a donated kidney came from a DCDD donor ranges from 1 in 45 donated kidneys at low-performing centers to 1 in 1.4 donated kidneys at high-performing centers. As discussed later in this chapter, while the possibility of acceptance of DCDD kidneys is often discussed at listing, the rate at which a transplant center accepts and uses medically complex organs, such as DCDD, is not usually discussed or made transparent to patients and families at the time of listing. As evidenced by the variation in procurement and use of DCDD organs across the country, an individual's access to a transplant can be greatly affected by the behaviors of the OPO and transplant center serving them.

---

[5] On the OPTN website, LifeLink of Puerto Rico does not have a DCDD row and did not report any 2021 DCDD data. See https://optn.transplant.hrsa.gov/data/view-data-reports/national-data (accessed January 14, 2022). Saade et al. (2005) provides a brief history of donation and transplantation in Puerto Rico.

[6] Based on committee analysis of OPTN data provided by SRTR; empirical Bayes estimates of the odds and 95% confidence intervals based on a mixed-effects logistic regression.

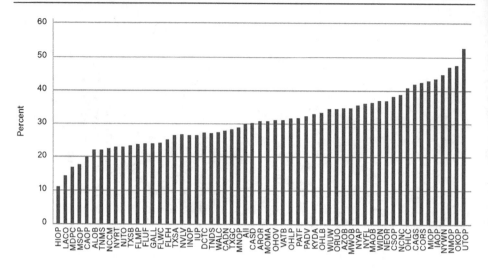

**FIGURE 6-3** Variability in percent of donation after circulatory determination of death (DCDD) donors by OPO.
NOTES: All donation services donors $n$ = 13,817. National average for all donation services areas in 2021 = 30 percent. DSA identifiers are identified by OPTN codes: the first two letters are the state where the OPO is headquartered, and the second two letters are related to what was submitted to CMS upon the original application. The full list of OPOs with key information can be found here: https://optn.transplant.hrsa.gov/about/search-membership/?memberType=Organ%20Procurement%20Organizations&organType=%27AL%27&state=0&region=0 (accessed January 25, 2022). PRLL DCDD donor percentage is not included in this figure.
SOURCE: Based on OPTN data as of January 10, 2022. https://optn.transplant.hrsa.gov/data/view-data-reports/national-data (accessed January 10, 2022).

## Special Considerations of DCDD Organs

Outcomes following transplantation with organs from DCDD donors are much improved when compared to remaining on the transplant waiting list without access to an organ. However, there are increased care requirements, higher costs, institutional difficulties, and stigmas related to use of DCDD organs that also must be considered. For kidney recipients, DCDD kidneys are associated with higher rates of delayed graft function (temporary requirement of dialysis after transplantation) compared with donation after neurological determination of death (DNDD) kidneys (Kim et al., 2020; Lia et al., 2021; van der Windt et al., 2021). DCDD lung transplant recipients may have a higher rate of renal dysfunction following transplantation, which could add to hospitalization length and potentially cost (Verzelloni Sef et al., 2021). For liver transplant recipients, the use of DCDD organs has traditionally been associated with increased risk of ischemic cholangiopathy, a devastating diagnosis that can result in multiple procedures, hospitalizations, and ultimately retransplant. The rates of ischemic cholangiopathy seem to be decreased with use of normothermic perfusion, but data are still forthcoming. Similarly, DCDD heart transplant has occurred in the setting of normothermic perfusion. Each of these potential complications is associated with increased costs of patient care for the transplant center and increased morbidity for the recipient. Some of these negative outcomes are being mitigated by normothermic perfusion and new pumping and perfusion approaches, but this technology is still novel and expensive (Padilla et al., 2021; Pearson et al., 2021). A new analysis of 136 individuals receiving heart transplants with DCDD hearts showed favorable outcomes and suggested an opportunity to increase adult heart transplantation volumes with DCDD hearts (Madan et al., 2022). Pagani (2022) notes that if DCDD heart transplantation continues to increase, clinical, economic, and ethical issues will need to be considered in order to construct a paradigm in which broader adoption of DCDD heart transplantation is possible. For example, the use of DCDD hearts will likely require changes in procedures and protocols for procuring these organs—including greater collaboration among thoracic and abdominal transplant procurement teams—as well as an increase in resources, as ex vivo perfusion equipment can cost $270,000, not including the time and materials required to use the console (Pagani, 2022).

Not only are transplant costs of care higher, there can also be higher costs for both OPOs and transplant centers in pursuit of DCDD donors. Not all DCDD donors have organs recovered because of variability in warm ischemic time, which leads to increased resource use for the OPO, and even the transplant centers pursuing these organs, potentially without any resultant organs. Additionally, while the committee feels strongly that every organ counts and is critical to pursue, DCDD donors yield fewer organs than DNDD donors, so the costs and efforts for recovery often result in fewer organs. Besides the direct costs to the OPO and transplant centers pursing the DCDD organs, there are added intangible burden and indirect costs from such things as staffing workload, administrative burden, and burnout that have not yet been comprehensively studied but may need to be considered (Kress et al., 2009). At the same time, there are OPOs and transplant centers that are successful high users of DCDD organs whose models should be shared, adapted, and used within the wider transplant community (see Chapter 7 for quality improvement initiatives). While there is the potential for increased costs to the patient, the transplant centers, and OPOs for procurement and use of DCDD organs, the pursuit and use of these organs is necessary to increase transplantation accessibility for all and improve patient outcomes.

## Relationship Between DCDD and DNDD Organs

There are important differences between DCDD and DNDD organs that complicate their procurement, use, and transplantation. DCDD donation requires circulatory cessation within a defined period of time. Prior to the increase in extra-renal transplantation of DCDD organs, 60 minutes warm ischemic time was acceptable (Kotloff et al., 2015). That time frame has shortened to 20–30 minutes as longer periods of warm time have been demonstrated to affect transplant outcomes, especially in liver transplantation (Kalisvaart et al., 2021). Predictive tools have had variable success in assessing the probability of circulatory cessation within defined time frames.

Determining neurological death is complex as well, and DNDD accounts for only approximately 2 percent of adult and 5 percent of pediatric in-hospital deaths in the United States (Greer, 2021). As with DCDD donor potential, standardized assessment of DNDD potential based on hospital-level data would be beneficial to better understand donor potential for each pathway of donation. The committee discussed concerns that the growth in DCDD was not at the expense of DNDD donors, and that it is not unusual for a DCDD donor to progress to DNDD status during the evaluation period. Growth in the recovery of organs from DNDD donors is also possible while increasing the recovery of DCDD donors. Attention is warranted to ensure that increases in DCDD procurements do not decrease DNDD procurement volume.

## Summary of DCDD Procurement and Transplantation

If the significant variations in DCDD procurement across the nation are not narrowed, there are life-threatening consequences for waiting recipients in the geographic areas served by low-performing OPOs and transplant centers with low use of DCDD organs. Overall system performance shows that the percentage of DCDD procured by the 57 OPOs of all deceased donors in 2021 was approximately 30 percent DCDD, and the highest-performing OPOs had approximately 53 percent of deceased donors from DCDD (see Figure 6-3). If all OPOs procured approximately 50 percent of donor organs from DCDD, it would be possible to double the number of DCDD donors overall to more than 6,000 donors, substantially increasing the supply of deceased donor organs for recipients on the waiting list. These key facts, together with the proven ability of the OPO and transplant community to achieve systematic improvement based on the experience of the highest performers in the system, inform the recommended national goals on DCDD outlined in Chapter 2. With the advent of normothermic perfusion of extra-renal organs in the last 3 years, utilization of livers, hearts, and lungs has increased and there are promising results for organ utilization and patient outcomes (Shah, 2021).

## Opportunities to Improve Recovery of Other Medically Complex Organs

In addition to DCDD organs, there are opportunities and initiatives to improve the recovery of other medically complex organs that were once considered off-limits, including from older donors, hepatitis C donors, HIV-positive donors, and donors with COVID-19. Organ recipients and their clinicians have always had to carefully weigh the costs and benefits of accepting medically complex organs: understanding the risk–benefit ratio of accepting and transplanting a less than perfect organ must be assessed against the possibility of receiving no transplant at all (see section on shared decision making).

### Older Donors

An area for opportunity and growth of the U.S. organ supply is ensuring recovery and use of organs that are donated from older donors. However, a recent review found that older donor age is associated with worse outcomes for liver, kidney, pancreas, heart, and lung transplantation; the donor age from which the negative survival effects start to become significant varies between organs (Dayoub et al., 2018). More organ-specific research on older deceased donors is needed. At the April 16, 2021 public webinar *International Examples of Organ Procurement, Allocation, & Distribution,*[7] Axel Rahmel, of Deutsche Stiftung Organ Transplantation, presented *Lessons from Eurotransplant* and described a successful "old for old" program where donors above 65 are preferentially allocated to recipients above 65; additionally, Beatriz Domínguez-Gil, of Organización Nacional de Trasplantes, presented data on the average age of deceased donors in Spain, with more than 50 percent over age 60, more than 30 percent over age 70, and more than 9 percent over age 80 (see section on international lessons learned for more information).

---

[7] See https://www.nationalacademies.org/event/04-16-2021/a-fairer-and-more-equitable-cost-effective-and-transparent-system-of-donor-organ-procurement-allocation-and-distribution-meeting-6 (accessed January 14, 2022).

## Hepatitis C Donors

The notion of knowingly giving an organ from an infected donor to an immunosuppressed transplant recipient may initially seem unthinkable. However, increased understanding of the diseases caused by certain pathogens, as well as the availability of new drugs to treat or prevent infections, mean that these medically complex organs can now be used successfully. In recent years, organ recipients treated prophylactically with new, highly effective hepatitis C virus (HCV) medications were protected from infection after receiving organs from HCV-infected donors for kidneys, hearts, lungs, and livers (Bethea at al., 2021; Madhusoodanan, 2021; Woolley et al., 2019). Transplanting kidneys from donors infected with HCV into patients without the virus was shown to have promising outcomes in recent single-center and multicenter studies (Goldberg et al., 2017; Sise et al., 2020). Additionally, the opioid epidemic has correlated with an increase in the supply of deceased organ donors, many of them infected with HCV; further research on HCV-positive donors is an important opportunity for increasing access to organs, particularly kidneys, for transplantation by using organs that were not often used in the past.

## HIV-Positive Donors

In transplant centers around the world, kidneys from deceased HIV-positive donors are increasingly being used for HIV-positive recipients, but the numbers are low. After they were pioneered in South Africa in 2008, surgeons have reported follow-up on 51 transplants. Since 2013, 25 have been reported in the United States (Thornton, 2021). Given advances in antiretroviral therapy, there are opportunities to explore transplanting HIV-infected organs to non–HIV positive recipients on the waiting list (Thornton, 2021).

## Donors Positive for COVID-19

While longitudinal studies have not been conducted owing to the novelty of COVID-19, there has been some early success in transplanting otherwise healthy organs from SARS-CoV-2-infected donors. One such study analyzed 10 kidney transplants from five deceased donors with new detection of SARS-CoV-2 RNA during donor evaluation in early 2021; with 8–16 weeks of follow-up, outcomes for all 10 patients and allografts had no signs or symptoms of donor-derived SARS-CoV-2 infection (Koval et al., 2021). More research is needed to understand the opportunities for organs transplanted from donors positive for COVID-19.

> Conclusion 6-2: Opportunities exist to improve the recovery of medically complex organs from older donors, hepatitis C donors, HIV-positive donors, and donors positive for COVID-19. While there are also challenges in transplant center acceptance of these organs, the challenges are similar to DCDD in terms of OPO recovery of these organs.

## Lessons from International Deceased Donor Organ Transplantation Systems

There are potential lessons to be gleaned from international deceased donor organ transplantation systems with a successful emphasis on equity. For example, Spain has implemented a comprehensive strategy to increase organ availability that may be instructive for improving organ availability in the United States (Matesanz et al., 2011). Spain's efforts include earlier referral of potential deceased donors to transplant coordination teams, benchmarking to identify success factors in donation after neurological death, family-based approaches and care methods for transplantation, and additional training for health care professionals (Matesanz et al., 2011). Other successful elements of the Spanish model include concerted efforts in professional training, active public outreach and engagement, and investment in infrastructure at the federal level. It has been proposed that a more aggressive approach to organ acceptance may benefit kidney transplant candidates in the United States.

A cohort study analyzing the use of deceased donor kidneys in the United States and France found that the kidney nonuse rate in the United States is nearly twice that of France (Aubert et al., 2019). Furthermore, a multicenter study of French donation centers found that donor kidney histology assessment, or biopsy, during allocation did not provide substantial incremental value in determining organ quality (Reese et al., 2021). Thus, the authors contended that many kidneys discarded in the United States owing to abnormal biopsies could instead be used to benefit patients on transplant waiting lists (see section on kidney biopsies for more information).

> *Conclusion 6-3: Greater than five-fold variation exists in the recovery of DCDD donors by OPOs across the country. Variation also exists in DCDD organ transplant rates by transplant centers across the country. Other nations transplant more DCDD donors than the United States with good outcomes. The committee concludes that an increase in the number of DCDD organs procured by OPOs, coupled with improved organ offer acceptance and use practices of transplant centers, would yield a significant number of organs for waiting candidates. With the innovation of ex vivo organ perfusion for liver, heart, and lungs, there is an increased opportunity to expand the donor pool with DCDD donation and increase the organs available that were not previously considered for transplant.*

## TRANSPLANT CENTER REGULATORY FRAMEWORK AND PERFORMANCE METRICS

Each of the approximately 250 transplant programs in the United States is subject to oversight by two federal entities. First, CMS has a long-term regulatory oversight perspective and the ability to decertify a transplant center if outcomes are not met.[8] Second, the OPTN uses its committee structure and responsibility for implementing NOTA and the OPTN Final Rule to frequently consider data on transplant center performance and to take corrective actions for individual transplant centers if needed.

### CMS Oversight of Transplant Centers

All transplant programs are housed within a hospital and since 2007 must comply with Medicare and specific hospital conditions of participation governing data submission, clinical experience, outcome, and process requirements for transplanting heart, lung, liver, kidney, pancreas, or intestine (CMS, 2020c). CMS relies on onsite evaluation of transplant programs, as well as data from the OPTN, to evaluate a transplant program's compliance with Medicare requirements. Transplant programs are required to maintain patient and graft

---

[8] CMS only has oversight over transplant programs that are certified for participation in Medicare. This is not a requirement, and there may be some transplant programs that are not certified by CMS. The OPTN has oversight over all transplant programs.

survival rates within CMS tolerance limits. In 2016, evidence indicated that transplant centers responded to the conditions of participation by removing sicker patients awaiting liver transplant to avoid harming the transplant center's performance according to CMS standards. The study also found that conditions of participation did not significantly affect 1-year posttransplant mortality as intended (Dolgin et al., 2016). In 2016, CMS noted that "we are concerned that transplant programs may avoid using certain available organs that they believe might adversely affect the program's outcome statistics" and revised its guidelines to broaden the acceptable "standard level" to include outcomes between 150 and 185 percent of the risk-adjusted expected number (CMS, 2016, p. 1).

## OPTN Oversight of Transplant Centers

The OPTN also has a role in overseeing transplant programs and requiring corrective action as needed. The OPTN Membership and Professional Standards Committee (MPSC), operating on behalf of the OPTN Board, is responsible for monitoring OPTN member compliance with membership criteria, OPTN policies, and the 2020 Final Rule. The SRTR contractor provides statistical and analytical support to the OPTN, as well as support in areas such as policy formulation and evaluation, system performance metrics, and economic analysis (SRTR, 2022a). SRTR's mission is to keep transplant programs, OPOs, policy makers, organ donors and families, and the public informed about the current state of solid organ transplantation in the United States. This is in alignment with the Final Rule, which states that the OPTN and SRTR "make available to the public timely and accurate program-specific information on the performance of transplant programs" and identify transplant programs and OPOs with better or worse outcomes.[9]

SRTR developed a five-tier outcome assessment system to present pre- and posttransplant performance metrics to make it easier for the public to understand and compare the outcomes of different transplant programs (SRTR, 2022b). Assessments are presented for three metrics: (1) survival on the waiting list (i.e., waiting list mortality rate), (2) getting a transplant faster (i.e., transplant rate), and (3) 1-year organ survival (i.e., first-year graft survival) (SRTR, 2022b). The SRTR performance assessment methodology calculates center performance for each statistic, producing a program score between 0 and 1 that is converted to one of five tier assignments, with higher scores and tiers indicating likely better performance (SRTR, 2022b). Transplant program-specific reports and OPO-specific reports are produced semiannually. CMS and the OPTN MPSC use the SRTR performance assessment methodology for 1-year organ survival to review transplant program performance (Kasiske et al., 2016).[10]

## Incentives in Transplant Center Performance

It is the committee's belief and experience that transplant providers intend to act in the best interests of their patients to review organ offers, accept the best organ for that patient, and perform a successful transplant. As indicated above, there is evidence to suggest that some transplant providers might be rejecting good organ offers that could benefit the recipient because of a reluctance to perform riskier surgeries (meaning procedures with either

---

[9] OPTN Final Rule 121.11(b)(iv), 2021.

[10] New transplant center performance metrics were approved by the OPTN Membership and Professional Standards Committee with implementation planned to begin in June 2022. See Chapter 7 for additional information, as well as https://optn.transplant.hrsa.gov/media/yctffgt2/20211206-bp-mpsc-enhnc-tx-prgrm-prfrmnc-mntrng-syst.pdf (accessed February 15, 2022).

medically complex organs or less than ideal patients) for fear it could damage the transplant center's statistics (Yasinski, 2016). As discussed earlier in this report, the OPTN oversight mechanisms for the organ transplantation system begin only at the time a patient is added to the waiting list. As one component of the system, transplant centers are currently only accountable for the patients that receive a transplant.

The current five-tier assessment system for transplant centers creates incentives and associated behaviors of transplant centers that are inconsistent with the Final Rule. If transplant programs are evaluated in terms of maximizing waiting list survival and 1-year organ survival, they will be incentivized to only accept what they believe to be the highest-quality organs and list the least severely ill patients. While this behavior may result in increased performance according to 1-year posttransplant survival, it will result in decreased survival benefit for patients who remain on the waiting list compared to receiving a transplant. Transplantation of more medically urgent patients who have decreased waiting list survival, yet still have excellent posttransplant survival, could save more lives. There is also concern that the current transplant center performance metrics will lead to increases, or at least not decreases, in the already high organ nonuse rate, and continued lack of equity for minority populations who, for example, have twice the accrued dialysis time upon entry to the waiting list.

Although CMS no longer uses 1-year posttransplant survival for either the patient or the graft as a metric for transplant center certification, publicly available data on transplant center performance relies heavily on this statistic (Yasinski, 2016). Every 6 months, the SRTR releases a publicly available assessment of each transplant center in the country, using 1-year posttransplant survival rates for patients or grafts as a key metric (Yasinski, 2016). However, the difference between performance tiers for transplant programs is often just a single point or two.

Some suggest that the current incentives for transplant centers push providers to keep older, sicker patients off the waiting list even if they would benefit from transplant, because transplanting these patients could be riskier than transplanting younger, healthier patients. Another way to correct poor performance ratings under the current system is for a transplant center to dramatically reduce the number of transplants performed. Reducing the number of transplants can increase posttransplant survival rates and therefore the center's rankings, allowing the center to remain in business. However, this approach limits access to lifesaving transplants to patients that a transplant center would have treated just a year or so before.

*Conclusion 6-4: The organ transplantation system is not accountable to all patients who need an organ transplant. A shift is needed toward policies that engender accountability to all patients in need of a transplant.*

*Conclusion 6-5: There is a need to create new performance metrics for transplant centers that go beyond one-dimensional evaluations of 1-year patient and graft survival. There is an opportunity to further improve transplant center performance metrics in order to capture factors that are critically important to patients, such as time waiting before transplant, likelihood of survival on the waiting list prior to transplant, and overall added benefit of the transplant in terms of survival over remaining on the waiting list. There is also a need for an independent assessment of any proposed performance metrics before adoption by the government, which would include a focus on equity in access to transplant referral and evaluation, as well as equity in access to transplant once evaluated and added to the waiting list.*

## KEY AREA FOR IMPROVEMENT FOR TRANSPLANT CENTERS: ORGAN USE

As noted throughout this report, the organ donation and transplantation system in the United States is the largest and most sophisticated system of its kind in the world. Countless hours and resources are expended by thoughtful and dedicated professionals to ensure compliance with NOTA and the Final Rule, to create organ allocation policies that are based on sound medical judgment, to seek to achieve the best use of donated organs, and to aim to achieve equitable allocation of organs among patients through distribution over as broad a geographic area as feasible and in order of decreasing medical urgency.[11] Using the combination of donor and candidate information, the OPTN computer system generates a "match run," which is a rank-order list of candidates to be offered each organ that is unique to each donor and each organ (UNOS, 2021a). The candidates who appear highest in the ranking are those who are in most urgent need of the transplant, and/or those most likely to have the best chance of survival if transplanted. While this process is well defined by policy, the actual acceptance and transplantation of an available organ to a recipient is much more complicated.[12]

The successful treatment of end-stage organ failure through transplantation continues to fuel demand for deceased donor organs, with the waiting list outpacing the number of transplants performed. However, in practice, many recovered organs are not used (SRTR, 2021). SRTR data show that in 2019, 14.3 percent of all recovered organs were not transplanted, an increase from the 13.2 percent reported in both 2017 and 2018 (Israni et al., 2021). There has been little movement in improving overall nonuse of recovered organs, and in 2019, 4,460 kidneys, 345 pancreata, 874 livers, 5 intestines, 31 hearts, and 338 lungs were not used compared to lower numbers in 2018—3,755 kidneys, 278 pancreata, 707 livers, 3 intestines, 23 hearts, and 317 lungs were procured but not transplanted (Israni et al., 2021). Thus, the nonuse problem is increasing in severity.

Compounding the problem of nonuse of organs is the size of the waiting list. The waiting list for kidneys is six times longer than the number of transplants performed, the liver waiting list is three times longer than the number of transplants performed, and the heart and lung waiting lists are double the number of transplants performed (OPTN, 2021a). Combining the year over year increase in the nonuse of recovered organs with organ demand exceeding supply, there is significant room for improvement in this area, especially in regard to kidneys, which represent 84.7 percent of the waiting list in February 2022.[13] As of September 2021, the proportion of kidneys from deceased donors that were recovered for transplant but ultimately not transplanted remains at approximately 20 percent (OPTN, 2021a; Stewart et al., 2017), with a projected 2021 rate of 23 percent (see Figure 6-4). This is representative of an upward trend, with a 91.5 percent increase in nonuse of deceased donor kidney between 2000 to 2015, despite organ quality remaining stable (King et al., 2021; Mohan et al., 2018).

---

[11] 63 FR 16332 Apr. 2, 1998, see https://www.ecfr.gov/current/title-42/chapter-I/subchapter-K/part-121 (accessed January 27, 2022).

[12] Patients and members of the public consider placement on the transplant waiting list to be an implicit promise of fair, unbiased treatment under a transparent allocation scheme; current practice may not be living up to that promise in a variety of ways (Segev et al., 2008).

[13] As of February 3, 2022, there were 90,315 candidates waiting for a kidney transplant out of a total of 106,616 candidates waiting for any type of organ transplant. 90,135/106,616 = 84.7 percent. https://optn.transplant.hrsa.gov/data/view-data-reports/national-data (accessed February 3, 2022).

As depicted in Figure 6-4, the nonuse of organs has increased, even as OPOs increased the number of donors over the same period (Mohan et al., 2021; OPTN, 2021a). This increase in nonuse of kidneys has sometimes been attributed to risk-averse behavior by transplant providers worried about the effect of transplanting medically complex organs, or concern over the effect of transplanting sicker patients, on the transplant center 1-year posttransplant survival metric. Although a factor, this explanation alone does not justify the variation seen in organ use and acceptance practices across transplant centers.

Mohan et al. (2021) reviewed data from 2000 to 2015 that confirmed an overlap in the quality of kidneys that are transplanted with those that are not used (Figure 6-5). While the nonuse of some kidneys may be unavoidable, the data suggest there are opportunities to facilitate increased use. Nonused kidneys are most likely to come from older, higher body mass index, black, female donors with comorbidities of diabetes and hypertension. The organ nonuse rate for livers increased from 8.6 percent in 2018 to 9.6 percent in 2019, driven by increased nonuse of grafts from donors aged 55 years or older and, to a lesser extent, those of donors aged 30–54 years. Livers recovered from DCDD donors remained four times more likely to *not* be used than livers recovered from DNDD donors (29.9 percent versus 7.1 percent, respectively) (Kwong et al., 2021; SRTR, 2019).

*Conclusion 6-6: Two facets of the organ transplantation system are in tension. Priority on each organ waiting list is based on formal, publicly announced policies, and organs are allocated by match-run algorithms; on the other hand, a patient's access to an organ offered depends on how the transplant professionals in the program caring for the patient exercise the discretion that the system gives them regarding when to accept or reject an organ for transplantation. This divergence—which is not transparent either to the general public or to all patients on the waiting list—has implications for equitable treatment of all patients, for adherence to the ethical principles of autonomy and beneficence, and for trust in the system.*

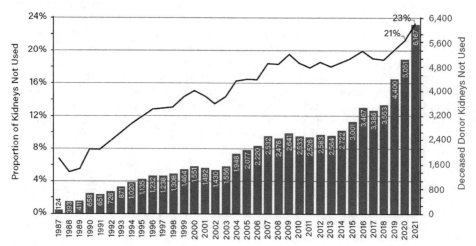

**FIGURE 6-4** Proportion and number of nonused deceased donor kidneys (1987–2021).
SOURCE: Mohan et al., 2021.
NOTE: 2021 rate is based on annualized OPTN data projected based on the first 8 months of 2021.

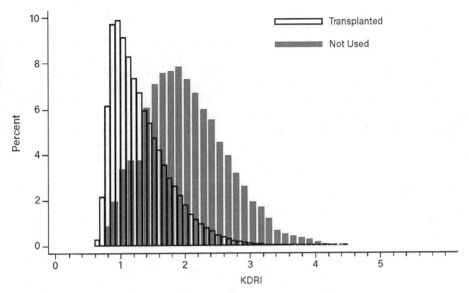

**FIGURE 6-5** Significant overlap exists in the quality of kidneys transplanted and not used.
NOTES: Percentage is calculated using data from 2000 through 2015. KDRI = kidney donor risk index.
SOURCE: Mohan et al., 2018.

## The Challenges of Use and Reasons for Nonuse

Policy prescriptions—administrative or organizational solutions within transplant programs—must mitigate against the ongoing increase in nonuse (King et al., 2019), and waiting patients should be informed of operational factors that are not related to organ supply that may affect their access to organs. There are numerous factors that may affect nonuse that are touched on briefly below.

### Donor Quality

Donor quality alone cannot explain the steady increase over time in the organ nonuse rate. Using a donor utilization index, Brennan et al. (2019) assessed 182 transplant centers' use practices with kidneys perceived as having a high risk from 2010 to 2016, and found that there was significant variation by OPTN region, revealing geographic trends in kidney use and nonuse. Similarly, an examination of regional changes in donor heart acceptance patterns found differences in acceptance and use patterns by geographic area, and suggested that these variations may reflect differences between transplant centers' willingness to accept donor hearts with higher risk,[14] differences in OPOs' cardiac evaluation and allocation practices, or a combination of both (Khush et al., 2015). When all organ allocation and distribution policies are fully migrated to the continuous distribution model, it will be

---

[14] In June 2020, the Centers for Disease Control and Prevention published a U.S. Health Service Guideline stating a change in terminology from *increased risk donor* to *risk criteria present for acute HIV, HBV and HCV infection*. See https://www.cdc.gov/mmwr/volumes/69/rr/rr6904a1.htm?s_cid=rr6904a1_w (accessed February 15, 2022).

important to continue monitoring the weight of the effects on organ acceptance and nonuse rates of policies not grounded in geography.

Transplant center size and regional competition may affect the variability of the nonuse rate. Volk et al. (2011) found that the transplant centers performing the most transplants and those with competing centers in their OPO were more likely to use increased risk organs,[15] particularly among recipients with lower Model for End-Stage Liver Disease (MELD) scores. Transplant centers using increased risk organs had equivalent waiting list mortality rates but tended to have higher posttransplant mortality. Future research on assessing the variabilities of nonuse rates across transplant centers, as well as potential interventions, is needed.

While the problem of demand exceeding the supply is a global issue, the deceased donor kidney nonuse rate in the United States is high relative to other similarly developed countries (Mohan et al., 2018; Stewart et al., 2017). By comparison, the nonuse rate in the United States is nearly twice that of France (Aubert et al., 2019). In fact, in a 2019 study, researchers found that 62 percent of kidneys not used in the United States would be successfully transplanted in France (Aubert et al., 2019). Sometimes, selectivity can also be a reason for organ nonuse rates. Li et al. (2021) reviewed the use of kidneys during the COVID-19 pandemic in 2020 and found that transplant centers that continued transplantation during the first surge used lower Kidney Donor Profile Index (KDPI) kidneys, while allowing the nonuse rate to rise. However, some of the high nonuse rate in the United States could be skewed by the common practice of recovering organs before obtaining transplant center acceptance. This is contrary to practices in areas such as the United Kingdom where "recovering [an organ] is conditional on acceptance. Hence, the United Kingdom discard rate reflects post-acceptance dynamics whereas U.S. [nonuse] rates reflect possibilities as well as kidneys that were recovered but not accepted by any U.S. transplant center" (Ibrahim et al., 2020). In the United States, donor hearts are not recovered until accepted for transplant, while kidneys are often recovered without acceptance for transplant and sometimes before the offers are sent to transplant centers. This could be an explanation for why nonuse rates are lower for hearts than other organs in the United States.

## Organ Biopsies

Mohan et al. (2018) analyzed the reported reasons for nonuse in over 36,000 kidney offers from 2000 to 2015, and "biopsy findings" made up 38 percent of responses, making it the most commonly cited reason for nonuse. Other commonly cited reasons for nonuse include

- "no recipient located," meaning an OPO was unable to find a willing transplant center to accept the organ (15 percent);
- "poor organ function" (10 percent);
- "donor history" (8 percent);
- "anatomical abnormalities" (7 percent); and
- "organ damage" (4 percent).

For over 20 years, biopsies have been the most frequently cited reason for kidney non-use, accounting for one-third of all kidneys not used (Stewart et al., 2017). There is growing evidence that biopsies may not significantly augment the prediction of outcomes beyond

---

[15] The phrase *increased risk* refers to the donor characteristics that could place the potential recipient at increased risk of disease transmission. See https://optn.transplant.hrsa.gov/governance/public-comment/guidance-on-phs-increased-risk-donor-organs (accessed February 15, 2022).

estimates using clinical criteria (e.g., age and KDPI) (Reese et al., 2021). This is a growing concern given that over 50 percent of all kidneys removed for transplant undergo biopsy. Lentine et al. (2021) called for a randomized controlled trial of biopsy use to determine if and when a procurement biopsy should be used in the decision to accept or decline an organ offer. The OPTN's Kidney Transplantation Committee has approved a Donor Criteria to Require Kidney Biopsy proposal for public comment in early 2022 (OPTN, 2021b).

In a retrospective study of prospectively collected data from the UNOS Standard Transplant Analysis and Research database, Steggerda et al. (2020) reviewed biopsies from deceased organ donors between 2006 and 2015 in order to consider higher macrosteatosis thresholds for liver transplantation. While it was a limited study, the results were able to identify a threshold macrosteatosis level for safe transplantation and characterize the donor and recipient factors that contribute to short- and long-term graft survival among steatotic allografts in the modern transplant era.

## Health Care Use and Organizational Issues

There are organizational and systemic factors that extend beyond organ quality that appear to also be contributing to the high rate of nonuse of deceased donor organs in the United States.

## Weekend Effect of Nonuse

There has been compelling research on the "weekend effect" for kidneys and livers. In SRTR data from 2000 to 2013, and compared with weekday kidneys, organs procured on weekends were significantly more likely to not be used (odds ratio: 1.16; 95% confidence interval: 1.13–1.19), even after adjusting for organ quality (adjusted odds ratio: 1.13; 95% confidence interval: 1.10–1.17) (see Figures 6-6 and 6-7) (King et al., 2019; Mohan et al., 2016). Program structure and staffing, particularly during weekends and in smaller programs,

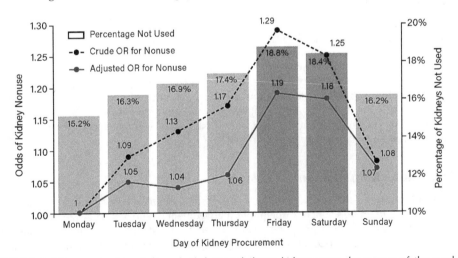

**FIGURE 6-6** Rate and odds of discard of deceased donor kidneys over the course of the week, 2000–2013.
NOTE: OR = odds ratio.
SOURCE: Mohan et al., 2016.

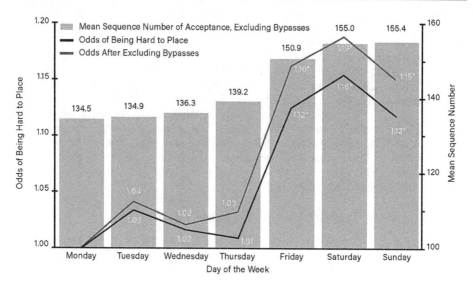

**FIGURE 6-7** Mean sequence number of accepted offer and adjusted odds of becoming a hard-to-place kidney (acceptance sequence number > 100) were higher on the weekend for transplanted deceased donor kidneys from 2008 to 2015.

NOTES: Day of the week refers to the day of the first offer for the kidney. Automatically bypassed offers are not included in the "excluding bypasses" calculations. Compared with kidneys offered on Mondays, kidneys offered on Fridays, Saturdays, and Sundays had a higher mean sequence number of accepted offer and adjusted odds of becoming a hard-to-place kidney (reference is Monday; adjusted for Kidney Donor Profile Index).

$P \leq .001$.

SOURCE: King et al., 2019.

affects kidney use and ultimately affects a patient's chances of receiving a transplant (King et al., 2019). This is unacceptable for a lifesaving surgical procedure such as transplantation.

Carpenter et al. (2019) observed that livers available for likely-weekend transplants were 11 percent more likely to be not used than their weekday counterparts, despite no differences in organ quality. This effect size was consistent and remained even after adjusting for other variables relating to donor, organ, and other factors. Rates of liver biopsy, macrosteatosis on biopsy, HCV-positive seropositivity, and donor risk factors were similar for both weekend and weekday transplants (Carpenter et al., 2019).

## Operations Management

Contributing to the "weekend effect" are hospital surgical scheduling and flow challenges where an entire science of operations management would help alleviate this universal issue. Systematic attention to operations management issues in nurse staffing, availability of rooms for surgical procedures, and availability of hospital beds posttransplant require collaboration and process change across the entire hospital enterprise. Litvak et al. (2021) describe an effective strategy to improve hospital efficiency, the quality of care, and timely access to care for emergent and urgent surgeries by classifying the time and resource needs of surgical patients and smoothing the flow of surgical admissions over all days of the week.

When organ nonuse is attributed to hospital operational management limitations rather than clinical quality or patient readiness, the result is a less equitable, less transparent, and less efficient organ transplantation system.

> *Conclusion 6-7: Nonuse of organs is higher on Fridays, Saturdays, and Sundays. This weekend effect can be mitigated through appropriate planning and surgical scheduling management, including issues related to nurse staffing, availability of hospital beds for patients receiving a transplant, and the availability of surgical units.*

The science of operations management has been used successfully to smooth surgical scheduling and better manage flow in multiple hospitals, including the Mayo Clinic of Florida, Boston Medical Center, Cincinnati Children's Hospital Medical Center, and Toronto's University Health Network (Litvak et al., 2021; Ryckman et al., 2009; Smith et al., 2013). This method requires first separating hospital resources (e.g., operating rooms) used for elective and unscheduled procedures and then ensuring that similar numbers of elective admissions occur in different hospital wards each day (Litvak and Fineberg, 2013).

Implementing proven processes to smooth surgical scheduling makes it possible for hospitals to have operating rooms, surgical staffing, ICU rooms, and other resources available to systematically deal with urgent, unscheduled surgeries when they arise (Litvak and Fineberg, 2013). Offers of lifesaving organs on Fridays, Saturdays, and Sundays provide a compelling example of the need for hospitals to properly plan for and ensure the availability of surgical capacity. A number of strategies to implement surgical schedule smoothing across hospitals with transplant centers could be used, including but not limited to systematic quality improvement to spread this known best practice; financial or payment incentives to hospitals that use these methods to ensure access to lifesaving, urgent surgical procedures such as transplants; and Conditions of Participation and/or Interpretive Guidelines by CMS surveyors to ensure that hospitals are properly managing surgical schedules to ensure access to emergency surgeries like transplants. In addition to ongoing commitment from hospital leaders, regulatory systems will need to support efforts to keep hospitals from overcrowding and improve patient morbidity and mortality (Kelen et al., 2021).

Not only does hospital flow affect the scheduling of organ transplants, it can also affect the timing of the organ donor procurement surgery. It is not uncommon for organ donor cases to be "bumped" to accommodate trauma or elective surgeries. The delay in the surgical recovery of deceased organs can lead to deterioration of organ function, making the organ less likely to be transplanted. An innovative solution for organ recovery are OPO-managed donor care units that do not depend on surgical suite availability and that offer improved transplant outcomes (see section on donor care units later in this chapter).

## Waiting List Management

Organ transplant waiting list management has become increasingly complex across all organ types, but especially in the kidney population. Large transplant programs report upwards of 1,000 or more kidney patients on their waiting list, underscoring the importance of assessing for transplant readiness, communication of waiting list status, and patient education. Husain et al. (2018) reported that nearly one in five kidneys is offered as a primary offer to a deceased patient on the waiting list, contributing to less efficiency in the process of organ offers, and perhaps contributing to organ nonuse. Understanding that 20 percent of kidney offers are to deceased individuals on the waiting list is exactly the type of situation that undermines public trust in the organ transplantation system. See Chapter 5 for more information.

## KEY AREA FOR IMPROVEMENT FOR TRANSPLANT CENTERS: ORGAN OFFER ACCEPTANCE

The U.S. organ transplantation system was built and designed primarily to maximize the ability of transplant centers and surgeons to exercise choice in accepting and transplanting organs. As stated earlier in this chapter, the system is *perfectly designed to achieve the results it gets*. For example, currently less than 1 percent of kidney offers are accepted (0.76 percent) (SRTR, 2021). Over 1.5 million offers were made to place the approximately 23,000 kidneys transplanted in 2019 (SRTR, 2021).

Understanding and improving variation in the acceptance of offered organs can decrease the nonuse rate if offers are purposefully made to programs likely to accept them. Standardizing and spreading best practices and improving allocation system efficiency will lead to a more fair, equitable, and transparent system. These opportunities are more fully outlined in Chapter 2 on goal setting and in Chapter 7 on quality improvement.

Each organ is "offered" to multiple transplant centers based on the formalized allocation systems previously designed and discussed in Chapter 5. The offers for a single organ are sent out sequentially based on a patient-by-patient basis to the transplant center where the patient is listed for transplant.

At the time of the organ offer, a transplant center assesses both the organ and the patient and determines if the organ is suitable for transplant for that patient at that moment at that center. A center can decline or accept an organ for each of its eligible patients in the sequence determined by the match run, or it can decline for all patients at their center. Reasons for offer declines are often multifactorial and are denoted by the center using refusal codes (discussed in detail below). The code categories include donor and candidate matching, organ specific, candidate specific, histocompatibility related, disease transmission risk, donor specific, and logistics, among other reasons (UNOS, 2021b). Like organ nonuse rates, the acceptance rates of organ offers vary significantly across transplant centers, and while the data are well documented, the behaviors that influence the decision-making process of accepting or declining an organ offer are less transparent and not well understood. The goal of allocation policy is to identify the best candidate for that organ and to have the transplant occur in a timely and efficient manner. Transplant centers receive many primary offers of organs for candidates on their waiting lists, and the offer may or may not be the best organ for that particular patient. There are significant data showing wide variation in acceptance rates across all organ types that result in inefficiency, potentially increasing the rates of nonused organs. Additionally, most of the primary organ offers are not accepted (Wolfe et al., 2007).

Mohan et al. (2021) present data that show the variability of nonuse that directly affects the probability of getting a kidney transplant within 3 years, and SRTR data confirm the variation in organ offer acceptance rates across all organs (King et al., 2020). This type of variation in performance across transplant centers results in severe consequences for those on waiting lists, including death. Organ offer acceptance ratios vary by more than 400 percent for kidneys, with similar levels of variation for other organ types (see Figure 6-8).

Variation in offer acceptance practices across transplant programs is larger than variation in other transplant program performance metrics, such as first-year outcomes, 3-year outcomes, waiting list mortality rate, or transplant rate. SRTR data suggest that there are programs accepting offers at rates about 80 percent lower than expected (ratios below 0.2), while other programs accept at rates 3.5 to 6 times the expected rate. These variations in organ offer acceptance practices reveal major differences in transplant center organ acceptance behavior, which impacts equitable access to transplant for waiting patients and can impact the efficient placement and ultimate acceptance of available organs. Figure 6-8 below details the variation in offer acceptance rates for all organ types, even after SRTR adjustments in the rates to account for differences in characteristics of candidates on their waiting list, quality of the offered organ, and geographic factors.

Choi et al. (2020) found that the rate at which U.S. heart transplant centers accepted a first-rank offer for a candidate on their waiting list varied significantly from 12.3 to 61.5 percent, with lower organ offer acceptance rates being associated with an increased risk of waiting list mortality. Additionally, another study observed marked variability in center practices regarding accepting livers allocated to the highest-priority patients, and that patients' odds of dying on the waiting list without a transplant were significantly increased by center-level decisions to decline organs (Goldberg et al., 2016). Mulvihill et al. (2020) also found that among 65 transplant centers, organ offer acceptance rates for lungs varied significantly, from 9 to 67 percent.

King et al. (2020) found geographic disparities in rates of kidney transplantation and concluded that practices in transplant centers versus differences in local organ supply and demand are unclear. Figure 6-9 compares the probability of receiving a deceased donor kidney transplant within 3 years of waiting list placement across centers. The variation is across all centers in the United States with a 16-fold variance between centers. Waiting patients at transplant centers with low offer acceptance rates have only a 4 percent chance of getting a transplant within 3 years. Conversely, patients waiting at transplant centers with high offer acceptance rates have a 65 percent chance of getting a transplant

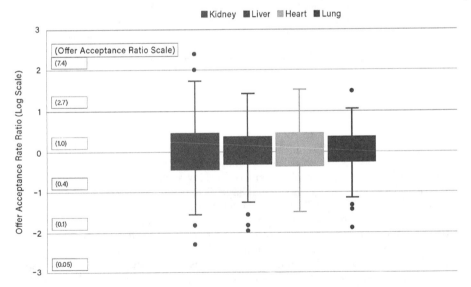

**FIGURE 6-8** Variation in offer acceptance rate ratios by organ type.
NOTE: The boxplots describe variation in offer acceptance practices within kidney, liver, heart, and lung transplant programs. Variation generally ranges from offer acceptance rate ratios of approximately 0.10 (90% lower offer acceptance rate than expected) to a high of approximately 5 (400% higher offer acceptance rate than expected). Offers between January 1 and December 31, 2020, were evaluated.
SOURCE: Scientific Registry of Transplant Recipients. Request for Information. Requested on October 5, 2021.

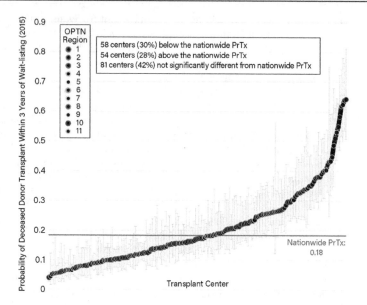

**FIGURE 6-9** The distribution of adjusted center-level probability of deceased donor kidney transplant within 3 years of wait listing in 2015 varied considerably nationwide, ranging from 4.0% to 64.2%.

NOTES: Probabilities are for the average patient (man, nonblack, PRA < 98%, no diabetes, nonobese, mean age and dialysis vintage at listing in the region). Each dot represents one center, and each color outline represents one OPTN region. Gray bars represent the 95% confidence intervals around each center's probability. Nationwide PrTx is the probability of deceased donor transplant within 3 years for all kidney transplant candidates in the United States added to the waiting list in 2015 in a national model.

SOURCE: King et al., 2020.

within 3 years (King et al., 2020). This is an inequitable and unacceptable level of variation in behavior and performance. Additionally, Figure 6-10 illustrates an up to 10-fold variation existing between transplant centers working with the same local organ supply (King et al., 2020). The authors suggest that large disparities between centers for likelihood of receiving a timely transplant may be related to center-level practice variations rather than geographic differences in underlying organ supply or patient case mix (King et al., 2020). These data challenge the conventional wisdom that variations in organ supply are the principal reason for geographic inequities in the ability of patients to get a transplant; instead, it points to the conclusion that the variations are largely a function of transplant center offer acceptance practices. As significant differences exist in the decision to accept an organ for transplant, standardizing center-level offer acceptance practices to the levels achieved by high-performing centers through further intervention has the potential to minimize waiting list mortality.

On average, patients who die waiting for a kidney had offers for 16 kidneys that were ultimately transplanted into other patients, indicating that many transplant centers refuse viable kidney offers on behalf of those on the waiting list (Husain et al., 2019).

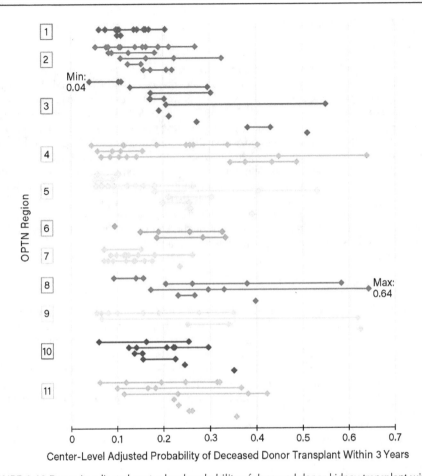

**FIGURE 6-10** Range in adjusted center-level probability of deceased donor kidney transplant within 3 years of wait listing in 2015 showing significant variation within and across DSAs.
NOTES: Each point represents one transplant center, and each level along the *y* axis represents one of the 58 DSAs, grouped by OPTN region. Each horizontal line illustrates the range in probability of transplant between centers in a given DSA. DSA = donation service area.
SOURCE: King et al., 2020.

It is important to note that programs have the option to apply broad organ offer filters (see section that follows on organ offer filters), ensuring that they do not receive organ offers that they believe they will not use. These programs do not get offers for organs in the filtered category for any of their patients. Programs applying filters may have higher organ offer acceptance rates than programs not utilizing filters because the "filtered" offers are not used in calculations of organ offer acceptance rates. Therefore, organ offer acceptance rates may not fully reflect accessibility to organs for patients on the waiting list at a particular center. As more organ offer filter options are developed, the interplay between filters, organ offer acceptance rates, and patient outcomes should be further evaluated.

# Understanding Organ Offer Tools

## Refusal Codes

Selectivity can be a reason for organ nonuse rates, and better information will inform understanding of the low rates of organ offer acceptance. The OPTN Final Rule requires transplant programs to provide the OPTN with "reasons for refusal" of organ offers made to candidates registered at their programs. The OPTN Policy *18.3, Recording and Reporting the Outcomes of Organ Offers,*[16] accordingly requires these reasons to be reported to the OPTN. Based on community feedback that codes from 2004 were outdated, too vague, and required clarification, new codes went into effect in December 2021. By providing more relevant and granular options, the insights gathered will improve upon the current list by reducing the overuse of the refusal code "donor age or quality," which accounted for 66 percent of the primary refusal reasons entered between July 2019 and June 2020.[17] These new codes are intended to provide better data for quality improvement, for retrospective reviews, and for deciding in real time whether to accept or decline an organ. The utility of the codes for these purposes depends upon transplant centers accurately reporting the reasons they refused the offered organ.

## Organ Offer Filters

Organ offer filters were first introduced by the OPTN in 2007 as a way to increase the efficiency of organ placement and to reduce the number of nonused kidneys. The concept was operationalized as a voluntary project where filters allowed a transplant center to screen out donor characteristics that would have little likelihood of being accepted for transplant, either for an individual patient or their entire waiting list. Filter settings include a broad range of characteristics, including medical history, intravenous drug use, age, history of diabetes, cold ischemia time, and pathway for determination of death (DCDD vs. DNDD).

In an analysis of organ offer filters from 2007 to 2019 in 175 kidney programs, King et al. (2022) noted that centers demonstrate a "fear of missing out" that has created less efficiency in the system, with very few centers having both restrictive filter settings and high offer acceptance. Over time, there has been an increase in the consideration of donors with a history of IV drug usage; however, more centers are unwilling to consider HCV+ donors, despite evidence in the safety of using these organs (see section on hepatitis C donors).

There are opportunities for refinement as current organ offer filters are not optimized to the fullest extent to increase organ allocation efficiency (Mohan et al., 2021) (see Box 6-3). In addition to whether a kidney transplant center optimizes the tool in organ acceptance practices, how the tool is structured and collected is not synchronized with available data analysis files, making it more difficult to understand how settings may impact actual transplant outcomes. The ability for a transplant center to bypass organ offers also raises the question about the variability in access to transplant for patients on the waiting list.

---

[16] See https://optn.transplant.hrsa.gov/media/4639/update_to_refusal_codes_mini-brief.pdf (accessed January 14, 2022) and 42 C.F.R. §121.7(b)(4).

[17] Based on OPTN data as of September 18, 2020. See https://optn.transplant.hrsa.gov/media/4639/update_to_refusal_codes_mini-brief.pdf (accessed February 16, 2022).

| BOX 6-3 | STRATEGIES TO IMPROVE THE USEFULNESS OF BYPASS FILTERS FOR THE ALLOCATION OF DECEASED DONOR ORGANS |
|---|---|

The OPTN could potentially encourage increased appropriate use of filters with the following strategies:

- Change default filter settings to reflect the prior calendar year behavior at the center while allowing centers to change those filters.
- Align the filters with available data so centers make informed choices about how restrictive they would like to be with respect to organ offers.
- Bypass filters should ideally apply to all organ offers and not just the small number that come through specific pathways.
- Provide centers with feedback reports similar to the organ offer report to help them understand the implication of their choices for their patients.
- Increased center-level transparency on how centers are setting their filters would allow patients to recognize centers that have choices that align with their preferences. Increased transparency of these settings is also likely to improve clinician judgment of the appropriate filter settings.

SOURCE: Mohan et al., 2021.

## Expedited Placement of Organs

Expedited placement can reduce delays in allocation by routing less-than-ideal organs to transplant centers with a proven willingness to use these organs (Mohan and Schold, 2021). Under the current system expedited placement (sometimes called "accelerated placement" or "out-of-sequence" allocation) allows an OPO to indicate exceptional circumstances in order to deviate from the policy-mandated match run that dictates patient priority for organ offers on the waiting list. When there are suboptimal donor characteristics related to donor disease or recovery-related issues, OPOs may turn to this discretionary tool of expedited placement to avoid nonuse of the organ (Giorgakis and Mathur, 2020; King et al., 2022). Expedited organ placement has been an important tool in organ allocation for many years as it allows OPOs to quickly place organs they believe are at risk of not being used for transplantation.

The committee heard testimony from international programs that have successful expedited placement strategies.[18] For example, both the Eurotransplant rescue allocation system and the UK Kidney Fast Track Scheme incorporate considerable flexibility for participating centers and have resulted in more than 50 percent of the organs that enter these pathways being transplanted (Callaghan et al., 2017).

While expedited placement can increase the use of organs, the necessary policy development and practice improvements to support expedited placement have generally lagged. Results remain to be evaluated for an expedited liver placement policy that went into effect

---

[18] See https://www.nationalacademies.org/event/04-16-2021/a-fairer-and-more-equitable-cost-effective-and-transparent-system-of-donor-organ-procurement-allocation-and-distribution-meeting-6 (accessed February 16, 2022).

in March 2021, providing guidance for OPOs and transplant centers, and instituting a consistent practice across the country for access to expedited offers. The 2019-2020 Kidney Accelerated Placement project implemented by the OPTN Organ Center offered kidneys with a high KDPI to transplant programs that had a history of accepting them. An evaluation of the project revealed there was no statistically significant change in the percentage of organ offer acceptances (Noreen et al., 2021).

Data suggest that a small number of transplant programs attract a large percentage of kidneys that are allocated through expedited placement. King et al. (2022) found that while the overall proportion of transplants from out-of-sequence allocation has remained stable over time, there are two outlier OPOs that use this discretionary tool more frequently than others. There are many reasons why OPOs may feel pressure to use out-of-sequence allocation—wide variation in local donation rates, donor quality, and transplant center acceptance behaviors are a few reasons (King et al., 2022). Expedited placement has the potential to result in disparities that result from routing organs only to transplant centers with greater resources, as well as concerns about further advantaging patients who have the means to be on multiple waiting lists in different areas of the country (Kinkhabwala et al., 2013; Mohan and Schold, 2021; Washburn and Olthoff, 2012). Out-of-sequence allocation is one tool for improving organ use rates and further study is warranted to understand if out-of-sequence allocation is associated with more successful and efficient organ placement and lower rates of organ nonuse. Perhaps most importantly, as out-of-sequence allocation relies on informal relationships between organizations and potentially concentrates a higher number of organs in a few transplant centers, the impact on disparities and equity will need to be closely monitored (King et al., 2022).

Key challenges to increase offer acceptances are noted in Box 6-4.

*Conclusion 6-8: Too many deceased donor organs are procured but not transplanted each year. It is too easy for transplant centers to decline usable organs, and account-ability for transplant center decision making is lacking. As demand for organs consistently exceeds supply, the continued underuse of available, usable, donated organs requires priority action.*

---

**BOX 6-4    CHALLENGES IN INCREASING OFFER ACCEPTANCES**

Several challenges must be overcome to increase organ offer acceptances. These include

- The transplantation system's deference to the flexibility of transplant centers and teams to exercise choice in accepting and transplanting organs.
- The organ allocation process often does not accurately identify, in a timely manner, the individuals who are not only the best match but also very likely to accept the organ.
- The organ offer process currently lacks accountability for transplant centers declining organs, thereby making it too easy for usable organs to be declined.
- Operations mismanagement, including the weekend effect.
- Less emphasis on shared decision making, affecting patient acceptance of medically complex organs.

## Summary of Maximizing Use

In a review of the data, the committee finds strong evidence that supports the need for improvement on many fronts in order to decrease the nonuse rate and involve patient preferences in the consideration of organ offers. While not all of the currently unused organs could be used, the persistence of this rate over time diminishes the fairness, equity, and transparency of the organ transplantation system.

The wide variation in nonuse and organ offer acceptance rates is the result of a combination of many factors that are within the control of the transplant center, as well as resulting from operational practices and behaviors that are not supported by evidence of geography, organ supply, or patient complexity. These operational issues must be resolved to improve the fairness, equity, and transparency of the organ transplantation system. The committee acknowledges that there are some factors, such as the medical complexities of an organ offer, that are not within the control of the transplant center. Many transplant centers are top performers and have found medical and operational solutions that are effective and maximize organ use. Donated organs that could be transplanted are not used for several reasons, prime among which is that the time involved each time an organ is offered but then rejected can reduce the viability of the organ, and the people to whom the organ is offered subsequently may regard it as undesirable because others have rejected it. Thus, greater use of donated organs depends on increasing the speed with which suitable organs are accepted by, and transplanted into, the patients to whom they are allocated and offered (see Box 6-5).

---

**BOX 6-5    OPPORTUNITIES TO INCREASE ORGAN USE**

Several changes could decrease the number of organs not used without precluding transplant professionals from exercising evidence-based clinical judgment regarding whether to accept or reject an organ offer:

- A more refined allocation algorithm could more accurately identify, in a timely manner, the patient for whom the organ is most likely to be accepted and successfully transplanted. Such an algorithm would incorporate more granular and up-to-date data about patients (e.g., medical condition or willingness to accept nonstandard organs), include all the aspects of organs that physicians usually take into account when deciding whether to accept an organ, and consider transplant programs' history of accepting or rejecting certain types of organs.
- Allocating more resources and personnel to managing patients awaiting transplants would not only improve average preoperative readiness for transplantation but also ensure that transplant programs can provide the OPTN more accurate, detailed, and current data about each patient, which will improve the precision of organ offers.
- Transplant centers are not currently accountable for their decisions to decline organs. It would be reasonable to require surgeons to explain their reasons for declining an organ offer.
- A transplant team can develop an understanding of each patient's individual preferences if, at the time the patient is first evaluated for a transplant and periodically thereafter, a member of the team explains the major factors that are considered when an organ is offered and shows the patient how survival benefits are calculated and how they can be compared when choosing among alternatives such as accepting a medically complex organ or waiting for another one.
- Once patients are on the waiting list, such discussions can also examine information about any organs that were offered to the patient and the reasons why the transplant team declined them, thereby allowing patients and their transplant team to come to a shared decision about the factors that the transplant program will submit to the OPTN and use in evaluating future organ offers.

*Conclusion 6-9: Some transplant programs state that they reject some medically complex organs because transplantation teams believe that transplants using such organs will negatively affect their program's performance metrics, as evaluated by 1-year patient and graft survival, which can result in financial penalties. Overcoming this problem involves both adjusting measures to better identify high-quality performance and conveying to teams how they can transplant medically complex organs without adversely affecting their performance data (e.g., by sharing the techniques used by programs that have actually improved their metrics while accepting many medically complex organs).*

## Patient Shared Decision Making

Shared decision making is a model of patient-centered care that enables and encourages people to play a role in the medical decisions that affect their health (AHRQ, 2020). There are opportunities to increase patient shared decision making in order to improve the fairness, equity, cost-effectiveness, and transparency of the nation's organ transplantation system. Ensuring patients are aware of all organs offered to them but declined by their transplant centers, and the reasons for the decline, will strengthen the patient-centered care that is an essential part of quality health care delivery.

### Relevant Reports

The National Academies (then IOM) led the development of important work to address patient safety in U.S. hospitals with its landmark *To Err Is Human* report (IOM, 2000). This report provided the foundation for a new and sustained national movement to improve safety in hospitals and still today has implications for ways to improve the organ transplantation system in the United States. *Crossing the Quality Chasm* (IOM, 2001) quickly followed with a review of the health care delivery system, specifically the provision of preventive, acute, chronic, and end-of-life health care for individuals. The theme of increasing patient involvement resulted in a recommendation that health care processes should be redesigned to

> share knowledge and the free flow of information, that patients should have unfettered access to their own medical information and to clinical knowledge. Furthermore, that clinicians and patients should communicate effectively and share information (IOM, 2001, p. 8).

Most recently, the World Health Organization has incorporated patient and family engagement as a key element to improve patient safety and for health care system improvement (WHO, 2021). These reports brought to light that patients were mostly unaware that hospital safety and health care quality were something to be concerned about, and most medical professionals were unaware of the scope of the problem. To the extent it was encountered, it was not discussed.

Although shared decision making has been examined in numerous clinical settings, it has received little attention from the organ transplantation system (Gordon et al., 2013). This chapter has discussed the need for transparency, where reasons for the thousands of organs recovered but not transplanted annually are not well understood.[19] When and why transplant centers accept or decline an organ offer is often opaque to the patients who are depending on transplant centers to make appropriate decisions for their circumstances (Mohan and

---

[19] See Chapter 3 for more information on increased transparency related to public trust and patient decision making, and see Chapter 5 on optimizing data for patient review in organ offers.

Schold, 2021). This is especially important because on average, patients who die waiting for a kidney had offers for 16 kidneys that were ultimately transplanted into other patients (Husain et al., 2019). The decision to take an offered kidney or wait for a "better" one is complex and individual to the specific patient and donated kidney pair. Characteristics of each patient—such as age and time on the waiting list—as well as characteristics of each donated kidney are variable and influence the outcome of any transplantation.

Acknowledging and incorporating patient preferences is important to facilitate decisions about whether accepting a specific kidney is the best choice for that patient. For most patients with significant waiting times, taking a higher KDPI kidney when it is offered leads to better survival benefit as compared to remaining on dialysis and waiting for a "better" offer. Figure 6-11 shows estimated survival for three scenarios: transplantation now, waiting and then undergoing transplantation with a lower KDPI kidney, and waiting indefinitely without transplantation. For this example, the hypothetical patient is 55 years old, does not have diabetes, has been on dialysis for 3.5 years, and has waited 809 days on the waiting list. In this case, accepting a 60 percent KDPI kidney now would increase survival by 57.5 days on average within the first 5 years following transplant, compared to waiting an additional 300 days for a 15 percent KDPI kidney. The probability the patient would die while waiting for the 15 percent KDPI kidney is 7 percent.

Figure 6-11 was created using one example of a web application to assist providers and patients in this type of shared decision making.[20] Use of this or a similar app would allow

---

[20] Available at https://wparker-uchicago.shinyapps.io/DDKT_survival_benefit_compare (accessed November 17, 2021).

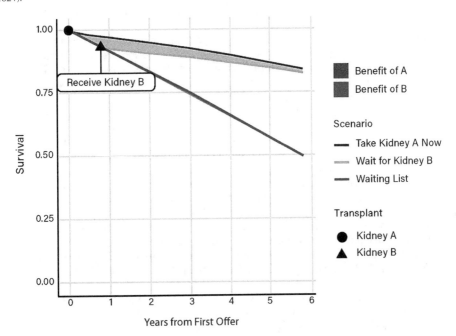

**FIGURE 6-11** Example of a tool estimating survival benefit of accepting an offered kidney versus waiting for a different offer to support incorporating patient preferences into decisions.
SOURCE: Parker et al., 2021.

patients to evaluate the difference in survival benefit associated with accepting a higher KDPI organ today versus waiting for an organ with lower KDPI at some point in the future. These parameters can be discussed in advance of an organ offer and updated over time as the patient remains on the waiting list and may experience changes in their preferences.

Shared decision making enables and encourages individuals to play a pivotal role in the medical decisions that affect their health, and the organ transplantation system can do this better with a focus on patient-centered care.

**Recommendation 9: Make it easier for transplant centers to say "yes" to organ offers. The OPTN should enhance organ allocation and distribution policies and processes to reduce nonuse of deceased donor organs and make it easier for transplant centers to say "yes" to organ offers. To improve the organ offer process, the OPTN should do the following:**

- Require the use of more refined filters for transplant centers to indicate their preferences for which kidneys will be accepted, if offered. The filters should especially focus on determining transplant center willingness to accept medically complex kidneys, akin to what is done in the UK's Kidney Fast Track Scheme.
- Implement expedited placement policies, at first offer, for offered and procured kidneys at high risk of nonuse to effectively direct difficult-to-place kidneys to transplant centers with a demonstrated history of using them.
- Since donations occur 7 days a week, the OPTN should require hospitals with transplant centers to smooth surgical scheduling using proven procedures in order to ensure the capability of organ procurement operations and organ transplants all 7 days of the week.
- Adapt the process of offering an organ to gradually increase the number of simultaneous offers of a given organ to save cold ischemic time and minimize herding effects.
- Review and standardize current requirements for organ quality assessments conducted by OPOs with the primary goal of helping transplant centers accept more organ offers by focusing on the following specific actions:
  - Develop evidence-based standards for organ quality assessment to be used by all OPOs prior to organ allocation. The standardized requirements for organ quality assessments should carefully consider the value of biopsies as it has been repeatedly shown that biopsy results deter organ acceptance, often inappropriately.
  - Develop clear guidelines for transplant centers to request any additional organ quality testing beyond the standardized requirements.

**Recommendation 10: Increase transparency and accountability for organ offer declines and prioritize patient engagement in decisions regarding organ offers. HHS should update the OPTN contract to require increased *transparency* around organ offer declines. The updated OPTN contract should do the following:**

- Require transplant centers to share with a patient and their family the number and context of organ offer declines for that individual on the waiting list during a defined period (e.g., every 3 to 6 months).
- Require the collection of more reliable, specific, and patient-centered data on reasons organ offers were declined through improvements in refusal codes. For example, require transplant centers to provide additional justification for declining

an offered kidney when survival benefit of the transplant is greater than staying on dialysis.
- Require investigation of approaches for shared decision making between patients and transplant teams in the organ offer process and implementation of models proven to be most useful and desirable.

**HHS should update the OPTN contract to require transplant center *accountability* for patient engagement and partnership between transplant center professionals and patients in deciding whether to accept or reject an offered organ. The updated OPTN contract should require**

- Close monitoring of any new transplant center performance metrics to ensure the desired outcomes are achieved and unintended consequences are avoided;
- Nudges in the form of reports showing a transplant center's decisions regarding offered organs, as well as comparisons to other transplant centers, to be proactively developed from SRTR data and shared with individual transplant centers on a monthly basis; and
- Transplant programs to document shared decision making that includes a discussion of survival benefit, relative to staying on the waiting list or dialysis, before deciding to accept or reject an offered deceased donor organ.

## DONOR CARE UNITS

In 2001, a significant innovation in the process of organ donation and recovery took place when Mid-America Transplant, the OPO located in St. Louis, Missouri, built a free-standing donor care unit (DCU),[21] and began transferring organ donors declared dead by neurological criteria for the purposes of donor medical management and organ procurement. Over the next 20 years, 11 OPOs built and managed free-standing DCUs that serve donation service areas ranging from heavily metropolitan to large rural geographies.

The original rationale for OPOs to build and manage DCUs has not changed: to increase the number of organs transplanted, improve and manage OPO cost-effectiveness, provide consistent and reliable organ donor processes, and enhance safety for local transplant teams (Englesbe and Merion, 2009; Moazami et al., 2007). Having dedicated space where medically managing and treating organ function in a deceased organ donor is a singular organizational focus means that donation can take place without the challenges and time constraints of a busy intensive care unit in either acute care hospitals or hospitals with less familiarity with organ donation. Similarly, the ability to rely on an operating room time that is not dependent on bumping scheduled cases, or delayed because of unexpected trauma cases makes the donation process more reliable and consistent. Moving the organ donor and not the DSA surgical team provides a level of safety that has become increasingly important. Finally, the ability for an OPO to improve cost-effectiveness related to donor management and surgical recovery remains a key factor in controlling costs.

---

[21] DCUs are also known as "Organ Recovery Centers," "Organ Procurement Organization Facilities," "Organ Procurement Centers," and "Specialized Donor Care Facilities."

## Description and Use of Donor Care Units

In general, a DCU is a facility built and managed by an OPO, under the guidance of the OPO's medical director, for the purposes of medically managing organ function and recovering organs for transplantation from deceased organ donors.[22] Because of legal requirements under state statute for hospital licensure, only donors declared dead by neurological criteria can be transferred to a DCU and not DCDD donors. After death is declared by neurological criteria in acute care or critical access hospitals, authorization for donation by the donor or surrogate decision maker has been obtained, the donor is hemodynamically stable, and approval for transfer has been given, the donor is moved by ground or air transport to the DCU. In the DCU, donor management takes place in a critical care setting where staff, monitored beds, and sophisticated imaging and diagnostic equipment such as X-ray, bronchoscopy, CT scanner, heart catheter, and point-of-care laboratory services are available onsite. The organ recovery procedure takes place in the same facility where large, state-of-the-art operating rooms can easily accommodate the multiple teams necessary for the surgical recovery of organs from multiorgan donors. With the advent of machine preservation for abdominal and thoracic organs, DCUs often house the equipment used to rehabilitate organs prior to transplantation. The ability to live stream the surgical procedure for distant surgeons and/or medical examiner/coroner/law enforcement via built-in high-resolution video cameras has provided a level of virtual hands-on experience not widely available in hospitals. Importantly, dedicated space is available for donor families to be with their loved ones, if they choose.

## Models of Donor Care Units

There are three distinct models of donor care units primarily in use across the country: OPO-managed DCUs ("free-standing recovery centers"), partnerships with community hospitals, and partnerships with transplant centers.

### *OPO-Managed DCUs*

OPO-managed DCUs, also known as free-standing recovery centers or organ procurement centers, are similar in structure, staffing, and available equipment to other DCUs, but they may differ in size of the facility and are located in the OPO building. Currently, there are OPO-managed DCUs in 11 cities in United States.[23] From a staffing perspective, OPO staff are trained to perform all donor management and testing procedures.

---

[22] Pediatric donor transfer practice varies by OPO due to equipment requirements. See Brockmeier presentation at the February 14, 2021, virtual workshop: https://www.nationalacademies.org/event/02-04-2021/a-fairer-and-more-equitable-cost-effective-and-transparent-system-of-donor-organ-procurement-allocation-and-distribution-a-virtual-workshop (accessed January 27, 2022).

[23] These include Mid-America Transplant, St. Louis, MO (2001); Gift of Life Michigan, Ann Arbor, MI (2010); Donor Alliance, Denver, CO (2012); Center for Organ Recovery & Education, Pittsburgh, PA (2014); Mississippi Organ Recovery Agency, Jackson, MS (2017); LifeBanc, Cleveland, OH (2017); One Legacy, Los Angeles, CA (2017); Louisiana Organ Procurement Agency, New Orleans, LA (2018); and Southwest Transplant Alliance, Dallas, TX (Under Construction). See Brockmeier presentation at the February 14, 2021, virtual workshop: https://www.nationalacademies.org/event/02-04-2021/a-fairer-and-more-equitable-cost-effective-and-transparent-system-of-donor-organ-procurement-allocation-and-distribution-a-virtual-workshop (accessed January 27, 2022).

## Partnerships with Community Hospitals

One large metropolitan OPO has developed a hybrid model of a DCU where, through an agreement with a community hospital, critical care beds and operating rooms are designated for donor management and the surgical recovery of organs. The staffing model for this type of DCU is similar to the donation process in donor hospitals—hospital staff provide bedside care and the OPO staff medically manage the donor.

## Partnerships with Transplant Centers

The advent of transplant hospitals building in-house capabilities came about initially as a result of the interpretation of the transplant center cost report, and subsequently, as a way to increase Medicare reimbursement for the transplant center. In this model, donors declared dead (by DCDD or DNDD criteria) within the transplant center may be moved to a dedicated bed or a dedicated space within the transplant center. It is also possible for the transplant center to have agreements with non–transplant center donor hospitals where, like the other models, after the declaration of death by neurological criteria, those donors are transferred from referring hospitals throughout the DSA to the DCU housed in the transplant center. The transplant hospital may assume all responsibility for staffing, or the OPO staff may provide those services.

## Key Benefits of Donor Care Units

DCUs have proven to be beneficial for both donor hospitals and donor families. In the DCU facility, private space for donor families include sleeping accommodations, internet access, restrooms, televisions, and landline use. Donor families are given the option to say their good-byes at the hospital, or move to the DCU. Under either scenario, "honor walks" and flag raising ceremonies still take place in the hospital ICU and all efforts are made to ensure that donation does not delay funeral ceremonies. Postdonation surveys consistently report high satisfaction with the DCU experience by donor families, with average results of 9.75 out of 10 for overall satisfaction (Doyle et al., 2016). Transferring donors to a DCU benefits hospitals by opening up bed space in busy ICUs and relieves staff in smaller hospitals who are less familiar with the donation process due to the infrequency of donation events. As mentioned earlier in this chapter, a DCU allows for stability in setting operating room times that will not be changed due to emergency admissions or other surgeries "bumping" organ procurement cases.

Importantly, DCUs have been cost effective in managing organ acquisition charges. The OPO pays a prorated reimbursement to donor hospitals that covers charges prior to the donor being transferred. After transfer to the DCU, the OPO assumes all expenses, which have been demonstrated to be lower than hospital charges. One OPO reported the average cost of donor recoveries between 2009 and 2014 51 percent lower when donors are transferred (hospital charges $33,161 compared to DCU costs of $16,153) (Doyle et al., 2016).

Several reports by the St. Louis group document a consistent and sustainable increase in organs transplanted, most notable with a 71 percent increase in lung transplantation when comparing two time periods (2001–2007 vs. 2009–2016) (Chang et al., 2018). From 2009 to 2014, the organ yield at the DCU was 6 percent higher in Standard Criteria Donors and 18 percent higher in Extended Criteria Donors (these donor categories are no longer used) compared to the national average of hospital recoveries (Doyle et al., 2016).

In addition to increased organ yield and decreased costs of organ procurements, DCUs have the potential to address provider burnout, the transplant surgery pipeline, and surgeon travel and allow for increased daytime operating (Doyle et al., 2016; Lindemann et al., 2019). Given the high-risk nature of air and ground transport to distant donor hospitals within a DSA, DCUs also provide an important element of greater safety for local transplant teams (Doyle et al., 2014). DCUs also have great potential for clinical research in organ dona-tion, given the collaborative environment that encourages academic inquiry and because a relatively uncommon population is referred to a single center (Bery et al., 2021; Marsolais et al., 2017).

An additional and unexpected benefit has been the increased collaboration between the OPOs with DCUs and the transplant centers in their DSA. The decision to build a DCU is one that requires careful collaboration between the OPO, donor hospitals, and transplant centers. The committee heard testimony of how OPOs garner support from stakeholders in their DSA in order for the DCU to be successful, and monitor satisfaction of hospital critical care staff, administration, physicians, and donor families to ensure that needs and expecta-tions are met. Based on committee testimony and shared satisfaction data, there have been no reported adverse effects to the donation culture within donor hospitals or any negative effect to donor families (Doyle et al., 2016).

## Potential Challenges of DCUs

With the emergence of DCUs, several concerns have been raised, including support from acute care and critical access hospitals to transfer donors, care of the donor family, and donor family satisfaction. Initially, medical and nursing staff expressed concern about losing a connection with the donation process; however, the implementation of high touch cer-emonies that include hospital staff (e.g., honor walks, flag raisings) have kept physician and nursing engagement high. As mentioned previously, care of the donor family has not been impacted by the presence of DCUs and donor families consistently report high satisfaction with their organ donation experience (Doyle et al., 2016). While OPO-managed DCUs rou-tinely survey donor family and donor hospital satisfaction, it is unclear if the same analysis is conducted by DCUs with partnerships in community hospitals and transplant centers and more qualitative data are needed.

Given the benefits covered in this section, why have the other 37 DSAs not incorporated a DCU? Challenges to wider application of DCUs include the OPO not being geographically located adjacent to major donor hospitals and transplant centers, transplant centers refusing to transfer donors due to significant cost report implications for reimbursement, perceptions by OPOs and their Boards that the undertaking in staff training and financial outlay is too difficult to manage given the size of the OPO, and loss of revenue to local hospitals. It may be that in parts of the country, regional DCUs would be an option to help mitigate these challenges, but the committee recognizes that they may seem daunting when initially con-sidered. Standardizing and spreading best practices of established DCUs will help mitigate these challenges.

## Committee Considerations

The financial arrangements surrounding the three DCU models described above include complex reimbursement structures negotiated between the relevant parties (OPOs, trans-plant centers, donor hospitals) and primarily, CMS. CMS has historically reimbursed donor hospitals that are also transplant centers for usable organs recovered from deceased donors at their facility. Currently, if a declared deceased donor at a donor hospital that is also a transplant center is transferred to a DCU for organ procurement, the transplant center can no longer receive reimbursement for recovering those organs and organs procured at a DCU are not counted toward the Medicare organ ratio, leading to a loss in Medicare reimbursement (Lindemann et al., 2019). This committee discussed that the potential for a significant financial effect on a transplant center's cost report has limited the willingness and ability of some transplant centers to transfer donors to DCUs and that changes in CMS or other reimbursement structures related to transferring donors to a DCU may be needed. For example, language around "excising organs" in the transplant center's cost report could be reconsidered to "identification and declaration (or pronouncement) of death." CMS may also consider ensuring that adequate volume exists within the OPO service area to ensure the efficient and safe operation of a DCU. In addition, capital investment, staff resourcing, and staff training would be important considerations in developing requirements for DCUs.

A December 2021 CMS Request for Information seeks public comments on a number of components of the transplantation system, including DCUs (referred to as organ recovery facilities by CMS). CMS expresses interest in learning about these facilities and the benefits and risks, particularly from a donor family and patient advocate perspective. As this committee discussed, and CMS also raises, it is possible that there will be a need for new specific health and safety requirements (possibly akin to ambulatory care center requirements) that would apply to DCUs.[24]

In developing Recommendation 11 below, the committee considered who is best to design, establish, and manage a DCU, and felt that OPOs were better suited for the responsibility of continuity of care with the deceased donor process. The committee concluded that CMS should review payment incentives for transplant centers such that the transplant center is neither financially punished nor excessively rewarded for performing deceased donor organ management and surgical recovery.

*Conclusion 6-10: Donor care units are an innovation in organ procurement and provide an opportunity to bring consistency and high-quality care to donor organ procurement and the donor family care experience.*

**Recommendation 11: Require the establishment and use of a donor care unit for each organ procurement organization.**
**To better serve donors and families, increase cost-effectiveness, and foster innovation in organ rehabilitation and donor intervention research, HHS should require each of the 57 OPOs to create, establish, and manage a DCU. Ensuring the success of donor care units at a national level will also require CMS to revise payment incentives for transplant centers such that the transplant center is neither financially punished nor excessively rewarded for performing deceased donor organ management and recovery. Specific actions include**

- For each DSA in the United States, HHS should require the OPO and transplant center(s) to collaborate on the development of a DCU that would be designed,

---

[24] See Federal Register Vol. 86, No. 230, of Friday, December 3, 2021. Request for Information; Health and Safety Requirements for Transplant Programs, Organ Procurement Organizations, and End-Stage Renal Disease Facilities (discussion of organ recovery facilities begins on page 68603). https://www.federalregister.gov/documents/2021/12/03/2021-26146/request-for-information-health-and-safety-requirements-for-transplant-programs-organ-procurement (accessed January 28, 2022).

established, and managed by the OPO, if one does not already exist, to serve that geographic area. Because multiple models of DCUs are in practice today, the committee recommends that HHS require the following attributes for each donor care unit:

- ○  Dedicated beds for deceased donors in a dedicated space;
- ○  Dedicated operating room with trained staff, reserved specifically for organ procurement surgery;
- ○  Dedicated space for donor families;
- ○  ICU-level care;
- ○  Oversight by a critical care physician;
- ○  Ability to conduct some in-house imaging and diagnostics of donors;
- ○  Ability to conduct organ rehabilitation and therapy;
- ○  Ability to conduct donor intervention research; and
- ○  Reasonable distance to an airport.

- CMS should adjust current reimbursement structures that create disincentives that dampen the willingness of some transplant centers to transfer donors to an OPO DCU. Transplant centers should not be disadvantaged financially by allowing a donor to be transferred to a DCU for donor management and organ recovery. Similarly, transplant centers should not excessively gain from transferring and managing already deceased donors from another hospital for the sole purpose of organ procurement.
- HHS should require hospitals to smooth surgical scheduling so that organ donation surgical procedures for DCDD donors and donors who cannot be transferred to a DCU can take place in a timely manner all 7 days of the week.

## REFERENCES

AHRQ (Agency for Health Care Research and Quality). 2020. *The SHARE Approach—Essential steps of shared deci-sionmaking: Quick reference guide.* https://www.ahrq.gov/health-literacy/professional-training/shared-decision/tools/resource-1.html (accessed January 26, 2022).

Aubert, O., P. P. Reese, B. Audry, Y. Bouatou, M. Raynaud, D. Viglietti, C. Legendre, D. Glotz, J.-P. Empana, X. Jouven, C. Lefaucheur, C. Jacquelinet, and A. Loupy. 2019. Disparities in acceptance of deceased donor kidneys between the United States and France and estimated effects of increased US acceptance. *JAMA Internal Medicine* 179(10):1365-1374.

Berwick, D. M. 1996. A primer on leading the improvement of systems. *BMJ Clinical Research* 312(7031):619-622.

Bery, A., G. Marklin, A. Itoh, D. Kreisel, T. Takahashi, B. F. Meyers, R. Nava, B. D. Kozower, H. Shepherd, G. A. Patterson, and V. Puri. 2021. Specialized donor care facility model and advances in management of thoracic organ donors. *Annals of Thoracic Surgery.* https://doi.org/10.1016/j.athoracsur.2020.12.026.

Bethea, E., A. Arvind, J. Gustafson, K. Andersson, D. Pratt, I. Bhan, M. Thiim, K. Corey, P. Bloom, J. Markmann, H. Yeh, N. Elias, S. Kimura, L. A. Dageforde, A. Cuenca, T. Kawai, K. Safa, W. Williams, H. Gilligan, M. Sise, J. Fishman, C. Kotton, A. Kim, C. C. Rogers, S. Shao, M. Cote, L. Irwin, P. Myoung, and R. T. Chung. 2020. Immediate administration of antiviral therapy after transplantation of hepatitis C-infected livers into uninfected recipients: Implications for therapeutic planning. *American Journal of Transplantation* 20(6):1619-1628.

Brennan, C., S. A. Husain, K. L. King, D. Tsapepas, L. E. Ratner, Z. Jin, J. D. Schold, and S. Mohan. 2019. A donor utilization index to assess the utilization and discard of deceased donor kidneys perceived as high risk. *Clinical Journal of the American Society of Nephrology* 14(11):1634-1641.

Callaghan, C. J., L. Mumford, L. Pankhurst, R. J. Baker, J. A. Bradley, and C. J. E. Watson. 2017. Early outcomes of the new UK deceased donor kidney fast-track offering scheme. *Transplantation* 101(12):2888-2897.

Carpenter, D. J., M. C. Chiles, E. C. Verna, K. J. Halazun, J. C. Emond, L. E. Ratner, and S. Mohan. 2019. Deceased brain dead donor liver transplantation and utilization in the United States: Nighttime and weekend effects. *Transplantation* 103(7):1392-1404.

Chang, S. H., D. Kreisel, G. F. Marklin, L. Cook, R. Hachem, B. D. Kozower, K. R. Balsara, J. M. Bell, C. Frederiksen, B. F. Meyers, G. A. Patterson, and V. Puri. 2018. Lung focused resuscitation at a specialized donor care facility improves lung procurement rates. *Annals of Thoracic Surgery* 105(5):1531-1536.

Choi, A. Y., M. S. Mulvihill, H.-J. Lee, C. Zhao, M. Kuchibhatla, J. N. Schroder, C. B. Patel, C. B. Granger, and M. G. Hartwig. 2020. Transplant center variability in organ offer acceptance and mortality among U.S. patients on the heart transplant waitlist. *JAMA Cardiology* 5(6):660-668.

CMS (Centers for Medicare & Medicaid Services). 2016. *Solid transplant programs - outcome thresholds - revised guidelines.* https://www.cms.gov/medicare/provider-enrollment-and-certification/surveycertificationgeninfo/downloads/survey-and-cert-letter-16-24.pdf (accessed November 4, 2021).

CMS. 2020a. *Organ procurement organization (OPO) conditions for coverage final rule: Revisions to outcome measures for OPOs cms-3380-f.* https://www.cms.gov/newsroom/fact-sheets/organ-procurement-organization-opo-conditions-coverage-final-rule-revisions-outcome-measures-opos (accessed November 4, 2021).

CMS. 2020b. *Medicare and Medicaid programs; organ procurment organizations conditions for coverage; revisions to the outcome measure requirements for organ procurement organizations.* A rule by the Centers for Medicare & Medicaid Services. https://www.federalregister.gov/d/2020-26329/p-195 (accessed February 2, 2022).

CMS. 2020c. *Transplant.* https://www.cms.gov/Medicare/Provider-Enrollment-and-Certification/Certificationand Complianc/Transplant (accessed November 4, 2021).

CMS. 2021. *HHS seeks public comments to advance equity and reduce disparities in organ transplantation, improve life-saving donations, and dialysis facility quality of care.* https://www.cms.gov/newsroom/press-releases/hhs-seeks-public-comments-advance-equity-and-reduce-disparities-organ-transplantation-improve-life (accessed January 26, 2022).

The Commonwealth Fund. 2020. *New international report on health care: U.S. suicide rate highest among wealthy nations.* https://www.commonwealthfund.org/press-release/2020/new-international-report-health-care-us-suicide-rate-highest-among-wealthy (accessed February 2, 2022).

Dayoub, J. C., F. Cortese, A. Anžič, T. Grum, and J. P. de Magalhães. 2018. The effects of donor age on organ transplants: A review and implications for aging research. *Experimental Gerontology* 110:230-240.

Dolgin, N. H., B. Movahedi, P. N. Martins, R. Goldberg, K. L. Lapane, F. A. Anderson, and A. Bozorgzadeh. 2016. Decade-long trends in liver transplant waitlist removal due to illness severity: The impact of Centers for Medicare and Medicaid Services policy. *Journal of the American College of Surgeons* 222(6):1054-1065.

Doyle, M. B. M., N. Vachharajani, J. R. Wellen, J. A. Lowell, S. Shenoy, G. Ridolfi, M. D. Jendrisak, J. Coleman, M. Maher, D. Brockmeier, D. Kappel, and W. C. Chapman. 2014. A novel organ donor facility: A decade of experience with liver donors. *American Journal of Transplantation* 14(3):615-620.

Doyle, M., V. Subramanian, N. Vachharajani, K. Collins, J. R. Wellen, E. Stahlschmidt, D. Brockmeier, J. Coleman, D. Kappel, and W. C. Chapman. 2016. Organ donor recovery performed at an organ procurement organization-based facility is an effective way to minimize organ recovery costs and increase organ yield. *Journal of the American College of Surgeons* 222(4):591-600.

Englesbe, M. J., and R. M. Merion. 2009. The riskiest job in medicine: Transplant surgeons and organ procurement travel. *American Journal of Transplantation* 9(10):2406-2415.

Gill, J. R., and M. E. DeJoseph. 2020. The importance of proper death certification during the COVID-19 pandemic. *JAMA* 324(1):27-28.

Giorgakis, E., and A. K. Mathur. 2020. Expedited placement to maximize utilization of marginal organs. *Current Opinion in Organ Transplantation* 25(6):640-646.

Goldberg, D. S., B. French, J. D. Lewis, F. I. Scott, R. Mamtani, R. Gilroy, S. D. Halpern, and P. L. Abt. 2016. Liver transplant center variability in accepting organ offers and its impact on patient survival. *Journal of Hepatology* 64(4):843-851.

Goldberg, D. S., P. L. Abt, E. A. Blumberg, V. M. Van Deerlin, M. Levine, K. R. Reddy, R. D. Bloom, S. M. Nazarian, D. Sawinski, and P. Porrett. 2017. Trial of transplantation of HCV-infected kidneys into uninfected recipients. *New England Journal of Medicine* 376(24):2394-2395.

Gordon, E. J., Z. Butt, S. E. Jensen, A. Lok-Ming Lehr, J. Franklin, Y. Becker, L. Sherman, W. J. Chon, N. Beauvais, J. Hanneman, D. Penrod, M. G. Ison, and M. M. Abecassis. 2013. Opportunities for shared decision making in kidney transplantation. *American Journal of Transplantation* 13(5):1149-1158.

Greer, D. M. 2021. Determination of brain death. *New England Journal of Medicine* 385(27):2554-2561.

Grinshteyn, E., and D. Hemenway. 2019. Violent death rates in the US compared to those of other high-income countries, 2015. *Preventive Medicine* 123:20-26.

Ho, J. Y. 2019. The contemporary American drug overdose epidemic in international perspective. *Population and Development Review* 45(1):7-40.

Husain, S. A., F. S. Winterhalter, and S. Mohan. 2018. Kidney transplant offers to deceased candidates. *American Journal of Transplantation* 18(11):2836-2837.

Husain, S. A., K. L. King, S. Pastan, R. E. Patzer, D. J. Cohen, J. Radhakrishnan, and S. Mohan. 2019. Association between declined offers of deceased donor kidney allograft and outcomes in kidney transplant candidates. *JAMA Network Open* 2(8):e1910312.

Ibrahim, M., G. Vece, J. Mehew, R. Johnson, J. Forsythe, D. Klassen, C. Callaghan, and D. Stewart. 2020. An international comparison of deceased donor kidney utilization: What can the United States and the United Kingdom learn from each other? *American Journal of Transplantation* 20(5):1309-1322.

IOM (Institute of Medicine). 1997. *Non-heart-beating organ transplantation: Medical and ethical issues in procurement.* Edited by J. T. Potts and R. Herdman. Washington, DC: National Academy Press.

IOM. 2000. *To err is human: Building a safer health system.* Edited by L. T. Kohn, J. M. Corrigan, and M. S. Donaldson. Washington, DC: National Academy Press.

IOM. 2001. *Crossing the quality chasm: A new health system for the 21st century.* Washington, DC: National Academy Press.

IOM. 2006. *Organ donation: Opportunities for action.* Edited by J. F. Childress and C. T. Liverman. Washington, DC: The National Academies Press.

IRODaT (International Registry in Organ Donation and Transplantation. 2021. *International registry in organ donation and transplantation.* https://www.irodat.org/?p=database (accessed January 7, 2022).

Israni, A. K., D. Zaun, J. D. Rosendale, C. Schaffhausen, W. McKinney, and J. J. Snyder. 2021. OPTN/SRTR 2019 annual data report: Deceased organ donors. *American Journal of Transplantation* 21(S2):567-604.

Kalisvaart, M., K. P. Croome, R. Hernandez-Alejandro, J. Pirenne, M. Cortés-Cerisuelo, E. Miñambres, and P. L. Abt. 2021. Donor warm ischemia time in DCD liver transplantation-working group report from the ILTS DCD, liver preservation, and machine perfusion consensus conference. *Transplantation* 105(6):1156-1164.

Karp, S., and G. Segal. 2021. *New regulation for organ procurement will improve equity and save lives.* https://www.thehastingscenter.org/new-regulation-for-organ-procurement-will-improve-equity-and-save-lives (accessed February 2, 2022).

Karp, S., G. Segal, and D. J. Patil. 2020. Fixing organ donation—what gets measured, gets fixed. *JAMA Surgery* 155(8):687-688.

Kasiske, B. L., N. Salkowski, A. Wey, A. K. Israni, and J. J. Snyder. 2016. Potential implications of recent and proposed changes in the regulatory oversight of solid organ transplantation in the United States. *American Journal of Transplantation* 16(12):3371-3377.

Kelen, G. D., R. Wolfe, G. D'Onofrio, A. M. Mills, D. Diercks, S. A. Stern, M. Wadman, and P. E. Sokolove. 2021. Emergency department crowding: The canary in the health care system. *NEJM Catalyst.* https://doi.org/10.1056/CAT.21.0217.

Khush, K. K., J. G. Zaroff, J. Nguyen, R. Menza, and B. A. Goldstein. 2015. National decline in donor heart utilization with regional variability: 1995-2010. *American Journal of Transplantation* 15(3):642-649.

Kim, D. W., D. Tsapepas, K. L. King, S. A. Husain, F. A. Corvino, A. Dillon, W. Wang, T. J. Mayne, and S. Mohan. 2020. Financial impact of delayed graft function in kidney transplantation. *Clinical Transplantation* 34(10):e14022.

King, K. L., S. A. Husain, D. J. Cohen, and S. Mohan. 2019. Deceased donor kidneys are harder to place on the weekend. *Clinical Journal of the American Society of Nephrology* 14(6):904-906.

King, K. L., S. A. Husain, J. D. Schold, R. E. Patzer, P. P. Reese, Z. Jin, L. E. Ratner, D. J. Cohen, S. O. Pastan, and S. Mohan. 2020. Major variation across local transplant centers in probability of kidney transplant for wait-listed patients. *Journal of the American Society of Nephrology* 31(12):2900-2911.

King, K. L., S. G. Chaudhry, L. E. Ratner, D. J. Cohen, S. A. Husain, and S. Mohan. 2021. Declined offers for deceased donor kidneys are not an independent reflection of organ quality. *Kidney360.* https://doi.org/10.34067/KID.0004052021.

King, K. L., S. A. Husain, A. Perotte, J. T. Adler, J. D. Schold, and S. Mohan. 2022. Deceased donor kidneys allocated out of sequence by organ procurement organizations. *American Journal of Transplantation.* https://doi.org/10.1111/ajt.16951.

Kinkhabwala, M., J. Lindower, J. F. Reinus, A. L. Principe, and P. J. Gaglio. 2013. Expedited liver allocation in the United States: A critical analysis. *Liver Transplantation* 19(10):1159-1165.

Kotloff, R. M., S. Blosser, G. J. Fulda, D. Malinoski, V. N. Ahya, L. Angel, M. C. Byrnes, M. A. DeVita, T. E. Grissom, S. D. Halpern, T. A. Nakagawa, P. G. Stock, D. L. Sudan, K. E. Wood, S. J. Anillo, T. P. Bleck, E. E. Eidbo, R. A. Fowler, A. K. Glazier, C. Gries, R. Hasz, D. Herr, A. Khan, D. Landsberg, D. J. Lebovitz, D. J. Levine, M. Mathur, P. Naik, C. U. Niemann, D. R. Nunley, K. J. O'Connor, S. J. Pelletier, O. Rahman, D. Ranjan, A. Salim, R. G. Sawyer, T. Shafer, D. Sonneti, P. Spiro, M. Valapour, D. Vikraman-Sushama, and T. P. Whelan. 2015. Management of the potential organ donor in the ICU: Society of Critical Care Medicine/American College of Chest Physicians/Association of Organ Procurement Organizations consensus statement. *Critical Care Medicine* 43(6):1291-1325.

Koval, C. E., E. D. Poggio, Y.-C. Lin, H. Kerr, M. Eltemamy, and A. Wee. 2021. Early success transplanting kidneys from donors with new SARS-CoV-2 RNA positivity: A report of 10 cases. *American Journal of Transplantation* 21(11):3743-3749.

Kress, J., D. L. Smith, P. C. Fehling, and E. J. Gordon. 2009. Improving the recruitment and retention of organ procurement coordinators: A survey study. *American Journal of Transplantation* 9(6):1451-1459.

Kwong, A. J., W. R. Kim, J. R. Lake, J. M. Smith, D. P. Schladt, M. A. Skeans, S. M. Noreen, J. Foutz, S. E. Booker, M. Cafarella, J. J. Snyder, A. K. Israni, and B. L. Kasiske. 2021. OPTN/SRTR 2019 annual data report: Liver. *American Journal of Transplantation* 21(S2):208-315.

Lentine, K. L., B. Kasiske, and D. A. Axelrod. 2021. Procurement biopsies in kidney transplantation: More information may not lead to better decisions. *Journal of the American Society of Nephrology* 32(8):1835-1837.

Li, M. T., K. L. King, S. A. Husain, J. D. Schold, and S. Mohan. 2021. Deceased donor kidneys utilization and discard rates during COVID-19 pandemic in the United States. *Kidney International Reports* 6(9):2463-2467.

Lia, D., P. Singer, V. Nair, J. Yang, L. Teperman, and E. Grodstein. 2021. DCD renal transplantation from donors with acute kidney injury. *Transplantation* 105(4):886-890.

Lindemann, J., L. A. Dageforde, N. Vachharajani, E. Stahlschmidt, D. Brockmeier, J. R. Wellen, A. Khan, W. C. Chapman, and M. M. Doyle. 2018. Cost evaluation of a donation after cardiac death program: How cost per organ compares to other donor types. *Journal of the American College of Surgeons* 226(5):909-916.

Lindemann, J., L. A. Dageforde, D. Brockmeier, N. Vachharajani, M. Scherer, W. Chapman, and M. B. M. Doyle. 2019. Organ procurement center allows for daytime liver transplantation with less resource utilization: May address burnout, pipeline, and safety for field of transplantation. *American Journal of Transplantation* 19(5):1296-1304.

Litvak, E., and H. V. Fineberg. 2013. Smoothing the way to high quality, safety, and economy. *New England Journal of Medicine* 369(17):1581-1583.

Litvak, E., S. Keshavjee, B. L. Gewertz, and H. V. Fineberg. 2021. How hospitals can save lives and themselves: Lessons on patient flow from the COVID-19 pandemic. *Annals of Surgery* 274(1):37-39.

Lynch, R. J., B. L. Doby, D. S. Goldberg, K. J. Lee, A. Cimeno, and S. J. Karp. 2021. Procurement characteristics of high- and low-performing OPOs as seen in OPTN/SRTR data. *American Journal of Transplantation.* https://doi.org/10.1111/ajt.16832.

Madan, S., O. Saeed, S. J. Forest, D. J. Goldstein, U. P. Jorde, and S. R. Patel. 2022. Feasibility and potential impact of heart transplantation from adult donors after circulatory death. *JACC* 79(2):148-162.

Madhusoodanan, J. 2021. Inner workings: Advances in infectious disease treatment promise to expand the pool of donor organs. *Proceedings of the National Academy of Sciences of the United States of America* 118(8):e2100577118.

Marsolais, P., P. Durand, E. Charbonney, K. Serri, A.-M. Lagacé, F. Bernard, and M. Albert. 2017. The first 2 years of activity of a specialized organ procurement center: Report of an innovative approach to improve organ donation. *American Journal of Transplantation* 17(6):1613-1619.

Matesanz, R., B. Domínguez-Gil, E. Coll, G. de la Rosa, and R. Marazuela. 2011. Spanish experience as a leading country: What kind of measures were taken? *Transplant International* 24(4):333-343.

McGivern, L., L. Shulman, J. K. Carney, S. Shapiro, and E. Bundock. 2017. Death certification errors and the effect on mortality statistics. *Public Health Reports* 132(6):669-675.

Moazami, N., O. H. Javadi, D. F. Kappel, J. Wagner, and M. D. Jendrisak. 2007. The feasibility of organ procurement at a hospital-independent facility: A working model of efficiency. *Journal of Thoracic and Cardiovascular Surgery* 133(5):1389-1390.

Mohan, S., and J. D. Schold. 2021. Accelerating deceased donor kidney utilization requires more than accelerating placement. *American Journal of Transplantation.* https://doi.org/10.1111/ajt.16866.

Mohan, S., K. Foley, M. C. Chiles, G. K. Dube, R. E. Patzer, S. O. Pastan, R. J. Crew, D. J. Cohen, and L. E. Ratner. 2016. The weekend effect alters the procurement and discard rates of deceased donor kidneys in the United States. *Kidney International* 90(1):157-163.

Mohan, S., M. C. Chiles, R. E. Patzer, S. O. Pastan, S. A. Husain, D. J. Carpenter, G. K. Dube, R. J. Crew, L. E. Ratner, and D. J. Cohen. 2018. Factors leading to the discard of deceased donor kidneys in the United States. *Kidney International* 94(1):187-198.

Mohan, S., S. L. Tummalapalli, and J. Schold. 2021 (unpublished). *Identifying innovative solutions to financial and policy barriers to increase deceased donor transplantation in the United States.* Paper commissioned by the Committee on a Fairer and More Equitable, Cost-Effective, and Transparent System of Donor Organ Procurement, Allocation, and Distribution, National Academies of Sciences, Engineering, and Medicine, Washington, DC.

Mulvihill, M. S., H. J. Lee, J. Weber, A. Y. Choi, M. L. Cox, B. A. Yerokun, M. A. Bishawi, J. Klapper, M. Kuchibhatla, and M. G. Hartwig. 2020. Variability in donor organ offer acceptance and lung transplantation survival. *Journal of Heart and Lung Transplantation* 39(4):353-362.

Noreen, S. M., D. Klassen, R. Brown, Y. Becker, K. O'Connor, J. Prinz, and M. Cooper. 2022. Kidney accelerated placement project: Outcomes and lessons learned. *American Journal of Transplantation* 22(1):210-221.

NQF (National Quality Forum). 2021. *How measures will serve our future.* https://www.qualityforum.org/Measuring_Performance/ABCs/How_Measures_Will_Serve_Our_Future.aspx (accessed November 3, 2021).

OPTN (Organ Procurement and Transplantation Network). 2021a. *National data.* https://optn.transplant.hrsa.gov/data/view-data-reports/national-data (accessed November 4, 2021).

OPTN. 2021b. *OPTN Kidney Transplantation Committee Meeting Summary: November 15, 2021.* https://optn.transplant.hrsa.gov/media/5lkpjmp2/20211115_kidney-committee_-meeting-summary.pdf (accessed January 27, 2022).

Padilla, M., E. Coll, C. Fernández-Pérez, T. Pont, Á. Ruiz, M. Pérez-Redondo, E. Oliver, L. Atutxa, J. M. Manciño, D. Daga, E. Miñambres, J. Moya, B. Vidal, J. M. Dueñas-Jurado, F. Mosteiro, A. Rodríguez-Salgado, E. Fernández-García, R. Lara, D. Hernández-Marrero, B. Estébanez, M. L. Rodríguez-Ferrero, M. Barber, F. García-López, A. Andrés, C. Santiago, A. Zapatero, R. Badenes, F. Carrizosa, J. J. Blanco, J. L. Bernal, F. J. Elola, C. Vidal, C. Terrón, P. Castro, J. Comas, and B. Domínguez-Gil. 2021. Improved short-term outcomes of kidney transplants in controlled donation after the circulatory determination of death with the use of normothermic regional perfusion. *American Journal of Transplantation* 21(11):3618-3628.

Pagani, F. D. 2022. Heart transplantation using organs from donors following circulatory death: The journey continues. *JACC* 79(2):163-165.

Parker, W. F., Y. Becker, and R. Gibbons. 2021 (unpublished). *Calculating the lives saved with deceased donor kidney transplantation.* Paper commissioned by the Committee on a Fairer and More Equitable, Cost-Effective, and Transparent System of Donor Organ Procurement, Allocation, and Distribution, National Academies of Sciences, Engineering, and Medicine, Washington, DC.

Pearson, R., C. Geddes, P. Mark, M. Clancy, and J. Asher. 2021. Transplantation of kidneys after normothermic perfusion: A single center experience. *Clinical Transplantation* 35(10):e14431.

POGO (Project on Government Oversight). 2021. *Re: First response to December 23, 2020 letter to AOPO.* https://www.documentcloud.org/documents/20529235-aopo-first-response-to-house-oversight-committee-final (accessed February 2, 2022).

Pritt, B. S., N. J. Hardin, J. A. Richmond, and S. L. Shapiro. 2005. Death certification errors at an academic institution. *Archives of Pathology and Laboratory Medicine* 129(11):1476-1479.

Reese, P. P., O. Aubert, M. Naesens, E. Huang, V. Potluri, D. Kuypers, A. Bouquegneau, G. Divard, M. Raynaud, Y. Bouatou, A. Vo, D. Glotz, C. Legendre, C. Lefaucheur, S. Jordan, J. P. Empana, X. Jouven, and A. Loupy. 2021. Assessment of the utility of kidney histology as a basis for discarding organs in the United States: A comparison of international transplant practices and outcomes. *Journal of the American Society of Nephrology* 32(2):397-409.

Ryckman, F. C., P. A. Yelton, A. M. Anneken, P. E. Kiessling, P. J. Schoettker, and U. R. Kotagal. 2009. Redesigning intensive care unit flow using variability management to improve access and safety. *Joint Commission Journal on Quality and Patient Safety* 35(11):535-543.

Saade, M., J. Davies, E. Torres, L. Morales-Otero, Z. Gonzalez-Caraballo, and E. A. Santiago-Delpin. 2005. A marked increase in organ donation in Puerto Rico. *Transplantation Proceedings* 37(9):3618-3620.

Segev, D. L., C. E. Simpkins, R. E. Thompson, J. E. Locke, D. S. Warren, and R. A. Montgomery. 2008. Obesity impacts access to kidney transplantation. *Journal of the American Society of Nephrology* 19(2):349-355.

Shafer, T. J., D. Wagner, J. Chessare, M. W. Schall, V. McBride, F. A. Zampiello, J. Perdue, K. O'Connor, M. J. Lin, and J. Burdick. 2008. U.S. organ donation breakthrough collaborative increases organ donation. *Critical Care Nursing Quarterly* 31(3):190-210.

Shah, A. S. 2021. Normothermic regional perfusion in donor heart recovery: Establishing a new normal. *Journal of Thoracic and Cardiovascular Surgery.* https://doi.org/10.1016/j.jtcvs.2021.11.084.

Sise, M. E., D. S. Goldberg, J. J. Kort, D. E. Schaubel, R. R. Alloway, C. M. Durand, R. J. Fontana, R. S. Brown, J. J. Friedewald, S. Prenner, J. R. Landis, M. Fernando, C. C. Phillips, E. S. Woodle, A. Rike-Shields, K. E. Sherman, N. Elias, W. W. Williams, J. L. Gustafson, N. M. Desai, B. Barnaba, S. P. Norman, M. Doshi, S. T. Sultan, M. J. Aull, J. Levitsky, D. S. Belshe, R. T. Chung, and P. P. Reese. 2020. Multicenter study to transplant hepatitis C–infected kidneys (MYTHIC): An open-label study of combined glecaprevir and pibrentasvir to treat recipients of transplanted kidneys from deceased donors with hepatitis C virus infection. *Journal of the American Society of Nephrology* 31(11):2678-2687.

Smith, C. D., T. Spackman, K. Brommer, M. W. Stewart, M. Vizzini, J. Frye, and W. C. Rupp. 2013. Re-engineering the operating room using variability methodology to improve health care value. *Journal of the American College of Surgeons* 216(4):559-568.

SRTR (Scientific Registry of Transplant Recipients). 2019. *2019 annual data report.* http://srtr.transplant.hrsa.gov/annual_reports/Default.aspx (accessed November 4, 2021).

SRTR. 2021. OPTN/SRTR 2019 annual data report: Preface. *American Journal of Transplantation* 21(S2):1-10.

SRTR. 2022a. *Guide to Key OPO Metrics.* https://www.srtr.org/about-the-data/guide-to-key-opo-metrics (accessed January 27, 2022).

SRTR. 2022b. *Calculating the 5-tier assesments: A guide for pre- and posttransplant metrics.* https://www.srtr.org/about-the-data/guide-to-using-the-srtr-website/txguidearticles/5-tier-outcome-assessment (accessed January 27, 2022).

Steggerda, J. A., M. B. Bloom, M. Noureddin, T. V. Brennan, T. Todo, N. N. Nissen, A. S. Klein, and I. K. Kim. 2020. Higher thresholds for the utilization of steatotic allografts in liver transplantation: Analysis from a U.S. national database. *PLoS ONE* 15(4):e0230995.

Stewart, D. E., V. C. Garcia, J. D. Rosendale, D. K. Klassen, and B. J. Carrico. 2017. Diagnosing the decades-long rise in the deceased donor kidney discard rate in the United States. *Transplantation* 101(3):575-587.

Thornton, J. 2021. Expanding HIV-positive organ donation. *Lancet* 397(10270):184-185.

Traino, H. M., A. J. Molisani, and L. A. Siminoff. 2017. Regional differences in communication process and outcomes of requests for solid organ donation. *American Journal of Transplantation* 17(6):1620-1627.

UNOS (United Network of Organ Sharing). 2020. *Establish better metrics for OPOs and transplant hospitals.* https://unos.org/news/media-resources/5-ways/establish-better-metrics-for-opos-and-transplant-hospitals (accessed November 4, 2021).

UNOS. 2021a. *How we match organs.* https://unos.org/TRANSPLANT/HOW-WE-MATCH-ORGANS/ (accessed November 17, 2021).

UNOS. 2021b. *Updated list of organ refusal reasons will go into effect on Dec. 2.* https://unos.org/news/updated-list-of-organ-refusal-reasons-will-go-into-effect-on-dec-2 (accessed February 4, 2022).

van der Windt, D. J., R. Mehta, D. R. Jorgensen, S. Hariharan, P. S. Randhawa, P. Sood, M. Molinari, M. Wijkstrom, A. Ganoza, and A. D. Tevar. 2021. Donation after circulatory death is associated with increased fibrosis on 1-year post-transplant kidney allograft surveillance biopsy. *Clinical Transplantation* 35(9):e14399.

Veatch, R. M. 2008. Donating hearts after cardiac death—reversing the irreversible. *New England Journal of Medicine* 359:672-673.

Verzelloni Sef, A., D. Sef, V. Trkulja, B. Raj, N. J. Lees, C. Walker, I. McGovern, J. Mitchell, F. De Robertis, and U. Stock. 2021. Postoperative acute kidney injury and renal replacement therapy after DCD lung transplantation. *Clinical Transplantation* 36(2):e14468.

Volk, M. L., H. A. Reichert, A. S. F. Lok, and R. A. Hayward. 2011. Variation in organ quality between liver transplant centers. *American Journal of Transplantation* 11(5):958-964.

Washburn, K., and K. Olthoff. 2012. Truth and consequences: The challenge of greater transparency in liver distribution and utilization. *American Journal of Transplantation* 12(4):808-809.

Wexelman, B. A., E. Eden, and K. M. Rose. 2013. Survey of New York City resident physicians on cause-of-death reporting, 2010. *Preventing Chronic Disease* 10:120288.

WHO (World Health Organization). 2018. *Global status report on road safety 2018: Summary.* Geneva: World Health Organization. https://www.who.int/publications/i/item/9789241565684 (accessed February 2, 2022).

WHO. 2021. *Global patient safety action plan 2021-2030.* https://www.who.int/publications/i/item/9789240032705 (accessed November 11, 2021).

Wolfe, R. A., F. B. LaPorte, A. M. Rodgers, E. C. Roys, G. Fant, and A. B. Leichtman. 2007. Developing organ offer and acceptance measures: When 'good' organs are turned down. *American Journal of Transplantation* 7(5 Pt 2):1404-1411.

Woolley, A. E., S. K. Singh, H. J. Goldberg, H. R. Mallidi, M. M. Givertz, M. R. Mehra, A. Coppolino, A. E. Kusztos, M. E. Johnson, K. Chen, E. A. Haddad, J. Fanikos, D. P. Harrington, P. C. Camp, and L. R. Baden. 2019. Heart and lung transplants from HCV-infected donors to uninfected recipients. *New England Journal of Medicine* 380(17):1606-1617.

Yasinski, E. 2016. *When donated organs go to waste.* https://www.theatlantic.com/health/archive/2016/02/when-donated-organs-go-to-waste/470838 (accessed November 17, 2021).

Yu, K., K. King, S. A. Husain, G. K. Dube, J. S. Stevens, L. E. Ratner, M. Cooper, C. R. Parikh, and S. Mohan. 2020. Kidney nonprocurement in solid organ donors in the United States. *American Journal of Transplantation* 20(12):3413-3425.

# 7

# Measuring and Improving
# System Performance

"The very first step is finding a hospital that will accept you and add you to its waiting list. My coverage determines which doctor or program I can even consult with."
—Fanny Vlahos, double lung transplant recipient,
Cystic Fibrosis Foundation, testimony to the committee
during July 15, 2021 public listening session

O ver the past 20 years, the U.S. health care system has undergone a significant transformation in defining, measuring, and reporting health care quality aimed at improving patient experiences and outcomes and decreasing health care costs. Measurement is a tool that can lead to better care by identifying opportunities for quality improvement, establishing transparency through public reporting, creating accountability for performance, and facilitating the identification and elimination of health disparities. Despite the exponential growth of health care quality measures over the past 2 decades, many parts of health care still face significant measurement challenges, thus limiting their ability to provide high-value and high-quality care.

In the case of the organ transplantation system, there is an impressive amount of data collected resulting in a body of measurement and public reporting. Compared to many other parts of American health care, the levels of measurement in the organ transplantation system are impressive. As one example, the Scientific Registry of Transplant Recipients (SRTR) website is an extraordinary national resource with extensive, publicly available data collected from transplant centers, organ procurement organizations (OPOs), and immunology laboratories on current and past organ donors, transplant candidates, transplant recipients, and transplant outcomes.[1]

---

[1] Scientific Registry of Transplant Recipients website: www.srtr.org (accessed November 2, 2021).

## OPTN MEASUREMENT CHALLENGES[2]

Despite its successes, the Organ Procurement and Transplantation Network (OPTN) still faces significant challenges regarding poor patient experience, overall access to available organs, long waiting list times, high rates of nonuse of procured organs, and high costs. Current data show racial, ethnic, gender, and geographical disparities in access, premature transplant failure and mortality, and reduced quality of life for living donors and recipients (Kulkarni et al., 2019; Puoti et al., 2016; Wesselman et al., 2021; Zhou et al., 2018). Adding a layer of complexity, the OPTN is a diverse ecosystem composed of various stakeholders (e.g., patients, physicians, policy makers, data intermediaries, and health systems) with varying objectives, levels of resources, and data infrastructure, all of which function across vastly different geographical areas. The differences in geography and resources across OPOs can result in varied quality of care and outcomes.

One systematic review found that out of the more than 300 transplant quality metrics reported in the literature, many were poorly defined, had inconsistent definitions, and focused primarily on safety and effectiveness with very few focusing on quality domains such as equity and patient-reported experience measures (Brett et al., 2018). As of 2018, existing transplant quality measures focus primarily on patient survival, transplant center volume, length of stay, and rehospitalization or unplanned return to the operating room. Other metrics include waiting list mortality, patient satisfaction, wait time for initial evaluation, in-hospital mortality, and infections (Brett et al., 2018). Out of all the organs, kidney transplantation has the most measures, and many of the metrics focus specifically on single organ transplant.

## Needed Improvements in OPTN Measurement

To address the numerous challenges facing the OPTN and its stakeholders, the committee has identified six key measurement challenges needing action:

1. Limited collection and use of disaggregated demographic data necessary to accurately track, understand, and eliminate disparities in procurement and transplantation;
2. Limited to no standardization of a short list of key process and outcome measures for assessing basic performance, especially for OPOs;
3. Gaps in standardized and publicly reported measurement related to patient referral, evaluation, and wait-listing at transplant centers;
4. Overemphasis by regulators, payers, and others on using only one or two measures to assess performance of OPOs (donation and transplant rates) and transplant centers (1-year graft survival);
5. Absence of established, consensus-based measurement development and endorsement processes such as those administered by the National Quality Forum; and
6. Limited use of patient-centric measures that address what matters most to patients, such as the odds of getting transplanted before death at one center compared to others.

Addressing these six key areas will help to improve systemwide measurement in ways that will inform quality improvement at the organizational and system levels, assist federal regulators with more thoughtful and comprehensive oversight of OPOs and transplant cen-

---

[2] Much of this section is excerpted or slightly modified from a paper commissioned by the committee for this study (Lantigua et al., 2021). Commissioned papers are in the study's public access file and are available upon request from the National Academies' Public Access Records Office (paro@nas.edu).

ters, better inform patient decision making and choices, and enable more robust understanding and interventions to address disparities, especially disparities in access to transplant.

> *Conclusion 7-1: Performance measures for donor hospitals, OPOs, and transplant centers need to be standardized and aligned to maximize donor referrals, evaluations, and organ procurements; optimize organ allocation; minimize organ nonuse rates and costs; and improve patient experiences and outcomes.*

## DASHBOARD OF STANDARDIZED, CONSENSUS-BASED PERFORMANCE MEASURES

Standardized performance measurement serves as a valuable method for identifying unwarranted variation in care, improving the quality and outcomes of health care services provided, and promoting interoperability and collaboration across organizations and systems. Additionally, standardized measures serve as a foundation for promoting transparency through public reporting and establishing accountability through pay-for-performance models. Standardized measures can also help to identify and eliminate health disparities by detecting differences in quality and access for specific populations or social groups.

Other areas of health care have successfully deployed integrated measurement dashboards to track progress, assess national performance, and guide improvement. One example is the Measure Applications Partnership (MAP) created in 2011 to fulfill a statutory requirement in which multistakeholder feedback is collected for the performance measures that the U.S. Department of Health and Human Services (HHS) is considering for public reporting and performance-based payment programs. The National Quality Forum created MAP as a pre-rulemaking process that allows room for dialogue, dissent, and consensus building to provide strategic input for federal quality programs, and specifically on the statutory measures under consideration by HHS.

Another integrated and comprehensive approach to national measurement is the Agency for Healthcare Research and Quality's (AHRQ's) National Scorecard on Hospital-Acquired Conditions. The AHRQ scorecard synthesizes information from multiple sources within the Centers for Medicare & Medicaid Services (CMS), the Centers for Disease Control and Prevention, and AHRQ to assess overall national progress in hospital patient safety. The scorecard focuses primarily on the 10 major forms of patient harm in hospitals (AHRQ, 2020). Other suites of measures used to track and assess performance include the CMS 5-Star Quality Rating System for Nursing Homes and the 5-Star Quality Rating System for Hospitals.

## Dashboard of Standardized Performance Metrics for the U.S. Organ Transplantation System

As described earlier in this report, there is an opportunity to move away from the current focus on a single metric, such as 1-year-graft survival for transplant centers or donation rates for OPOs, and move toward an interrelated and integrated approach to measurement and performance. Emphasizing the standardization of metrics as a central element can help make the transplantation system become more equitable, transparent, and effective. Established, consensus-based processes facilitated by organizations such as the National Quality Forum can be used to develop measure frameworks that identify the largest needs; define policy gaps through the identification of disparities in care; support accreditation, regulation, and patient choice by identifying areas that are most meaningful to care; and reduce opportunities for manipulation of the system (Obadan-Udoh et al., 2019). For example, some physicians may escalate care to transplant candidates on the waiting list in order to increase their priority in the formalized allocation system (OPTN, 2018).

To help mitigate these measurement challenges and address the six areas for improvement outlined above, the committee recommends the creation of an integrated dashboard of standardized metrics built upon consensus-based measures to holistically track, assess, and guide the full spectrum of the organ transplantation system (see Recommendation 12). The committee believes a dashboard of standardized metrics will help move the organ transplantation system toward an integrated systems approach to measurement, improvement, operations, and results, thereby improving the quality and outcomes of health care services provided in the organ transplantation system.

The suggested standard dashboard does not need to be created from scratch and should be built upon existing extensive OPTN and SRTR measures to the maximum extent possible. Accurate and robust data are needed to have valid and reliable quality measures. Incomplete information and inadequate information exchange can create considerable challenges for care delivery, quality measurement, and health care payment. The committee's recommendation calls for the creation of standardized performance measures that should be included in the dashboard, but the ultimate quality measures chosen need to be based on a consensus-driven process and not impose undue data collection or reporting burden on health professionals or patients. Data registries support efficient measurement with limited data collection burden. Studies have shown that the use of data registries, electronic health records, and health information exchanges help to regulate data collection, facilitate data exchange across multiple institutions, and allow for national benchmarking (Blumenthal, 2018; D'Amore et al., 2021). Data intermediaries—organizations that import data from disparate sources—calculate and report back quality measures that can also help lower the burden of measurement (Ahmad and Tsang, 2012).

In many cases, the standardized measures would replace existing measures, rather than increase the existing burden. For example, OPOs currently track important information like authorization rates. However, the current challenge is that there is no standardized approach to this tracking, which makes it difficult to compare performance, identify low and high performers, appropriately apply incentives and disincentives, guide improvement, or perform other work that requires standardized measurement. The committee's recommended dashboard should also minimize measurement burden by drawing on existing work, such as the OPTN metrics dashboard and access to transplant dashboard.[3]

The OPTN Membership and Professional Standards Committee has proposed four new metrics for evaluating transplant center performance. Two pretransplant measures for transplant centers are the rate of pretransplant deaths and the ratio of organ offers made to and accepted for candidates, as well as two posttransplant metrics of 90-day graft survival and 1-year graft survival conditional to the 90-day period. Implementation of these new measures is expected to be staged, with conditional posttransplant graft survival effective June 2022, followed by offer acceptance by July 2023, and pretransplant (waiting list) mortality by July 2024. As discussed previously, the committee supports the idea of using a more holistic approach—more than a singular metric to evaluate transplant program performance—and applauds the rationale behind these proposed measures. At the same time, the committee believes a more robust set of performance measures, including measures related to access *prior to wait-listing* (i.e., number of patients referred to the center for evaluation and number

---

[3] The OPTN metrics dashboard and Equity in Access dashboard are available at https://optn.transplant.hrsa.gov/data (accessed November 12, 2021).

of referred patients who were evaluated), need to be included in the dashboard of metrics in order to move the transplantation system toward a more equitable and transparent system. Figure 7-1 contains the committee's suggestions for the elements of the proposed standardized performance metrics for transplant centers to be included in the dashboard.

## Referring Organizations & Transplant Centers

**Novel measurements**

- Access: Number of Patients Referred to the Center for Evaluation
- Access: Number of Referred Patients Who Were Evaluated
- Access: Number of Evaluated Patients Who Were Listed
- Number of Organs Offered to Patients That Were Declined
- Survival benefit

**Exsisting measurements**

- Number of Listed Patients Who Died Waiting
- Number of Listed Patients Who Were Transplanted
- 1 Year Graft Survival of Transplanted Patients
- 5 Year Graft Survival of Transplanted Patients

## Donor Hospitals & OPOs

**Novel measurements**

- Number of Ventilated Deaths within 1 Hour of Extubation
- Number of Deaths Medically Suitable for Donation
- Number of Referred Deaths Responded to by OPO
- Number of Authorizations

**Exsisting measurements**

- Number of Total Deaths
- Number of Organs Transplanted
- Number of Deaths Referred by Hospitals to OPO

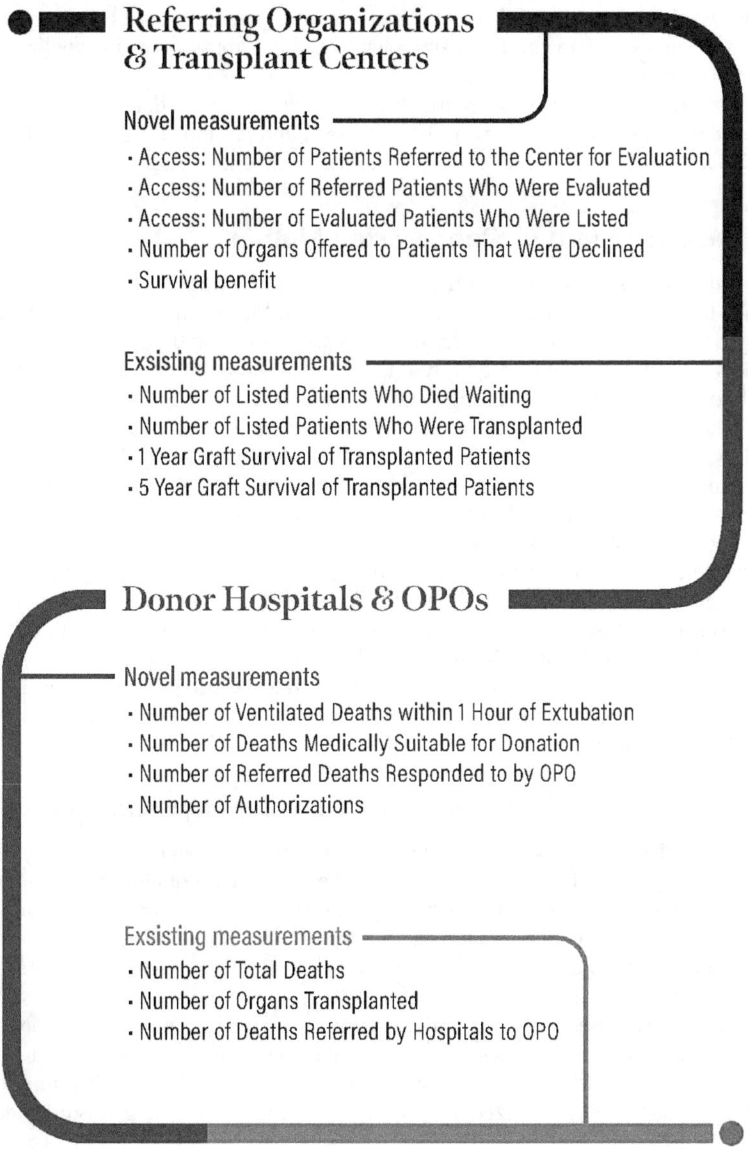

**FIGURE 7-1** Recommended measurement elements for referring organizations, transplant centers, donor hospitals, and OPOs.

## Measurement Elements of the Recommended Dashboard of Standardized Performance Metrics

The dashboard of standardized metrics would include existing measures (i.e., number of listed patients who died waiting and number of total deaths), as well as several novel measures, including those that can close gaps related to disparities and equity—particularly related to access to the waiting list. Additionally, the standardized dashboard would permit the consideration and potential use of patient-centric measures, such as waiting time for transplant, chances of dying on the waiting list, and the number of organs declined on behalf of waiting patients.

The committee suggests measurements to be included in the dashboard of standardized metrics for referring organizations and transplant centers, and donor hospitals and OPOs (Figure 7-1).

## Using the Dashboard of Standardized Metrics

The data included in the standard dashboard should be publicly available and up to date to remain transparent, accountable, and helpful to relevant organizations. The committee envisioned that the standardized performance metrics could be used first as quality improvement tools and, if successful, in quality improvement efforts, then the metrics can be used as standards of performance with regulatory implications.

Audiences and users of the dashboard include individual organizations (e.g., donor hospitals, OPOs, referring organizations, and transplant centers) to gauge their own overall performance, to identify variation within their own organization, and to target areas of improvement in quality and outcomes. Patients and families seeking to make informed choices about transplant access and care would also use the dashboard. Researchers as well as federal regulators who seek consensus measures that have been endorsed and affirmed by organizations like the National Quality Forum and the regulated community of practice would also use the dashboard. For patients, having standardized process and outcome metrics for the organ transplantation system would contribute mightily as a source of information that likely would be applied in ways other than as a dashboard, such as via applications that package key elements of the data and make it available either proactively, via nudging and other means, or reactively.

### *Importance of the Patient Voice in Measure Development and Use*

In the past decade, the health care enterprise has shifted from patients being passive care recipients to empowered active participants in their care, with quality measurement following this critical shift. Collaboration between patients, caregivers, and health care providers can improve cost and health outcomes. To ensure that standardized measures matter to patients, patients and families need to be engaged in identifying where measures should be used, which measures are most meaningful to them, and where new measures are needed to assess important aspects of care. Patients can be engaged in the development and use of standardized performance measures through patient and family advisory councils, quality improvement teams, and on governing and leadership boards. Creating avenues for patients to inform the use of standardized performance measures can help ensure measures are meaningful and useful.

## A Path Forward

Standardized performance measures, derived through a consensus-based process, can serve as a powerful tool in ensuring that the U.S. transplantation system is efficient, fair, equitable, and of high value. This can be accomplished by identifying how to best maximize donor referrals, evaluations, and the procurement and allocation of organs while minimizing nonuse rates and overall costs. The U.S. transplantation system currently faces challenges similar to other sectors of health care regarding disparities in access and outcomes, inefficiencies, and high costs. However, unlike many other areas of health care, the OPTN is well positioned to develop, select, and implement standardized performance measures to drive high-quality, high-value care. Specifically, the OPTN has the existing infrastructure to support standardized measurement, including robust data collection, clear identified partners, and available evidence-based guidelines. Existing partners already formulate and evaluate data for policy and organ allocation system performance metrics and can be engaged alongside other relevant stakeholders to identify process gaps and targets for measurement.

Standardized performance measures would facilitate a better understanding of the geographical- and patient-level challenges facing the organ transplantation system and enable the implementation of data-driven quality improvement to create lasting change. The development of a consensus-based measurement framework for the organ transplantation system can help create a transparent process that incorporates broad stakeholder input, maximizes trust in the associated processes, and encourages buy-in from the field. Additionally, a consensus-based framework can help to advance patient-centered care by centering the patient voice, identifying existing quality gaps and disparities, harmonizing existing and future measurement, and ultimately helping to improve the effectiveness and equity of the organ transplantation system.

*Conclusion 7-2: The performance of the U.S. organ transplantation system, and its component parts, is highly variable and often inexplicable, with little understanding or justification for areas of variation that are acceptable or unacceptable. There is a need to reduce variations in the performance of donor hospitals, OPOs, and transplant centers in order to increase equity, efficiency, usefulness, reliability, predictability, and trustworthiness of the transplantation system. Creating standardized, consensus-based metrics to compare performance of donor hospitals, OPOs, and transplant centers needs to be a priority for HHS and the OPTN. Federal agencies overseeing the transplantation system will need to collaborate on data collection, even for the parts of the system they do not oversee, to ensure relevant, accurate, and timely data are available about the transplantation system.*

**Recommendation 12: Create a dashboard of standardized metrics to track performance and evaluate results in the U.S. organ transplantation system.**

**HHS should use a combination of currently collected data and new data elements specifically related to access to transplant to create a publicly available dashboard of standardized metrics to measure the performance of the organ transplantation system. The metrics in the dashboard should be developed to be meaningful to donor families, individuals with chronic disease or organ failure, transplant candidates, and individuals on the waiting list and their families, and to ensure accountability and partnership across the components of the system. The metrics should be used for quality improve-**

ment, and once they are deemed valid and reliable, they should be used for regulatory purposes. Specific actions HHS should take include the following:

- Establish standardized data collection requirements, with an emphasis on timeliness of reporting, for donor hospitals, OPOs, and transplant centers. All data points collected should reflect demographics—that is, the most updated way of capturing race, ethnicity, and language, as well as socioeconomic factors, disability status, a social deprivation index based on geography, and other factors to better document, understand, reduce, and eventually eliminate disparities.
- Require collaboration among the federal agencies with oversight of the transplantation system on data collection to ensure relevant, accurate, and timely data are available about the transplantation system.
- Collaborate with an organization like the National Quality Forum to develop consensus measures and measure specifications to evaluate and improve the performance of the organ transplantation system in a standardized way. Recommended data points needed from donor hospitals, OPOs, referring organizations, and transplant centers are detailed in Figure 7-1.
- Create a publicly available dashboard of standardized metrics to provide a complete human-centered picture of the patient experience—from patient referral for transplant evaluation, time on the waiting list, to posttransplant quality of life—managed by the SRTR or a similar entity.

## QUALITY IMPROVEMENT IN ORGAN DONATION AND TRANSPLANTATION

Over the last 30 years principles of quality improvement (QI) pioneered in manufacturing have been applied in health care to improve patient care and outcomes. While the application of the methods has been uneven across systems and regions, a great deal has been learned about principles of quality improvement and their value. Coupled with the QI movement in health care has been the study of how to take learning and improvement from one location, such as a hospital or clinic, to another setting. The success in improvements in patient safety in the United States in the 1990s and 2000s generated an interest in their application across the health system and social sector in subsequent years. Lessons from this application of improvement methods at a large scale, built on the foundation of improvement science and methods, has great potential to further improve the organ transplantation system in the United States.

In 2003, the organ transplantation system began work to employ these methods that were used to great success, initially to increase the rate of organ donation across the country (Shafer et al., 2008), and subsequently to improve organ recovery after circulatory death and to increase kidney transplants (OPTN, 2020; Tosoc-Haskell et al., 2019). While demonstrating a promising foundation upon which to build, tremendous variation and continued potential for improvement persist among donor hospitals, OPOs, referring organizations, and transplant centers.

### Challenges and Opportunities in Quality Improvement

Typically, where systems struggle is not in the generation of ideas and successful practices but in effectively spreading those practices to all who could benefit from a broader execution. QI methods can successfully facilitate the broad adaptation and adoption of successful practices through an emphasis on execution.

For people to change they must have the desire to change or demonstrate a will to change, as commonly referenced in QI literature (Nolan, 2007). How to encourage change and generate the will for change is therefore an important undertaking. The psychologist Jonathan Haidt uses the metaphor of a "divided mind" in which human behavior can be understood as a rider on top of an elephant. The rider, representing logical thought, acts as an advisor to the elephant it is riding. The elephant can be understood as human emotion, which in contrast to the rider is larger and seemingly has a disproportionate share of the say in which direction the rider will go (Haidt, 2006). While humans often know what they ought to do, this metaphor illustrates why rational thought and emotions do not always align to produce the desired or expected results. Quality improvement principles described by Deming underscore the importance of psychology and recognizing how and why humans are motivated to change. This understanding is critical to the success or failure of improvement initiatives.

In successful quality improvement, changes must be adopted over time across a desired population. Therefore, it is useful to understand demographically the different "personalities" as they pertain to receptiveness to change. In considering the diffusion of innovation, one must consider the types of people involved and their receptivity to an innovation (Dearing and Cox, 2018). These categories are helpful for change leaders to understand as they consider strategies to build the will for change within their organizations and across entire networks and systems. Different strategies will work for different people, and change leaders need to be prepared to understand the heterogeneity among their audiences and what will compel changes among different categories and individuals.

Improvements in the health care system will almost always require complex behavior change, and successful QI efforts must employ an intentional strategy for spreading changes. As appealing as the concept of natural diffusion sounds, complex behavior change requires active efforts to facilitate the adaptation or adoption of new ideas and practices. McCannon et al. (2007) elaborate that

> Good ideas, even when their value is thoroughly demonstrated in one place, will not reliably spread into action through normal communication channels at a pace truly responsive to the enormous health care challenges.

This is also applicable to the U.S. organ transplantation system. Fortunately, strategies to support active dissemination and use of complex changes have been well documented in health care settings. The strategies combine principles from quality improvement, network management, social psychology, and logistics, and apply them to large-scale change efforts. These disciplines come together to form a method, or multitude of methods, by which change is facilitated.

## Systematic Quality Improvement Options

Effective systems will have the infrastructure in place to identify what is working on an ongoing basis ("bright spotting") and to couple that identification with the ability to test, adapt, and spread what works across the entire network (Sutton and Rao, 2014). This process requires support with the tools and resources to make change and track whether the change is leading to improvement. In executing successful changes at scale, three large-scale-change networked learning models may apply to the organ donation system: (1) collaboratives; (2) behavior change campaigns; and (3) mandates, policy, and regulation.

## Collaboratives

A collaborative, also called a breakthrough series collaborative, is a results-oriented model designed to spread a change when there is a gap between current practice and desired results with an evidence-based intervention (or set of interventions) that are known to be effective in closing the gap. This method is frequently used when piloting or spreading practices and can be used with groups ranging from the tens to thousands. Collaboratives were developed by the Institute for Healthcare Improvement (IHI) and have been used nationally and internationally. Hallmarks of collaboratives are shared, time-bound aims across the network of participants, a core group of participants who take part in group activities and are responsible for taking on the role of change agents within their home organization, a shared set of standardized measures, and a shared set of interventions being adapted and spread across the network. There is a rhythm to the work wherein participating teams attend meetings that provide just-in-time subject matter and QI information, then apply the newly gained knowledge at their home organization(s) while measuring progress, and then attend a meeting that provides additional knowledge and support. This cycle continues multiple times within a year. Peer-to-peer sharing and transparency are emphasized so results can be known and understood, successes and failures can lead to learning, and progress can be spread and celebrated.

The Health Resources and Services Administration (HRSA) within the U.S. Department of Health and Human Services led the U.S. Organ Donation Breakthrough Collaborative from 2003 to 2007 which was not only successful in increasing the number of eligible organ donors across the country, but also spurred subsequent collaboratives for the next decade that together have yielded positive changes among donor services. The collaborative set a shared aim of increasing the organ donation rate in the country from 46 percent of all eligible donors to 75 percent among the nation's 500 largest trauma centers. Using a shared set of changes and measures and the collaborative model described above, the organ donation rate increased by 10.8 percent in 2004 with continuing increases in subsequent years (IHI, 2003, 2021a). The collaborative helped to redesign the organ donation system (Shafer et al., 2006), and the effect of the collaborative on the number of monthly U.S. organ donors can be seen in Figure 7-2. In the month following the first learning session of the collaborative in September 2003, the number of U.S. organ donors increased compared to the same month of the prior year for 35 of the next 39 months. The collaborative also had a positive return on investment with an estimated 41,000 life-years gained and $2.5 billion saved in the years since the initiation of the collaborative, while the cost of running the collaborative was just $2.5 million (Schnitzler, 2021).

Subsequent collaboratives in the organ donation community have continued a steady trajectory of improvement within parts of the system. Numerous OPOs have become skilled systems improvers through the use of QI methods that form the foundation of collaborative improvement. Transplant centers have been involved in QI efforts to a lesser degree. However, building on the success of OPO improvement initiatives, the participation of transplant centers in similar initiatives could lead to comparable improvement in the U.S. organ transplantation system.

Notably, in 2020 CMS and HRSA launched a transplant learning collaborative, aimed at reducing the national nonuse rate of procured kidneys from 19 to 15 percent and increasing annual growth in the number of deceased donor kidneys transplanted from 5 to 15 percent (HRSA, 2020). The project aims to build on the best practices of high performers within the U.S. transplantation system and is informed by the work of the OPTN's Collaborative Innovation and Improvement Network (Wey et al., 2020).

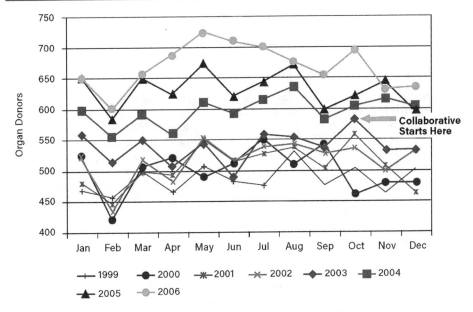

**FIGURE 7-2** Monthly U.S. organ donor rate, 1999–2006, reflecting effect of the Organ Donation Breakthrough Collaborative.
SOURCE: Reproduced with permission from Shafer et al., 2008. https://journals.lww.com/ccnq/Abstract/2008/07000/US_Organ_Donation_Breakthrough_Collaborative.2.aspx (accessed January 27, 2022).

## Behavior Change Campaigns

Behavior change campaigns borrow principles of how to reach large audiences from political campaigns and apply them to behavior change. The approach was developed through the 100,000 Lives Campaign and the 5 Million Lives Campaign operated by IHI, and has now been applied successfully both within health care and the social sector (IHI, 2021b; McCannon et al., 2006). Additional successful examples include the 100,000 Homes Campaign, which led to 100,000 homeless people across the country finding permanent housing, and the Partnership for Patients, led by CMS and HHS (Bornstein, 2014; CMS, 2021c). Campaigns are appropriate when trying to reach large audiences with one or a set of simple, highly vetted interventions with well-understood application. For instance, the 100,000 Lives Campaign sought to prevent instances of harm in U.S. hospitals by spreading six evidence-based interventions such as one to prevent surgical site infections, in order to save 100,000 lives (McCannon et al., 2006). Campaigns are built around compelling aims and rely on local infrastructure such as existing networks or "field offices" to support application at a local level.

A campaign could be used effectively in the organ transplantation system if, for instance, high leverage and well-understood interventions from the Organ Donation Breakthrough Collaborative can be distilled with an aim to spread their use further or increase uptake of their use. Similarly, a campaign could take straightforward practices that result in successful organ transplant waiting list management in some regions and spread them to regions that could benefit from improvement while using local infrastructure for the support and management of the change efforts. Because many OPOs have some QI skills already, they could be prime candidates to help with the local management of such efforts.

## Mandates, Policy, and Regulation

Mandates, policies, and regulations are often the logical output of the approaches described above. Rather than being the starting point, they can be used effectively to leverage change once an intervention has been well characterized, spread to many locations, and the intricacies of its effect in numerous settings are well understood. All too often these approaches are used as a first line to stimulate change rather than using awareness-raising and will-building strategies. When this is done, there is a risk of unintended consequences because the intervention's effect is not yet fully understood in certain situations and the nuance of spreading change is overlooked. When planned and timed well, mandates, policies, and regulations can have a significant effect.

> *Conclusion 7-3: The committee concludes widespread variation in practices and performance among donor hospitals, OPOs, referring organizations, and transplant centers shows there is a need to support and expand the use of proven systemwide quality improvement methods used in other areas of health care and that have successfully been used in the past to improve organ donation.*

**Recommendation 13: Embed continuous quality improvement efforts across the fabric of the U.S. organ transplantation system.**

**HHS should take actions to reduce variations in the performance of donor hospitals, OPOs, and transplant centers and increase the reliability, predictability, and trustworthiness of the U.S. organ transplantation system through implementing and sustaining continuous quality improvement efforts across the system. HHS should hold the component parts of the organ transplantation system accountable for achieving demonstrable performance improvement. With government leadership, quality improvement efforts should create greater systemness and accountability for the highest possible performance among all donor hospitals, OPOs, and transplant centers. Special attention and focus should be given to spreading best practices in organ procurement and transplantation that reduce and eliminate inequities and disparities. The following are specific actions HHS should take in this regard:**

- Sustain continuous quality improvement work on a national scale over time as a long-term investment in lifesaving transplants.
- Align quality improvement efforts with the performance goals for the U.S. organ transplantation system (see Recommendation 1). Quality improvement efforts should improve the prework that includes identifying who would possibly benefit from a transplant and also the postwork of caring for people who receive a transplant.
- Deploy quality improvement techniques that focus on behavior change tools, implementation science, nudging, and education theory to realize uptake of best practices for organ procurement, use, and transplantation across donor hospitals, OPOs, and transplant centers.
- Promote the development, systematic sharing, adaptation, and use of best practices in areas such as rapid referral and early response by donor hospitals and OPOs,

increasing donation authorization rates among diverse populations, pursuit of all possible organ donors, how to have culturally sensitive conversations with all families about organ donation, intensive waiting list management, successful use of medically complex organs, and how best to communicate with patients about organ offers.

- Urge hospitals to smooth surgical scheduling to both enable organ donation surgical procedures, and to ensure the hospital's capability to accept and use organ offers, regardless of which day of the week the gift of donation occurs.
- Explore additional tools and approaches for promoting innovation in the organ transplantation system, including the following:
  - Launch a nationwide learning process improvement collaborative to address deceased organ donors, waiting list management, the acceptance of offered organs, transplant rate, and automated organ referrals.
  - Encourage preapproved controlled experiments by OPOs and transplant centers to allow experimentation with innovation and the development of evidence to support widespread adoption of best practices.
  - Incentivize transplant centers, donor hospitals and OPOs to actively participate in the kidney transplantation collaborative sponsored by CMS and HRSA.
  - Require the OPTN to implement an organized system of proactive communication or nudges in the form of special messages or brief reports aimed at calling attention to outlier performance by OPOs and transplant centers, based on SRTR data. Nudges should be sent to both high and low performers. For example, OPOs with a low percentage of donation after circulatory determination of death (DCDD) donors in their deceased donor organ pool could receive a special message or brief report calling attention to their current performance in comparison to other OPOs.

## ALIGNING INCENTIVES TO MAXIMIZE ORGAN USE

The committee was tasked with making recommendations to better align the performance metrics or incentives of various stakeholders within the OPTN, specifically donor service areas, OPOs, and transplant centers, to maximize donor referrals, evaluations, procurement, and organ placement and allocation while minimizing organ nonuse rates (see Chapter 1 for the full Statement of Task).

Building on the previous report chapters and the committee's focus areas of equity, system performance, and maximizing the use of procured organs, the remainder of Chapter 7 includes the committee's analysis of the evidence around financial incentives and the identification of opportunities to improve alignment of incentives in the organ transplantation system. In addition to the stakeholders referenced in the study task, the committee considers dialysis centers, donor hospitals, and physicians (primary care and specialists such as nephrologists) responsible for referring transplant candidates for evaluation as core participants in the transplantation system. Therefore, the committee considered financial incentives related to these stakeholders as well. As described earlier in the report, the organ transplantation system is complex and the component parts of the system—including payers such as CMS, the Veterans Health Administration, and private payers—do not currently operate as a fully integrated system accountable for achieving predictable, consistent, and equitable results.

*Conclusion 7-4: The authority of federal payers and the power of private insurers to set eligibility requirements and payment rates in the organ transplantation system greatly influences who obtains a transplant and when that occurs. Donors, families, hospitals, OPOs, transplant centers, and patients awaiting a transplant depend on these public and private payers to act in ways that will promote rather than retard steps, such as those recommended in this report, aimed at increasing the number and the equitable distribution of organ transplants.*

## Select CMS Initiatives in Organ Transplantation Reimbursements

CMS provides federal leadership on reimbursement policies for Medicare-eligible patients in need of transplantation, and in particular individuals needing kidney transplants. Since 1972, Medicare benefits have been provided to individuals with end-stage kidney (renal) disease regardless of age and without a waiting period to enroll in Medicare. The benefits support dialysis or kidney transplant. As discussed in previous chapters, CMS also sets conditions for coverage for OPOs and conditions of participation for transplant programs and donor hospitals—setting requirements that must be met for OPOs, transplant programs, and donor hospitals to receive Medicare and Medicaid payment.

CMS requests that dialysis centers inform new patients of their transplant options, which can potentially lead to referral for transplant evaluation before dialysis even begins (Waterman et al., 2015). Strategies are needed to reduce existing disparities in referral for transplant evaluation, however. In the United States, black patients are less likely to be put on a waiting list for transplant before beginning dialysis than white patients, but early, predialysis discussions about transplantation can improve waiting list placement among black patients (Kutner et al., 2012). Transplant education and engagement activities for dialysis facility staff and patients have also been associated with increased kidney transplant evaluation referrals and improved equity in the referral process in a randomized controlled trial among patients receiving dialysis at facilities in Georgia (Patzer et al., 2017).

The CMS Innovation Center has had an active role in testing different funding models for treatment options for end-stage kidney disease. For example, three relevant activities in the past 5 years include the following:

- The End-Stage Renal Disease (ESRD) Treatment Choices Model began in January 2021 and encourages dialysis facilities and health care providers, through payment adjustments, to decrease disparities in the rates of home dialysis and kidney transplantation among end-stage kidney disease patients with lower socioeconomic status. The test model is mandatory for the dialysis facilities randomly selected by CMS to participate and accounts for 30 percent of all end-stage kidney disease facilities and managing clinicians (Medicare-enrolled physicians and nonphysicians that care for one or more end-stage kidney disease beneficiaries) in the United States (CMS, 2021a).
- The Kidney Care Choices model began in January 2022 and focuses on financial incentives for health care providers—dialysis facilities, nephrologists, and other health care providers—to manage the care for Medicare beneficiaries with chronic kidney disease (stages 4 and 5) and end-stage kidney disease (CMS, 2021b). The goal is to delay the onset of dialysis and incentivize kidney transplantation. One of the payment incentives in the model is a $15,000 bonus payment for Medicare patients that receive a kidney transplant and do not return to dialysis. The payment is made to nephrologists who partner with transplant providers, and possibly dialysis facilities and other providers, to incentivize supporting Medicare patients through the transplant process, including continued care management posttransplant. The $15,000

payment is disbursed in smaller amounts for each year posttransplant, and the payments must be shared with partners (e.g., transplant teams, OPOs) (CMS, 2019a).

- A learning collaborative through the CMS ESRD Treatment Choices Model was established in 2020 to operate as a voluntary learning system focused on reducing the kidney nonuse rate, and increasing the availability of deceased donor kidneys for transplantation. The learning system includes model participants and other stakeholders such as transplant centers, OPOs, and large donor hospitals, and uses learning and QI techniques to systematically spread the best practices of the highest performers (CMS, 2019b).

## Donor Hospital Conditions of Participation

The cooperation and involvement of donor hospitals and medical personnel is an essential function of the organ transplantation system. Shortly after the enactment of the National Organ Transplant Act, Prottas (1998) described the relationship thus,

> the primary factor affecting the supply of transplantable organs is the cooperation of health professionals. OPOs must obtain timely access to potential donors who are mainly identified and contacted by the nurses and neurophysicians in ICUs [intensive care units]. The discretion of medical personnel is limited to their judgment about medical suitability for donation while required request laws ensure that the family is offered the option of organ donation.

Over the past 30 years, there have been numerous iterations of state and federal statutes and regulations that have addressed this fundamental relationship between donor hospitals and OPOs. Two effective regulatory and statutory requirements for increasing organ donation have been (1) the timely referral of all individuals whose death is imminent or who died in the hospital, and (2) first person authorization.

The committee received public comments regarding the outdated nature of CMS Interpretive Guidelines (IGs) for hospital conditions of participation, which have been in place since 2008. There is an opportunity to improve alignment in hospital regulations related to organ donation. Current IGs lack sufficient detail and direction in addressing hospital practices related to the timely referral of donors, the ability to pronounce death timely, authorization by first person or legal next of kin, DCDD as a pathway to donation, or physiologically maintaining donors until the OPO can test and allocate organs. The IGs are also silent in requiring the measurement of hospital performance against the conditions of participation.

Updated CMS guidance in the Interpretive Guidelines would more effectively integrate hospital and OPO systemness, fairness, equity, and the transparency necessary for improvements in organ donation, and ultimately transplantation. The following elements could be considered in updating CMS guidance and survey procedures to enhance clarity for hospitals and OPO performance:

- Require hospitals to create electronic or automated referral processes with the OPO to ensure timely referrals of potential donors, and provide patient-level information necessary to determine donor potential. Ideally, this information would also be reported electronically to CMS as part of the calculations used to assess the number of eligible donors.
- Require honoring first person authorization, and establish processes for OPO and hospital responsibilities when there is initial opposition to the donor registry.
- Address several processes essential to DCDD donation: require hospitals to participate in DCDD donation; provide guidance addressing DCDD referral triggers, which may be dif-

ferent than for donation after neurological determination of death (DNDD); and require hospital support in the declaration of death, whether in the ICU, emergency department, operating room, or elsewhere in the hospital.

- Strengthen the requirements that hospitals maintain potential donors while necessary testing and placement of organs takes place, including the declaration of DNDD or DCDD.
- Require trained OPO staff to approach donor families, eliminating the provision for hospital-designated requestors. Hospital staff would serve in a supportive capacity in all family conversations related to donation.
- Update areas where ventilator support might be used, and donors supported, beyond the ICU or emergency department.
- Include in the CMS survey procedures the addition of a policy or process map showing integration of the OPO into the hospital quality assurance and performance improvement process, including an interview with OPO staff to verify.
- Survey hospital compliance against top-line measures of 100 percent timely referral of all deaths, and determine compliance with measurable elements of hospital agreements with OPOs.
- Hold hospitals accountable for smoothing surgical scheduling to ensure the capacity to recover and transplant donated organs 7 days a week.

*Conclusion 7-5: The CMS Interpretive Guidelines and survey processes for donor hospitals need updating to reflect changes that have taken place in medical practice and processes related to the relationship between donor hospitals and OPOs in order to maximize every donation opportunity.*

## Opportunities to Align Reimbursement Incentives

In considering opportunities to improve alignment of reimbursement incentives for stakeholders in the organ transplantation system, the committee explored the following areas:

- Referrals for transplant evaluation;
- Reimbursement to transplant centers for transplanting medically complex organs and caring for patients who receive these transplants;
- Intensive waiting list management;
- Enhanced communication and education with patients on the waiting list;
- Medical care and support for waiting list patients, including those with complex needs; and
- Innovative technology to maximize organ use.

The remainder of this chapter discusses these opportunities for improved alignment, reflects on differing viewpoints within the committee regarding the appropriate role of financial incentives in changing behaviors, and ends with the committee's recommendations for aligning reimbursement and programs with desired outcomes and behaviors (Recommendation 14).

### Referrals for Transplant Evaluation

For patients with advanced chronic kidney disease and end-stage kidney disease, kidney transplantation is the treatment of choice. As described in Chapter 2, transplantation is superior to dialysis in improving both patient survival and quality of life (OPTN, 2015). Additionally, kidney transplantation is also the most cost-effective treatment for end-stage kidney disease, although the extent of cost savings vary by quality of the donor organ. Clinical practice guidelines indicate all patients with advanced chronic kidney disease (stages 4 and 5) and end-stage kidney disease need to be referred for transplant evaluation, as should certain patients with a higher level of kidney function. Among the benefits of early referral are the opportunity to provide more comprehensive patient education about transplant options and potentially intervene earlier in the course of disease. To improve the quality of care for patients with kidney disease, strategies are needed to incentivize nephrologists and dialysis centers to educate and refer patients for transplant evaluation.

## Reimbursement for Medically Complex Cases

As stated previously, compared to dialysis, kidney transplantation increases overall survival rates and improves quality of life for patients with end-stage kidney disease, in addition to being cost effective. An economic assessment of kidney transplant practice found that compared to dialysis, all transplantation types were associated with improved survival and were cost effective regardless of donor type, despite the higher costs associated with the use of medically complex organs and living donors. Compared to dialysis, the authors found cost savings with living donor and low–Kidney Donor Profile Index (KDPI) deceased donor transplantations, while transplantations using high-KDPI deceased donors, ABO-incompatible living donors, or human leukocyte antigen-incompatible living donors were found to be cost effective (less than $100,000 per quality-adjusted life year) (Axelrod et al., 2018).

In the inpatient prospective payment system Final Rule for 2021, CMS recognized that increasing the range of donated organs used in transplantation to include more medically complex organs can result in some patients requiring more medical support. For example, the two new Diagnosis Related Group (DRG) codes created for kidney transplant patients who require dialysis posttransplant and for such patients with major complications and comorbidities are, respectively, 15 and 40 percent higher than the DRG payment for uncomplicated kidney transplants. Likewise, the new DRG for simultaneous kidney and pancreas transplants where the patient needs dialysis is 23 percent higher than what is paid when that form of posttransplant care is not required.

The Donor Risk Index (DRI), a measurement of donor organ quality, was developed to quantitatively assess risk of graft failure following liver transplant (Feng et al., 2006). Increasing DRI is correlated with risk of organ failure. DRI is also an independent predictor of the perioperative and postoperative costs of liver transplant. A retrospective database analysis of the interactions between donor characteristics, recipient liver disease severity, and total inpatient costs of liver transplantation found that the donors in the highest DRI quartile added nearly $12,000 to the cost of transplantation and nearly $22,000 to posttransplantation cost compared to the lowest-risk donors (Salvalaggio et al., 2011). The confluence of these factors may be particularly effective on transplant centers in competitive regions where liver transplant patients with higher Model for End-Stage Liver Disease scores receive organs with high DRI (Salvalaggio et al., 2011).

## Intensive Waiting List Management

Optimizing transplant waiting list management is critical for maintaining candidacy of kidney transplant recipients and effectively managing the waiting list as organs become available. A novel kidney transplant waiting list management strategy called Transplant Readiness

Assessment Clinic (TRAC), was developed to support active management for patients whose Kidney Allocation Scores exceeded a certain threshold (Cheng et al., 2018). The use of TRAC resulted in a higher proportion of patients being actively managed at 18 months. An aggressive waiting list management protocol was designed and tested in two hospital settings, finding that the costs associated with this aggressive protocol were offset by the economic benefits of increased transplantation and reduced time lost in the allocation of deceased donor organs (Grafals et al., 2014). Improving waiting list management requires more clarity about waiting list inactivity prior to kidney transplantation, which is known to affect clinical outcomes. For instance, a study of adult kidney transplant patients in the United States found that inactive periods on the waiting list were predictive of increased pre- and posttransplantation mortality (Norman et al., 2013).

## Enhanced Communication and Education with Patients on the Waiting List

The provision of kidney transplant education is associated with higher rates of transplant (Balhara et al., 2012). Patients who initiate the process of transplant evaluation with greater transplant knowledge and motivation tend to be more likely to receive successful transplants years later (Rodrigue et al., 2014). Educational materials about transplantation—including information about waiting list practices and organ offers and declines—need to be presented to waiting list patients in a broadly accessible manner using clear communication strategies.

Transplant education is of particular importance within the dialysis center context, as 70 percent of ESRD patients are on dialysis (Waterman et al., 2020). Dialysis centers that have higher referral rates and transplant wait-listing rates tend to use multiple patient education strategies (Waterman et al., 2015). Education strategies that have been associated with increased transplant waiting list rates include distribution of print education and use of more than one intensive education practice within dialysis centers (Waterman et al., 2020). According to a survey of nephrologists, most respondents (81 percent) reported that patients at dialysis centers should receive at least 20 minutes of education; however, less than half reported actually spending more than 20 minutes educating individual patients and their families (Balhara et al., 2012).

It is critical to identify and mitigate ways that disparities in the provision of transplant education contribute to disparities in access to transplantation. An evaluation of the association between transplant education practices and access to transplantation analyzed United States Renal Data System data from 2005 to 2007 (Kucirka et al., 2012). Patients who were older, obese, uninsured, Medicaid insured, and patients at for-profit centers were less likely to be assessed at all; women were more likely to be deemed medically unfit; and black patients were more likely to be assessed as psychologically unfit. Moreover, the readability of educational materials can impede access to transplant among patients with lower levels of health literacy if the materials are not easy to understand (Bababekov et al., 2017).

## Medical Care and Support for Waiting List Patients, Including Those with Complex Needs

Many transplant candidates have multiple physical and mental health comorbidities that can affect their clinical outcomes and quality of life while they are wait-listed. For example, conditions such as diabetes, hypertension, and obesity can contribute to the development of ESRD—which itself is a risk factor for comorbidities such as cardiovascular disease—and the number of comorbidities among kidney transplant recipients has increased substantially in recent years (Wu et al., 2020). A prospective cohort study that analyzed the relationship between donor kidney recipient comorbidity and survival outcomes in the United Kingdom found that heart failure and diabetes were associated with poorer transplant survival among living donor kidney transplant recipients (Wu et al., 2020). Comorbidity assessment is of particular importance among patients with ESRD being evaluated for kidney transplantation, because comorbidities can accelerate the progression of ESRD and reduce the chance of survival (Fernández et al., 2019). A study evaluating the association between comorbidity and waiting list mortality among frail and nonfrail kidney transplantation candidates found that nonfrail candidates with high comorbidity burdens at kidney transplant evaluation have increased risk of waiting list mortality (Fernández et al., 2019). New care modalities such as remote video monitoring may contribute to improved patient safety and satisfaction, as has been demonstrated in lung-transplant candidates with multiple comorbidities (Zubrinic et al., 2019).

Many organ transplant recipients experience mental health conditions both pre- and posttransplant. For example, depression is thought to affect up to 60 percent of solid organ transplant recipients (Corbett et al., 2013). Mental health comorbidities can affect these patients' clinical outcomes and undermine their quality of life; however, when properly supported, transplant patients with mental health conditions have outcomes similar to the general transplant population (Corbett et al., 2013). Therefore, potential transplant candidates should be assessed for mental health issues, as well as preexisting medical conditions that mimic mental health problems, so that pharmacological treatment and other interventions can be offered to patients while they are on the waiting list (Corbett et al., 2013; Crawford et al., 2013). In solid organ transplant patients, feeling a sense of control has been associated with positive health outcomes (Crawford et al., 2013).

A randomized trial investigated the effects of two health educational models on the psychology and nutrition of patients waiting for deceased donor kidney transplantation (Ye et al., 2011). The observational group had lower self-rated anxiety and depression after the intervention as well as higher triceps skinfold thickness, hemoglobin, and albumin. These findings suggest that comprehensive health education methods can contribute to alleviating mental stress, improving nutrition, and contributing to better quality of life for patients awaiting kidney transplantation.

Pretransplant psychosocial vulnerability factors are associated with negative outcomes for transplant patients, including higher infection rates, reduced treatment adherence, increased rejection episodes, acute late rejection, hospital readmission, increased cost of care, posttransplant malignancies, graft loss, and decreased transplant survival (Maldonado, 2019). A cross-sectional survey on the concerns and anxiety of patients awaiting organ transplant was conducted in Hong Kong, revealing the importance of providing sufficient psychosocial support to those awaiting organ transplantation (Li et al., 2012). To better support patients, a psychosocial pretransplant evaluation could help to identify and provide care for mental health issues the patient may have, as well as helping to strengthen the patient's support system (Maldonado, 2019).

A patient's social support is often used as a factor for determining transplant eligibility in the United States, despite limited supporting evidence, the subjectivity and variability of its assessment, vague regulatory guidance, and low provider confidence (Berry et al., 2019; Ladin et al., 2019). According to a survey that measured the use of social support to determine transplant eligibility, respondent transplant providers estimated that almost 10 percent of patients evaluated during the survey year were disqualified based on the inadequacy of their social support (Ladin et al., 2019). This suggests the need to reevaluate social support criteria and examine its potential contribution to inequities and disparities, including biased wait-listing processes (Berry et al., 2019; Ladin et al., 2019).

## *Innovative Technology to Maximize Organ Use*

Recent innovations in methods for preserving organs prior to transplant have the potential to substantially expand the volume of the donor organ pool, mitigate organ injury, improve the quality of donated organs, and contribute to maximizing the use of solid organs (Petrenko et al., 2019; Salehi et al., 2018; Tatum et al., 2020). For instance, advances in organ perfusion technology have led to increases in the transplantation of medically complex donor organs (Chew et al., 2019). In the case of transplants using hearts donated after cardiac death, *ex vivo* blood-based perfusion technology is increasingly being introduced into clinical practice (Saemann et al., 2020). This technology has allowed cardiac allografts to be procured from greater distances than would be possible using cold static storage; the process also provides nutrients that reduce the risk of ischemic injury for functional preservation (Chew et al., 2019). In the field of liver and kidney transplantation, a clinical trial of *ex vivo* hypothermic oxygenated perfusion was conducted using organs from medically complex donors after brain death (Ravaioli et al., 2020). The clinical outcomes suggest that machine perfusion is a safe and effective system to reduce ischemic preservation injuries in kidney and liver transplants. A meta-analysis found hypothermic machine perfusion to be superior to static cold storage in deceased donor kidney transplantation in terms of reducing the risk of delayed graft function; it was also cost-saving at 1 year compared to cold storage (Tingle et al., 2020).

## Committee Considerations

In considering the alignment of incentives in the organ transplantation system, including the appropriate role of financial incentives, members of the committee held differing views. Some believe that transplant centers face higher costs if they provide wait-listed patients intensive management and take on especially complicated cases (e.g., using more medically complex organs, treating them to improve their usefulness, and transplanting patients with extensive medical and social needs), and they will therefore be disinclined to follow this report's recommendation that they take on more such cases unless they are reimbursed at an appropriately higher rate. Other members pointed out that increased payment should not be necessary since some high-performing transplant centers are already able to excel in meticulously managing their waiting list and in handling a large number of complicated cases within the current regulatory and payment structures. For example, if one transplant center can accept and successfully transplant a high number of medically complex organs under current rules and payment structures, then other transplant centers should be able to reach a similarly high level of performance without increased payment. Under this reasoning, quality improvement efforts and the sharing of best practices across transplant centers, rather than increased payments, are the right way to increase the number of organs used and the diversity of patients successfully transplanted. In the end, the committee agreed on the following conclusions and recommendation:

> *Conclusion 7-6: This report presents a number of conclusions and recommendations that aim to provide more transplants more fairly, such as by making better use of donated organs; by increasing the number of organs obtained and the proportion treated to improve their suitability for transplantation; by broadening the pool of patients who are referred, evaluated, and listed for a transplant; and by better management of patients on the waiting list. Implementing the committee's recom-*

*mendations will require changes in policies and practices, and some—particularly those recommendations that entail using more medically complex organs or treating organs more extensively to improve their usefulness for transplantation—are likely to have financial costs.*

*Conclusion 7-7: OPOs or transplant centers are less likely to implement recommended changes in policies and practices—such as using more medically complex organs or transplanting patients with more serious comorbidities—when they involve added financial costs that are not specifically covered.*

*Conclusion 7-8: When considering any reductions in the formulas used to pay transplant centers and OPOs of the sort proposed, but not adopted, in the CMS FY 2021 IPPS rule, CMS could use the Innovation Center's testing authority to fully explore the potential effect of such changes to avoid unintentionally interfering with the implementation of policies, such as those recommended by the committee, that aim to alleviate problems with the fairness, efficiency, and transparency of the organ transplantation system.*

**Recommendation 14: Align reimbursement and programs with desired behaviors and outcomes.**
    **CMS should align payment and other policies to meet the national performance goals for the organ transplantation system (see Recommendation 1). Within 2 years, CMS should**

- Continue and expand funding, as needed, for the current quality improvement initiative aimed at reducing the kidney nonuse rate, and pursuing simultaneous expansion of kidney donation by spreading the best practices of transplant centers and OPOs.
- Sustain and expand current work in the End-Stage Renal Disease program to
  - refer more eligible patients for transplant,
  - help referred patients to get both evaluated and listed by transplant centers,
  - assist patients in fully understanding and engaging with transplant centers when organs that are offered are declined on their behalf, and
  - work with Congress to update and increase the existing and outdated dialysis withholding payment to fund ESRD quality improvement activities.
- Sustain and expand model tests and other payment policies to increase reimbursement for nephrologists and dialysis centers to educate and refer patients for transplant evaluation.
- Increase reimbursement for referral for transplant evaluation for all organ types, and in the case of kidney transplant, even before dialysis begins.
- Update the CMS Interpretive Guidelines to reflect current practices and promote a collaborative relationship between the donor hospital and OPO, and institute measurable reporting mechanisms for donor hospital data. Address this systematically as part of both CMS hospital surveys and surveys by deemed organizations such as The Joint Commission.
- Explore financial incentives and make changes to Interpretive Guidelines to make hospitals accountable for smoothing surgical scheduling to ensure the capacity to recover and transplant donated organs 7 days a week.

**HHS, CMS, and other payers should consider new opportunities to increase the use of organs. HHS, CMS, and other payers should take the following steps:**

- Increase payment for improving the procurement and transplantation of all types of organs, as CMS did in the 2021 IPPS Final Rule when it created new DRGs with higher payments for kidney transplants that required a higher level of medical care.
- Incentivize OPOs and transplant centers to learn from the organizations and centers that already make extensive use of medically complex organs, and actively work to spread the practices for obtaining and transplanting these organs have proven to be most successful and cost effective.
- Within the next 2 years, the CMS Innovation Center should design and implement one or more model tests to assess the effects of additional increased payments to address the added costs of rehabilitating and using more organs that are medically complex and increasing equitable access to a broader pool of patients. These model tests should also measure the potential improvement in health care quality and financial savings of providing transplants more quickly to patients who would otherwise require continued extensive medical support, such as an artificial organ or hospitalization.

## REFERENCES

Ahmad, F., and T. Tsang. 2012. The melody of quality measures: Harmonize and standardize. *Health Affairs Blog.* https://www.healthaffairs.org/do/10.1377/hblog20120221.017126/full (accessed November 2, 2021).

AHRQ (Agency for Healthcare Research and Quality). 2020. *AHRQ National scorecard on hospital-acquired conditions.* https://www.ahrq.gov/hai/pfp/index.html (accessed November 2, 2021).

Axelrod, D. A., M. A. Schnitzler, H. Xiao, W. Irish, E. Tuttle-Newhall, S.-H. Chang, B. L. Kasske, T. Alhamad, and K. L. Lentine. 2018. An economic assessment of contemporary kidney transplant practice. *American Journal of Transplantation* 18(5):1168-1176.

Bababekov, Y. J., B. Cao, F. C. Njoku, Y.-C, Hung, J. T. Adler, J. J. Pomposelli, C. D. Chang, and H. Yeh. 2017. Readability of patient education websites of liver transplant centers—A barrier to the waitlist? *Journal of the American College of Surgeons* 225(4):e78.

Balhara, K. S., L. M. Kucirka, B. G. Jaar, and D. L. Segev. 2012. Disparities in provision of transplant education by profit status of the dialysis center. *American Journal of Transplantation* 12(11):3104-3110.

Berry, K. N., N. Daniels, and K. Ladin. 2019. Should lack of social support prevent access to organ transplantation? *American Journal of Bioethics* 19(11):13-24.

Blumenthal, S. 2018. Improving interoperability between registries and EHRs. *American Medical Informatics Association Joint Summits in Translational Science Proceedings* 2018:20-25. https://www.ncbi.nlm.nih.gov/pmc/articles/PMC5961768 (accessed February 1, 2022).

Bornstein, D. 2014. The push to end chronic homelessness is working. *New York Times.* https://opinionator.blogs.nytimes.com/2014/05/28/the-push-to-end-chronic-homelessness-is-working/ (accessed November 2, 2021).

Brett, K. E., L. J. Ritchie, E. Ertel, A. Bennett, and G. A. Knoll. 2018. Quality metrics in solid organ transplantation: A systematic review. *Transplantation* 102(7):e308.

Cheng, X. S., S. Busque, J. Lee, K. Discipulo, C. Hartley, Z. Tulu, J. D. Scandling, and J. C. Tan. 2018. A new approach to kidney wait-list management in the kidney allocation system era: Pilot implementation and evaluation. *Clinical Transplantation* 32(11):e13406.

Chew, H. C., P. S. Macdonald, and K. K. Dhital. 2019. The donor heart and organ perfusion technology. *Journal for Thoracic Disease* 11(6):S938-S945.

CMS (Centers for Medicare & Medicaid Services). 2019a. *Kidney Care Choices (KCC) Model: Request for Applications (RFA).* https://innovation.cms.gov/files/x/kcc-rfa.pdf (accessed November 10, 2021).

CMS. 2019b. *Medicare programs; Specialty care models to improve quality of care and reduce expenditures.* https://www.federalregister.gov/documents/2020/09/29/2020-20907/medicare-program-specialty-care-models-to-improve-quality-of-care-and-reduce-expenditures#p-2346 (accessed November 11, 2021).

CMS. 2021a. *ESRD Treatment Choices (ETC) Model.* https://innovation.cms.gov/innovation-models/esrd-treatment-choices-model (accessed November 10, 2021).

CMS. 2021b. *Kidney Care Choices (KCC) Model*. https://innovation.cms.gov/innovation-models/kidney-care-choices-kcc-model (accessed November 10, 2021).

CMS. 2021c. *Innovation models: Partnership for patients*. https://innovation.cms.gov/innovation-models/partnership-for-patients (accessed November 2, 2021).

Corbett, C., M. J. Armstrong, R. Parker, K. Webb, and J. M. Newberger. 2013. Mental health disorders and solid-organ transplant recipients. *Transplantation* 96(7):593-600.

Crawford, I., T. Hogan, and M. J. Silverman. 2013. Effects of music therapy on perception of stress, relaxation, mood, and side effects in patients on a solid organ transplant unit: A randomized effectiveness study. *The Arts in Psychotherapy* 40(2):224-229.

D'Amore, J. D., L. K. McCrary, J. Denson, C. Li, C. J. Vitale, P. Tokachichu, D. F. Sittig, A. B. McCoy, and A. Wright. 2021. Clinical data sharing improves quality measurement and patient safety. *Journal of the American Medical Informatics Association* 28(7):1534-1542.

Dearing, J. W., and J. G. Cox. 2018. Diffusion of innovations theory, principles, and practice. *Health Affairs* 37(2):183-190.

Feng, S., N. P. Goodrich, J. L. Bragg-Gresham, D. M. Dykstra, J. D. Punch, M. A. Debroy, S. M. Greenstein, and R. M. Merion. 2006. Characteristics associated with liver graft failure: The concept of a donor risk index. *American Journal of Transplantation* 6(4):783-790.

Fernández, M. P., P. M. Miguel, H. Ying, C. E. Haugen, N. M. Chu, D. M. Rodriguez-Puyol, L. Rodriguez-Manas, S. P. Norman, J. D. Watson, D. L. Segev, and M. A. McAdams-DeMarco. 2019. Comorbidity, frailty, and waitlist mortality among kidney transplant candidates of all ages. *American Journal of Nephrology* 49(2):103-110.

Grafals, M., M. Rogers, P. Weems, J. Moore, J. Verbesey, A. Gilbert, E. Gonzales, R. Ghasemian. D. Zwerski, T. Fishbein, and M. Cooper. 2014. Kidney transplant wait list management optimization: Abstract A450. *Transplantation* 98:810.

Haidt, J. 2006. *The happiness hypothesis: Finding modern truth in ancient wisdom*. New York: Basic Books.

HRSA (Health Resources and Services Administration). 2020. *Advisory Committee on Organ Transplantation (ACOT): April 2020 meeting minutes*. https://www.hrsa.gov/sites/default/files/hrsa/advisory-committees/organ-transplantation/acot-april-2020-meeting-minutes.pdf (accessed February 1, 2022).

IHI (Institute for Healthcare Improvement). 2003. *The breakthrough series: IHI's collaborative model for achieving breakthrough improvement*. Boston, MA: Institute for Healthcare Improvement. http://www.ihi.org/resources/Pages/IHIWhitePapers/TheBreakthroughSeriesIHIsCollaborativeModelforAchievingBreakthroughImprovement.aspx (accessed November 2, 2021).

IHI. 2021a. *Improvement stories: Organ donation breakthrough collaborative*. http://www.ihi.org/resources/Pages/ImprovementStories/OrganDonationBreakthroughCollaborative.aspx (accessed November 2, 2021).

IHI. 2021b. *Overview: 5 million lives campaign*. http://www.ihi.org/Engage/Initiatives/Completed/5MillionLives Campaign/Pages/default.aspx (accessed November 2, 2021).

Kucirka, L. M., M. E. Grams, K. S. Balhara, B. G. Jaar, and D. L. Segev. 2012. Disparities in provision of transplant information affect access to kidney transplantation. *American Journal of Transplantation* 12(2):351-357.

Kulkarni, S., K. Ladin, D. Haakinson, E. Greene, L. Li, and Yanhong Deng. 2019. Association of racial disparities with access to kidney transplant after the implementation of the new kidney allocation system. *JAMA Surgery* 154(7):618-625.

Kutner, N. G., R. Zhang, Y. Huang, and K. L. Johansen. 2012. Impact of race on predialysis discussions and kidney transplant preemptive wait-listing. *American Journal of Nephrology* 35(4):305-311.

Ladin, K., J. Emerson, K. Berry, Z. Butt, E. J. Gordon, N. Daniels, T. A. Lavelle, and D. W. Hanto. 2019. Excluding patients from transplant due to social support: Results from a national survey of transplant providers. *American Journal of Transplantation* 19(1):193-203.

Lantigua, C., K. Ibarra, A. Herr, K. Giblin, and C. Queram. 2021 (unpublished). *An approach to developing a framework for consensus-based standardized performance metrics in the United States transplant system*. Paper commissioned by the Committee on a Fairer and More Equitable, Cost-Effective, and Transparent System of Donor Organ Procurement, Allocation, and Distribution, National Academies of Sciences, Engineering, and Medicine, Washington, DC.

Li, P. K., K. H. Chu, K. M. Chow, M. F. Lau, C. B. Leung, B. C. H. Kwan, Y. F. Tong, C. C. Szeto, and M. M. M. Ng. 2012. Cross sectional survey on the concerns and anxiety of patients waiting for organ transplants. *Nephrology (Carlton)* 17(5):514-518.

Maldonado, J. R. 2019. *Why it is important to consider social support when assessing organ transplant candidates?* Abingdon-on-Thames, UK: Taylor & Francis.

McCannon, C. J., M. W. Schall, D. R. Calkins, and A. G. Nazem. 2006. Saving 100,000 Lives in US Hospitals. *BMJ* 332:1328-1330.

McCannon, C. J., D. M. Berwick, and M. R. Massoud. 2007. The science of large-scale change in global health. *JAMA* 298(16):1937-1939.

Nolan, T. W. 2007. *Execution of strategic improvement initiatives to produce system-level results*. IHI Innovation Series white paper. Cambridge, MA: Institute for Healthcare Improvement.

Norman, S. P., M. Kommareddi, and F. L. Luan. 2013. Inactivity on the kidney transplant wait-list is associated with inferior pre- and post-transplant outcomes. *Clinical Transplantation* 27(4):E435-E441.

Obadan-Udoh, E. M., J. M. Calvo, S. Panwar, K. Simmons, J. M. White, M. F. Walji, and E. Kalenderian. 2019. Unintended consequences and challenges of quality measurements in dentistry. *BMC Oral Health* 19(1).

OPTN (Organ Procurement and Transplantation Network). 2015. *Educational guidance on patient referral to kidney transplantation (OPTN minority affairs committee)*. https://optn.transplant.hrsa.gov/resources/guidance/educational-guidance-on-patient-referral-to-kidney-transplantation (accessed November 10, 2021).

OPTN. 2018. *Manipulation of the organ allocation system waitlist priority through the escalation of medical therapies*. https://optn.transplant.hrsa.gov/media/2500/ethics_whitepaper_201806.pdf (accessed November 17, 2021).

OPTN. 2020. *OPTN to launch a collaborative improvement project to increase recovery of DCD organs*. https://optn.transplant.hrsa.gov/news/optn-to-launch-a-collaborative-improvement-project-to-increase-recovery-of-dcd-organs (accessed November 2, 2021).

Patzer, R. E., S. Paul, L. Plainga, J. Gander, L. Sauls, J. Krisher, L. L. Mulloy, E. M. Gibney, T. Browne, C. F. Zayas, W. M. McClellan, K. H. Arriola, and S. O. Pastan. 2017. A randomized trial to reduce disparities in referral for transplant evaluation. *Journal of the American Society of Nephrology* 28(3):935-942.

Petrenko, A., M. Carnevale, A. Somov, J. Osorio, J. Rodriguez, E. Guiber, B. Fuller, and F. Froghi. 2019. Organ preservation into the 2020s: The era of dynamic intervention. *Transfusion Medicine and Hemotherapy* 46(3):151-172.

Prottas, J. 1998. Shifting responsibilities in organ procurement: A plan for routine referral. *JAMA* 260(6):832-833.

Puoti, F., A. Ricci, A. Nanni-Costa, W. Ricciardi, W. Malorni, and E. Orona. 2016. Organ transplantation and gender differences: A paradigmatic example of intertwining between biological and sociocultural determinants. *Biology of Sex Differences* 7:35.

Ravaioli, M., V. De Pace, A. Angeletti, G. Comai, F. Vasuri, M. Baldassarre, L. Maroni, F. Odaldi, G. Fallani, P. Caraceni, G. Germinario, C. Donadei, D. Malvi, M. Del Gaudio, V. R. Beruzzo, A. Siniscalchi, V. M. Ranieri, A. D'Errico, G. Pasquinelli, M. C. Morelli, A. D. Pinna, M. Cescon, and B. La Manna. 2020. Hypothermic oxygenated new machine perfusion system in liver and kidney transplantation of extended criteria donors: First Italian clinical trial. *Scientific Reports* 10(1):1-11.

Rodrigue, J. R., M. J. Paek, O. Eguna, A. D. Waterman, J. D. Schold, M. Pavlakis, and D. A. Mandelbrot. 2014. Making house calls increases living donor inquiries and evaluations for blacks on the kidney transplant waiting list. *Transplantation* 98(9):979-986.

Saemann, L., Y. Guo, Q. Ding, P. Zhou, M. Karck, G. Szabo, and F. Wenzel. 2020. Machine perfusion of circulatory determined death hearts: A scoping review. *Transplantation Reviews (Orlando)* 34(3):100551.

Salehi, S., K. Tran, and W. L. Grayson. 2018. Focus: Medical technology: Advances in perfusion systems for solid organ preservation. *Yale Journal of Biology and Medicine* 91(3):301.

Salvalaggio, P. R., N. Dzebisashvili, K. E. MacLeod, K. L. Lentine, A. Gheorghian, M. A. Schnitzler, S Hohmann, D. L. Segev, S. E. Gentry, and D. A. Axelrod. 2011. The interaction among donor characteristics, severity of liver disease, and the cost of liver transplantation. *Liver Transplantation* 17(3):233-242.

Schnitzler, M. A. 2021. *How much could we invest in deceased donor organ procurement?* Presentation during February 3–4, 2021 public workshop for the Committee on a Fairer, More Equitable, Cost-Effective, and Transparent System of Donor Organ Procurement, Allocation, and Distribution. https://www.nationalacademies.org/event/02-04-2021/a-fairer-and-more-equitable-cost-effective-and-transparent-system-of-donor-organ-procurement-allocation-and-distribution-a-virtual-workshop (accessed November 11, 2021).

Shafer, T. J., D. Wagner, J. Chessare, F. A. Zampiello, V. McBride, and J. Perdue. 2006. Organ donation breakthrough collaborative: Increasing organ donation through system redesign. *Critical Care Nurse* 26(2):33-48.

Shafer, T. J., D. Wagner, J. Chessare, M. W. Schall, V. McBride, F. A. Zampiello, J. Perdue, K. O'Connor, M. J-Y. Lin, and J. Burdick. 2008. US organ donation breakthrough collaborative increases organ donation. *Critical Care Nursing Quarterly* 31(3):190-210.

Sutton, R. I., and H. Rao. 2014. *Scaling up excellence: Getting to more without settling for less*. New York: Crown Business.

Tatum, R., T. J. O'Malley, A. S. Bodzin, and V. Tchantchaleishvili. 2020. Machine perfusion of donor organs for transplantation. *Artificial Organs* 45(7):682-695.

Tingle, S. J., R. S. Figueiredo, J. A. Moir, M. Goodfellow, E. R. Thompson, I. K. Ibrahim, L. Bates, D. Talbot, and C. H. Wilson. 2020. Hypothermic machine perfusion is superior to static cold storage in deceased donor kidney transplantation: A meta-analysis. *Clinical Transplantation* 34(4):e13814.

Tosoc-Haskell, H., K. Sisaithong, and R. Carrico. 2019. The collaborative improvement and innovation network project to drive quality improvement. *Current Opinion in Organ Transplantation* 24(1):73-81.

Waterman, A. D., J. D. Peipert, C. J. Goalby, K. M. Dinkel, H. Xiao, and K. L. Lentine. 2015. Assessing transplant education practices in dialysis centers: Comparing educator reported and Medicare data. *Clinical Journal of the American Society of Nephrology* 10(9):1617-1625.

Waterman, A. D., J. D. Peipert, H. Xiao, C. J. Goalby, S. Kawakita, Y. Cui, and K. L. Lentine. 2020. Education strategies in dialysis centers associated with increased transplant wait-listing rates. *Transplantation* 104(2):335-342.

Wesselman, H., C. G. Ford, Y. Leyva, X. Li, C. C. H. Chang, M. A. Dew, K. Kendall, E. Croswell, J. R. Pleis, Y. H. Ng, M. L. Unruh, R. Shapiro, and L. Myaskovsky. 2021. Social determinants of health and race disparities in kidney transplant. *Clinical Journal of the American Society of Nephrology* 16(2):262.

Wey, A., J. Foutz, S. K. Gustafson, R. J. Carrico, K. Sisaithong, H. Toscoc-Haskell, M. McBride, D. Klassen, N. Salkowski, B. L. Kasiske, A. K. Israni, and J. J. Snyder. 2020. The Collaborative Innovation and Improvement Network (COIIN): Effect on donor yield, waitlist mortality, transplant rates, and offer acceptance. *American Journal of Transplantation* 20(4):1076-1086.

Wu, D. A., M. L. Robb, J. L. R. Forsythe, C. Bradly, J. Cairns, H. Draper, C. Dudley, R. J. Johnson, W. Metcalfe, R. Ravanan, P. Roderick, C. R. V. Tomson, C. J. E. Watson, J. A. Bardley, and G. C. Oniscu. 2020. Recipient comorbidity and survival outcomes after kidney transplantation: A UK-wide prospective cohort study. *Transplantation* 104(6):1246-1255.

Ye, H. J., L.-J. Hu, Y.-Y. Yao, and J.-H. Chen. 2011. The effects of two health education models on psychological and nutritional profile of patients waiting for kidney transplantation. *Zhonghua Nei Ke Za Zhi* 50(10):845-847.

Zhou, S., A. B. Massie, X. Luo, J. M. Ruck, E. K. H. Chow, M. G. Bowring, S. Bae, D. L. Segev, and S. E. Gentry. 2018. Geographic disparity in kidney transplantation under KAS. *American Journal of Transplantation* 18(6):1415-1423.

Zubrinic, M., N. Marks, L. Brzozowski, J. Qiu, D. Lin, K. Wang, J. De Romana, L. Singer, and S. Keshavgee. 2019. Prelung transplant waitlist mortality rate reduction using remote video monitoring technology. *Journal of Heart and Lung Transplantation* 38(4):S199.

# Appendix A

# Public Meeting Agendas

This appendix includes public meeting agendas for the committee's first meeting (December 10, 2020), workshop (February 4–5, 2021), webinar (April 16, 2021), and listening session (July 15, 2021). These meeting agendas are listed in chronological order.

## FIRST VIRTUAL COMMITTEE MEETING
### Thursday, December 10, 2020

11:00 a.m.     **Welcome and Opening Remarks to Public Audience**
KENNETH W. KIZER, *Committee Chair*

11:15 a.m.     **Delivery of Study Charge and Q&A/Discussion with Committee**
Objectives:
- Receive study background and charge from NIH.
- Discuss study task with the sponsor, and determine scope of committee's work (i.e., what is in and what is out).
- Clarify issues identified by the committee, and seek answers to questions.
- Discuss report audience and expected products.

JONAH ODIM, Section Chief, Clinical Transplantation Section, NIAID

Discussants:
- NEIL AGGARWAL, Branch Chief, Lung Biology and Disease Branch, NHLBI
- KEVIN ABBOTT, Program Director, Division of Kidney, Urologic, and Hematologic Diseases, NIDDK
- AFSHIN PARSA, Program Director, Division of Kidney, Urologic, and Hematologic Diseases, NIDDK

11:30 a.m.      **Discussion with Committee**

12:30 p.m.      **Study Context and Overview of OPTN Allocation Policies**
                BRIAN SHEPARD, CEO, United Network for Organ Sharing (UNOS) and
                Executive Director, Organ Procurement and Transplantation Network
                (OPTN)

12:45 p.m.      **Discussion with Committee**

1:30 p.m.       **Adjourn Open Session**

# VIRTUAL PUBLIC WORKSHOP
## February 4 and 5, 2021
## DAY 1: Thursday, February 4, 2021

10:00 a.m.      **Introduction and Charge to the Workshop Speakers and Participants**
                KENNETH W. KIZER, *Committee Chair*
                Chief Healthcare Transformation Officer
                Senior Executive Vice President
                Atlas Research

                **SESSION I. BIOETHICAL CONSIDERATIONS OF FAIRNESS, EQUITY,
                AND TRANSPARENCY**
                Session Chair: Kenneth W. Kizer, *Committee Chair*

                Session Objectives:
                • Discuss the bioethical considerations of fairness, equity, and transparency in deceased donor organ procurement, allocation, and distribution.
                • Consider what the terms *fairness, equitable,* and *transparency* currently mean when applied to the deceased donor transplant system.

10:05 a.m.      **Bioethical Underpinnings of a Fair, Equitable, and Transparent Deceased Donor Organ Procurement, Allocation, and Distribution System**
                JAMES CHILDRESS
                Professor Emeritus, University Professor and John Allen Hollingsworth
                Professor of Ethics, and Professor of Religious Studies
                University of Virginia

10:15 a.m.      **Examining the Legal Underpinnings of the Transplant System—Are There Inherent Barriers to Fairness, Equity, and Transparency?**
                ALEXANDRA GLAZIER
                CEO
                New England Donor Services

10:25 a.m.      **Discussion with Committee** (20 mins)

## SESSION II. THE U.S. ORGAN PROCUREMENT SYSTEM
Session Chair: SUE DUNN, *Committee Member*

Session Objectives:
- Discuss OPO processes and systems that ensure fairness and equity in organ donation.
- Describe innovative OPO practices that have led to increased organ donation and transplant.

10:45 a.m.     **Overview of the Organ Procurement Process**
HOWARD NATHAN
CEO
Gift of Life (Philadelphia)

SUSAN GUNDERSON
CEO
LifeSource (Minneapolis)

11:05 a.m.     **Discussion with Committee** (15 mins)

11:20 a.m.     **Organ Use—OPO Challenges and Approaches**
KEVIN O'CONNOR
CEO
LifeCenter Northwest (Seattle)

RICHARD PEREZ
Medical Director, Transplant Center
University of California, Davis

11:40 a.m.     **Discussion with Committee** (15 mins)

11:55 a.m.     **Panel Discussion: Innovation in the Organ Procurement Process**

Panel Objectives:
- Explore the role of OPOs in community acceptance of organ donation to help address inequities and disparities within the system.
- Discuss a range of innovative practices within OPOs to increase donations and transplants.
- Discuss challenges that OPOs face and potential solutions for overcoming those barriers.

Moderator: SUE DUNN, *Committee Member*

Panelists:
JOE FERREIRA
President, Association of Organ Procurement Organizations
CEO, Nevada Donor Network

ALEXANDRA GLAZIER
CEO
New England Donor Services

DIANE BROCKMEIER
President and CEO
Mid-America Transplant

12:20 p.m.     **Discussion with Committee** (15 mins)

12:35 p.m.     **Break** (15 mins)

**SESSION III. TRANSPLANT CENTER OPERATIONS AND
ORGAN ACCEPTANCE DECISIONS**
Session Chair: LEIGH ANNE DAGEFORDE, *Committee Member*

Session Objective: Discuss the opportunities and challenges facing transplant centers, and explore what is working and not working in terms of
accessing organs, considering organ offers, managing waiting lists, and
optimizing the use of available organs.

12:50 p.m.     **A Moderated Discussion on the Challenges and Opportunities for
Improving Organ Use at the Transplant Center Level**
Moderator: LEIGH ANNE DAGEFORDE, *Committee Member*

Panelists (5 minutes of remarks each):
RICHARD HASZ
Vice President, Clinical Services
Gift of Life Donor Program, Philadelphia

ALEXANDRE LOUPY
Professor of Nephrology and Epidemiology
Paris University

SUMIT MOHAN
Associate Professor of Epidemiology and Medicine
Columbia University Medical Center

BRIGITTE SULLIVAN
Executive Director
NYU Langone Transplant Institute

KELLY WATSON
Transplant Coordinator, Lung Transplant
University of North Carolina

1:45 p.m.      **Discussion with Committee** (20 mins)

## SESSION IV. DATA COLLECTION AND MODELING
Session Chair: DORRY SEGEV, *Committee Member*

Session Objective: Examine the current approach to modeling proposed organ allocation policy changes (e.g., simulated allocation models), including successes and limitations, and consider new opportunities for improving organ allocation models.
Moderator: DORRY SEGEV, *Committee member*

2:05 p.m.    **The Role of Modeling in Proposed Organ Allocation Policy Changes**
DAVID MULLIGAN
President, Organ Procurement and Transplantation Network/United Network for Organ Sharing
Professor of Surgery (Transplant); Section Chief, Transplantation Surgery and Immunology
Yale University

2:15 p.m.    **Simulated Allocation Models and Their Strengths and Limitations Including Data Availability**
JON SNYDER
Director
Scientific Registry of Transplant Recipients (SRTR)

2:25 p.m.    **Envisioning the Future—Opportunities for Improving Organ Allocation Models**
NIKHIL AGARWAL
Associate Professor, Economics
MIT

2:35 p.m.    **How Well Do Organ Allocation Policies Correlate to Models—A Case Study**
MICHAEL GIVERTZ
Medical Director, Heart Transplant and Mechanical Circulatory Support
Brigham and Women's Hospital
Harvard University

2:45 p.m.    **Discussion with Committee** (15 mins)

3:00 p.m.    **Break** (10 mins)

## SESSION V. PUBLIC COMMENT PERIOD
Moderator: KENNETH W. KIZER, *Committee Chair*

3:10 p.m.    **Receive Comments from Individuals Registered in Advance (2 minutes each)**

3:55 p.m.          **Reflections on Day 1 and Preview of Day 2**
                   KENNETH W. KIZER, *Committee Chair*
                   Chief Healthcare Transformation Officer
                   Senior Executive Vice President
                   Atlas Research

4:00 p.m.          **Adjourn Workshop Day 1**

# DAY 2: Friday, February 5, 2021

10:00 a.m.         **Welcome and Overview of Day 2**
                   KENNETH W. KIZER, *Committee Chair*
                   Chief Healthcare Transformation Officer
                   Senior Executive Vice President
                   Atlas Research

                   **SESSION VI. EXPLORING DISPARITIES AND ACCESS ISSUES IN
                   ORGAN PROCUREMENT, ALLOCATION, AND DISTRIBUTION**
                   Session Chair: JEWEL MULLEN, *Committee Member*

                   Session Objectives:
                   • Explore what is known about inequities and disparities in deceased
                     donor organ procurement, allocation, and distribution.
                   • Discuss which communities are affected and examine the effect of dis-
                     parities on those communities.
                   • Learn about successful efforts to mitigate these disparities and inequities.
                   Moderator: JEWEL MULLEN, *Committee Member*

10:10 a.m.         **Inequities and Disparities in Deceased Donor Organ Procurement,
                   Allocation, and Distribution**
                   KIMBERLY JACOB ARRIOLA
                   Professor, Rollins School of Public Health
                   Emory University

10:25 a.m.         **The Role of Communication Dynamics in Organ Procurement,
                   Allocation, and Distribution**
                   LAURA SIMINOFF
                   Dean, College of Public Health
                   Temple University

10:40 a.m.         **Panel Discussion: Perspectives on Disparities and Access Issues**
                   Moderator: ELISA GORDON, *Committee Member*

                   Panelists (5 minutes of remarks each):
                   MARYAM VALAPOUR
                   Senior Staff for Lung Transplantation
                   Scientific Registry of Transplant Recipients (SRTR)
                   Staff, Respiratory Institute, Cleveland Clinic

BURNETT "BEAU" KELLY
Surgical Director
Dialysis Clinic Inc. Donor Services

LILIA CERVANTES
Associate Professor of Medicine
University of Colorado

AARON WIGHTMAN
Pediatric Nephrologist and Bioethicist
University of Washington

KEREN LADIN
Associate Professor, Public Health and Community
Tufts University

11:20 a.m.    **Discussion with Committee** (30 mins)

11:50 a.m.    **Break** (20 mins)

**SESSION VII. DECEASED DONOR FAMILY PERSPECTIVES**
Session Chair: CHARLES BEARDEN, *Committee Member*

Session Objective: Receive the perspectives of family members of deceased organ donors.

12:10 p.m.    **Panel Discussion: Perspectives from the Family Members of Organ Donors**
Moderator: CHARLES BEARDEN, *Committee Member*

Panelists:
GABRIELA LANDEROS-WILLIAMS
Donor Family Member

DEANNA SANTANA
Donor Family Member

KENNETH MORITSUGU
Donor Family Member

12:40 p.m.    **Discussion with Committee** (20 mins)

1:00 p.m.     **Break** (10 mins)

**SESSION VIII. TRANSPLANT RECIPIENT PERSPECTIVES**
Session Chair: KENNETH W. KIZER, *Committee Chair*

Session Objectives: Receive the perspectives of individuals who have received a donor organ, and explore the factors that played into their decision-making process.

1:10 p.m.    **Moderated Panel Discussion with Donor Organ Recipients**
Moderator: KENNETH W. KIZER, *Committee Chair*

Panelists:
ALEXIS CONELL
Member, Community Advisory Council
APOLLO Research Study

HALA DURRAH
Patient Family Engagement Consultant and Advocate, and Parent of a Liver
Transplant Recipient

RICHARD KNIGHT
President
American Association of Kidney Patients
Transplant Recipient

ROBERT MONTGOMERY
Chair, Department of Surgery
NYU Langone Transplant Institute

1:40 p.m.    **Discussion with Committee** (20 mins)

**SESSION IX. COSTS AND OTHER ECONOMIC FACTORS**
Session Chair: DENNIS WAGNER, *Committee Member*

Session Objectives: Consider the economic costs of the organ procurement,
allocation, and distribution systems, and determine who is paying those
costs and if there are opportunities to reduce costs.

2:00 p.m.    **Moderated Panel Discussion with Select Speakers**
Moderator: DENNIS WAGNER, *Committee Member*

MARK SCHNITZLER (7 mins)
Director of Outcomes Research and Quality for Transplantation
Saint Louis University

DAVID AXELROD (7 mins)
Professor, Kidney, Pancreas, and Living Donor Transplantation Surgical
Director, Fellowship Director, Transplant
University of Iowa

***Synthesis and Reaction***: MARIO MACIS, *Committee Member*

CHARLES ROSEN (7 mins)
Professor of Surgery, Division of Transplantation Surgery
Medical Director, Department of Contracting and Payer Relations
Mayo Clinic

Sara Eve Shaeffer (1 min)
Executive Director, ESRD NCC
Health Services Advisory Group, Inc.

Christopher Zinner (6 mins)
Managing Director
Accenture Federal Services

**Synthesis and Reaction**: Neil Powe, *Committee Member*

2:35 p.m.   **Discussion with the Committee** (15 mins)

2:50 p.m.   **Reflections on Day 2**
Kenneth W. Kizer, *Committee Chair*

3:00 p.m.   **Adjourn Workshop**


## VIRTUAL PUBLIC WEBINAR
## Friday, April 16, 2021

11:00 a.m.   **Welcome and Introduction**
Kenneth W. Kizer, *Committee Chair*
Chief Healthcare Transformation Officer
Senior Executive Vice President
Atlas Research

### SESSION I: INTERNATIONAL EXAMPLES OF ORGAN PROCUREMENT, ALLOCATION, AND DISTRIBUTION

Session Objectives:
- Discuss lessons the United States can learn from global transplant leaders about more efficient distribution, increased use, and more equitable allocation of deceased donor organs.
- Identify specific policies, practices, and incentives used successfully by other countries that could potentially be adapted to improve the U.S. organ transplant system.

Questions for Speakers:
- *Policy making*: Who is responsible for policy making around deceased donor organ procurement, allocation, and distribution in your country? How are policies developed and any disagreements among stakeholders addressed?
- *Increasing transplants*: How has your country responded to the challenge of increasing the number of organs available for transplant?

- *Allocation*: How are deceased donor organs allocated among individuals on the waiting list in your country? How is equity considered in allocation schemes?
- *Use*: How are deceased donor organs determined as acceptable to use in your country? Do individual physicians and hospitals consider organ offers individually for each patient?
- *Implementation*: What were the barriers to implementing organ allocation policies in your country? What implementation barriers would you see in the United States?

Moderator: KENNETH W. KIZER

| | |
|---|---|
| 11:10 a.m. | **Lessons from Canada**<br>JOHN GILL<br>Professor of Medicine<br>University of British Columbia<br>President-Elect, American Society of Transplantation |
| 11:25 a.m. | **Lessons from Israel**<br>JACOB LAVEE<br>Director, Heart Transplant Unit<br>Sheba Medical Center<br>Professor of Surgery<br>Tel Aviv University |
| 11:40 a.m. | **Discussion with Committee** (20 minutes) |
| 12:00 p.m. | **Lessons from the UK**<br>GABRIEL ONISCU<br>Director, Edinburgh Transplant Centre<br>Consultant Transplant Surgeon and Honorary Reader in Transplantation<br>Royal Infirmary of Edinburgh |
| 12:15 p.m. | **Lessons from Eurotransplant**<br>AXEL RAHMEL<br>Medical Director<br>Deutsche Stiftung Organtransplantation |
| 12:30 p.m. | **Lessons from Spain**<br>BEATRIZ DOMINGUEZ-GIL<br>Director General<br>Organización Nacional de Trasplantes |
| 12:45 pm. | **Discussion with Committee Members** (20 minutes) |
| 1:05 p.m. | **Session Wrap-Up**<br>KENNETH W. KIZER, *Committee Chair*<br>Chief Healthcare Transformation Officer<br>Senior Executive Vice President<br>Atlas Research |

1:10 p.m.    **Break** (40 minutes)

### SESSION II: EXPLORING DISPARITIES AND INEQUITIES IN PATIENT REFERRAL, EVALUATION, AND WAITING LIST MANAGEMENT PRACTICES

Session Objectives:
- Examine how patients get referred to organ transplant specialists, evaluated by specialists, and placed on a waiting list for a deceased donor organ.
- Explore the areas along this clinical pathway where barriers and biases exist, and discuss possible solutions to making the process more equitable.

Questions for Speakers:
- Is the process of patient referral for organ transplant equitable, and if not, which populations experience adverse disparities? Where exactly in the process are patients from these populations not referred for transplants, and why? What system-level actions could be taken to prevent disparities in referrals and mitigate inequitable outcomes?
- Once patients have been referred to a transplant program, do similar problems occur in the process of evaluating and listing them as candidates for transplantation?
- Are any of the disparities and inequities in patient referral and evaluation for a transplant organ specific?
- What role does implicit bias play in patients having trouble gaining access to an organ transplant waiting list and actually receiving a transplant? How can such biases be addressed?
- How does waiting list management by transplant centers and referring hospitals and physicians affect underrepresented groups' access to transplantation? Could particular policies and practices be adopted to manage waiting lists more efficiently and effectively and also contribute to alleviating disparities in access to organ transplant?

Moderator: KENNETH W. KIZER

1:50 p.m.    **Working Toward a More Equitable Patient Referral and Waiting List System for Kidney Transplantation**
AMY WATERMAN
Professor in Residence, Division of Nephrology
UCLA Health

2:05 p.m.    **Working Toward a More Equitable Patient Referral and Waiting List System for Liver Transplantation**
MALAY SHAH
Surgical Director, Liver Transplant Program
University of Kentucky, School of Medicine

| | |
|---|---|
| 2:20 p.m. | **Bias Associated with Allocation of Heart Transplant and Other Advanced Heart Failure Therapies** <br> KHADIJAH BREATHETT <br> Assistant Professor <br> University of Arizona, School of Medicine |
| 2:35 p.m. | **Discussion with Committee Members** (20 minutes) |
| 2:55 p.m. | **Waiting List Management Techniques—Experience from the COIIN Project and Beyond** <br> ANDREA TIETJEN <br> AVP, Transplant Administrative Services <br> Saint Barnabas Medical Center |
| 3:10 p.m. | **Addressing Inequities Through Improved Waiting List Management** <br> GISELLE GUERRA <br> Medical Director, Kidney Transplant Program <br> Miami Transplant Institute |
| 3:25 p.m. | **Discussion with Committee Members** (20 minutes) |
| 3:45 p.m. | **Session Wrap-Up and Adjourn** <br> KENNETH W. KIZER, Committee Chair <br> Chief Healthcare Transformation Officer <br> Senior Executive Vice President <br> Atlas Research |

## VIRTUAL PUBLIC LISTENING SESSION

## Thursday, July 15, 2021

| | |
|---|---|
| 11:00 a.m. | **Welcome and Introductions** <br> KENNETH W. KIZER, Committee Chair <br> Chief Healthcare Transformation Officer <br> Senior Executive Vice President <br> Atlas Research |
| 11:05 a.m. | **Creating a Fairer and More Equitable System—Are There Structural Barriers Embedded in the Path to an Organ Transplant in the United States? (5 minutes each)** <br> • DONNA HANDY, Patient, Massachusetts General Hospital <br> • ASHLEY HELSING, Director of Government Relations, National Down Syndrome Society <br> • ROBERT HIGGINS, Director of the Department of Surgery, Johns Hopkins University School of Medicine <br> • KELLY ISRAEL, Policy Associate, Autistic Self-Advocacy Network <br> • JAYME LOCKE, Director, UAB Comprehensive Transplant Institute |

- JERRY MCCAULEY, Medical Director of Transplantation Services, Thomas Jefferson University; Vice President, United Network for Organ Sharing (UNOS)
- BRIAN SHEPARD, CEO, UNOS
- SRIDHAR TAYUR, University Professor of Operations Management, Carnegie Mellon University
- FANNY VLAHOS, Attorney; double-lung transplant recipient; Member of the Lung Transplant Initiative and Guidelines Committee, Cystic Fibrosis Foundation
- JANET WEINER, Board Member, Cystic Fibrosis Foundation, Washington, DC, chapter
- CHARLOTTE WOODWARD, Community Outreach Associate, National Down Syndrome Society

12:00 p.m. **Clarifying Questions from the Committee**

12:10 p.m. **Maximizing Public and Professional Trust—What Steps Can Be Taken to Build a More Transparent and Accountable System? (5 minutes each)**
- DAVID GOLDBERG, Associate Professor of Medicine, University of Miami
- MARTIN HATLIE, President and CEO, Project Patient Care
- EMILY LARGENT, Emanuel and Robert Hart Assistant Professor of Medical Ethics and Health Policy, University of Pennsylvania
- RAYMOND LYNCH, Associate Professor of Surgery and Director of Public Policy and Community Relations, Emory Transplant Center
- VIRGINIA (GINNY) MCBRIDE, Executive Director, OurLegacy
- CONSTANCE MOBLEY, Associate Director of Liver Transplantation, Houston Methodist J.C. Walter Jr. Transplant Center
- BLAIR SADLER, Senior Fellow, Institute for Healthcare Improvement
- GREG SEGAL, CEO, Organize
- MARION SHUCK, President, Association for Multicultural Affairs in Transplant (AMAT)

12:55 p.m. **Clarifying Questions from the Committee**

1:05 p.m. **BREAK**

1:25 p.m. **Aligning Incentives—What Can Be Done to Increase the Efficiency and Effectiveness of the Organ Transplant System? (5 minutes each)**
- CLIVE CALLENDER, Professor of Surgery, Howard University of Medicine
- A. OSAMA GABER, Chair, Houston Methodist Department of Surgery and Incoming President, American Society of Transplant Surgeons
- MICHELE BRATCHER GOODWIN, Director, Center for Biotechnology and Global Health Policy, University of California, Irvine School of Law
- PAUL MYOUNG, Senior Administrative Director, Massachusetts General Hospital
- HOWARD NATHAN, President, Gift of Life Donor Program
- MARTY SELLERS, Associate Professor of Surgery, Emory University; Associate Medical Director, LifeLink
- JANICE STARLING, Founder, All Kidney Patients Support Group

2:00 p.m.          **Clarifying Questions from the Committee**

2:10 p.m.          **Increasing Rates of Organ Donation and Acceptance—What Steps Would Save More Lives of Those on the Waiting List? (5 minutes each)**
- JENNIFER ERICKSON, Innovation Fellow, Federation of American Scientists
- RICHARD FORMICA, Past President, American Society of Transplantation
- KEVIN FOWLER, Consultant, The Voice of the Patient, Inc.
- KEVIN LONGINO, CEO, National Kidney Foundation
- JEROLD MANDE, Visiting Fellow, Tisch College of Civic Life, Tufts University
- MELISSA MCQUEEN, Transplant Families
- PATTI NILES, CEO, Southwest Transplant Alliance
- VELMA SCANTLEBURY, Professor of Surgery, University of North Texas Health Science Center
- QUIN TAYLOR, Founder, Tayloring Gratitude
- JANICE WHALEY, President and CEO, Donor Network West

3:00 p.m.          **Clarifying Questions from the Committee**

3:10 p.m.          **Closing Comments**
KENNETH W. KIZER, *Committee Chair*
Chief Healthcare Transformation Officer
Senior Executive Vice President
Atlas Research

3:15 p.m.          **Adjourn**

# Appendix B

# IOM and National Academies Solid Organ Transplantation Reports

The Institute of Medicine (IOM) and the National Academies of Sciences, Engineering, and Medicine (the National Academies) published several reports addressing solid donor organ recovery and transplantation. This section provides an overview of the key findings and recommendations included in those reports that are most relevant to the current study.

## NON–HEART-BEATING ORGAN TRANSPLANTATION: MEDICAL AND ETHICAL ISSUES IN PROCUREMENT

In 1997, amid efforts to broaden the pool of organ donors, the U.S. Department of Health and Human Services (HHS) requested a report expressing concern about the limited supply of organs for transplantation into patients with terminal organ failure (IOM, 1997). HHS raised questions as to whether (1) interventions undertaken prior to declaration of death might prevent damage to potential donor organs, and (2) interventions to improve organ quality and supply may also hasten the death of potential donor patients. The report recommended that IOM should consider approaches to organ supply interventions that maximize the availability of organs without violating ethical norms regarding the rights or welfare of potential donors. This guidance was issued at a time when there was great interest in expanding donation after circulatory determination of death (DCDD) solid organ donation (IOM, 1997).

## NON–HEART-BEATING ORGAN TRANSPLANTATION: PRACTICE AND PROTOCOLS

A follow-up report published in 2000 focused on developing consensus and consistency for non–heart-beating donation practices and protocols (IOM, 2000). It was intended to help improve organ transplant system integrity and sustain public support for and interest in organ donation (IOM, 2000). The committee clarified non–heart-beating donor (NHBD) donation practices, reviewed similarities and differences among donor protocols, developed and implemented protocols, and reviewed impediments to developing consensus on NHBD organ donation practices. This report and its preceding 1997 reports are critical in the consideration of DCDD, especially as greater focus continues to be placed upon DCDD to increase the availability of organs without compromising procured donor organ performance quality.

## ORGAN PROCUREMENT AND TRANSPLANTATION: ASSESSING CURRENT POLICIES AND THE POTENTIAL EFFECT OF THE HHS FINAL RULE

In 1999, IOM convened the Committee on Organ Procurement and Transplantation Policy to review HHS' Final Rule, which proposed to (1) make changes to the organ allocation system, (2) correct apparent geographic disparities in the amount of time individuals waited for an organ, and (3) ensure equitable access for minorities[1] and the economically disadvantaged (IOM, 1999). At the time, transplant centers and organ procurement organizations (OPOs) had varying policies—official and unofficial—regarding priority assignment and waiting list access for these patients, and the committee recommended the removal of waiting time as a determinant of waiting list priority. The committee found that the major factors producing geographic disparity in transplantation were the size of the population served by the OPO and the volume of patients transplanted, leading to their key recommendation that organ allocation for livers be based on broader sharing of organs within regions consisting of a minimum of 9 million people. HHS immediately adopted the committee's recommendations, but the implementation of these recommendations was stifled by political factors and the replacement of the head of HHS.

Six years later, the Scientific Advisory Board of HHS found that under the local system, patients were being transplanted with Model for End-Stage Liver Disease (MELD) scores that led to decreased posttransplant survival relative to what they would have experienced by remaining on the waiting list. This revealed that when limited to small geographic areas (e.g., OPOs), improved risk stratification can still lead to inefficient allocation. OPOs with small and medium volume (i.e., less than 75 transplants per service area per year) were significantly more likely to transplant less severely ill patients (status 2B and 3) than OPOs that averaged more than 75 transplants per year. Based on these findings, broader regional sharing of livers was adopted at various MELD score thresholds.

## ORGAN DONATION: OPPORTUNITIES FOR ACTION

In 2006, IOM published a report focusing on opportunities for action to improve quality, coordination, and reliability among the multiple organizations and systems involved in organ donation, thus addressing the gap between supply and demand of transplantable organs (IOM, 2006). Further, the report considered the potential for broader policies and practices to reduce the gap in organ donation: for instance, by bolstering preventive health efforts to reduce the need for transplantation; by ensuring equitable access to transplantation by negating current financial and insurance constraints; and by providing ongoing access

---

[1] The report noted that while African Americans had equal likelihood of receiving a liver transplant once listed, this group was less likely to be referred for evaluation and placed on the waiting list than white patients.

to immunosuppressive medications to ensure that each donated organ is used in an optimal care environment that includes proper follow-up.

The report recommended the development of improved systems to support organ donation and the implementation of mandates to develop continuous quality improvement initiatives for OPOs and organ transplant centers. However, the report also cautioned against the undesirable consequences of interventions when evaluating perspectives and principles of opportunities for action in the organ donation process. For example, implementing policies in only a few select states may result in adverse negative spillover effects on public attitudes, potentially eroding public support for organ donation—negative perceptions may be very difficult, if not impossible, to reverse. The report also examined the use of financial incentives (i.e., cash payments or tax deductions) and preferential access to health care for donors and potential donors to see if they would provide additional increases in the rates of organ donations; ultimately, hard data on this concept are lacking and may need further research. However, the report did recommend that the use of financial incentives to increase organ transplants should not be promoted at the time of its writing. Finally, the report strongly recommended redoubling efforts to encourage and reduce barriers to live donor organ donation.

## OPPORTUNITIES FOR ORGAN DONOR INTERVENTION RESEARCH: SAVING LIVES BY IMPROVING THE QUALITY AND QUANTITY OF ORGANS FOR TRANSPLANTATION

In 2017, the National Academies of Sciences, Engineering, and Medicine published a report on organ donor intervention research as a potential way to improve the quality and increase the number of transplantable organs, including organs that might be otherwise discarded that focused on solid organ transplantation (NASEM, 2017). To this end, it emphasized the need to

- Improve transparency and public trust in the donation process for research followed by transplantation.
- Improve coordination and information sharing of donor preferences.
- Clarify legal guidance on organ donation.
- Promote informed consent for organ recipients in organ donor intervention research.
- Establish centralized management and oversight of organ donor intervention research to ensure equitable, transparent, and high-quality research.
- Promote transparency on organ donor intervention research (NASEM, 2017).

It recommended that the Organ Procurement and Transplantation Network, OPOs, the Health Resources and Services Administration, advocacy organizations, and professional associations explore, develop, test, and implement communication strategies that effectively explain organ donor intervention research. Moreover, the report called for improved coordination and sharing of information about donor and potential recipient preferences regarding research on organ donors and donor organs procured.

## REFERENCES

IOM (Institute of Medicine). 1997. *Non-heart-beating organ transplantation: Medical and ethical issues in procurement*. Washington, DC: National Academy Press. https://doi.org/10.17226/6036.

IOM. 1999. *Organ procurement and transplantation: Assessing current policies and the potential impact of the DHHS Final Rule*. Washington, DC: National Academy Press. https://doi.org/10.17226/9628.

IOM. 2000. *Non-heart-beating organ transplantation: Practice and protocols*. Washington, DC: National Academy Press. https://doi.org/10.17226/9700.

IOM. 2006. *Organ donation: Opportunities for action*. Washington, DC: The National Academies Press. https://doi.org/10.17226/11643.

NASEM (National Academies of Sciences, Engineering, and Medicine). 2017. *Opportunities for organ donor intervention research: Saving lives by improving the quality and quantity of organs for transplantation*. Washington, DC: The National Academies Press. https://doi.org/10.17226/24884.

# Appendix C

# Biographical Sketches of Committee Members and Staff

## COMMITTEE MEMBERS

**Kenneth W. Kizer, M.D., M.P.H. (NAM)** (*Chair*), currently serves as the Chief Health Care Transformation Officer and Senior Executive Vice President for Atlas Research. He has been elected to both the National Academy of Medicine and the National Academy of Public Administration. Dr. Kizer is a highly experienced physician executive whose diverse professional experience includes senior leadership positions in the public and private sectors, academia, and philanthropy. He has previously served as founding president and chief executive officer of the National Quality Forum; Under Secretary for Health, United States Department of Veterans Affairs, and chief executive officer of the nation's largest health care system, during which time he engineered the internationally acclaimed transformation of the Veterans Healthcare System in the late 1990s; founding Chairman, President, and CEO, Medsphere Systems Corporation, a leading commercial provider of subscription-based health information technology; founding Director, Institute for Population Health Improvement and Distinguished Professor, University of California, Davis; inaugural Chief Medical Officer, California Department of Managed Health Care; Director, California Department of Health Services; and Director, California Emergency Medical Services Authority, where he was the architect of the state's EMS and trauma care systems in the early 1980s. During his record tenure as California's top health official he won high praise for orchestrating the state's response to the then new HIV/AIDS epidemic, implementing California's famed Tobacco Control Program and the '5-a-Day' for Better Nutrition Program that was later adopted for national implementation, pioneering Medicaid managed care, and restructuring many of the state's public health programs. He also has served on the U.S. Preventive Services Task Force and as chairman of The California Wellness Foundation. Dr. Kizer has long-standing interests in organ transplantation stemming from his experience as a practicing emergency physician, public health official, and health system leader, as well as his personal experiences as the husband of a multiple times organ transplant recipient. He has a deep understanding of the anxieties and difficulties families experience while waiting for an organ.

**Itai Ashlagi, Ph.D.,** is an associate professor at the Management Science and Engineering Department at Stanford University. Dr. Ashlagi's research interests include game theory and the design and analysis of marketplaces. He specializes in matching markets, such as kidney paired donation, organ allocation, school choice, and the National Resident Matching Program. Dr. Ashlagi is a recipient of the National Science Foundation CAREER award and is recognized as a Franz Edelman Laureate for his outstanding contribution to kidney paired donation. Before joining Stanford University, he was an assistant professor of operations management at the Massachusetts Institute of Technology's Sloan School of Management and, prior to that, a postdoctoral researcher at Harvard Business School. Dr. Ashlagi received his Ph.D. in operations research from the Technion-Israel Institute of Technology. Dr. Ashlagi serves as a consultant for Rejuvenate Healthcare, LLC, a company working with health care providers, payers, and patients to facilitate kidney transplants.

**Charles Bearden, P.A., CPTC,** has been a practicing PA for over 48 years. He has the distinction of being the longest practicing organ recovery/transplant coordinator in the United States with 44 years of coordinating over 2,500 heart, lung, liver, kidney, pancreas, and intestinal organ transplants. Mr. Bearden is currently an advisory board member for Clinical Consulting Associates. Prior to beginning his physician associate studies, Mr. Bearden worked as a cardiovascular technician at Grady Memorial Hospital in Atlanta, GA, and trained under Dr. J. Willis Hurst. Dr. Hurst was starting the PA Program at Emory and encouraged him to apply to the first physician associate program class at the Emory University School of Medicine in 1971. He was accepted and at the age of 19 began his PA education. He served as class vice president and graduated in 1973. He made the highest score in his class on the first National Board of Medical Examiners (NBME) Certifying Examination for PAs held in 1973. In 1974, Mr. Bearden served on the NBME Committee to validate the first PA National Board Examination. He was certified by the National Commission on Certification of Physician Assistants in both primary care in 1975 and in surgery in 1980. In 1978 he co-founded and co-directed the first Organ Bank in Atlanta and remained with the Atlanta branch of DCI until 1988 when he relocated to their Chattanooga, TN office. Mr. Bearden remained with DCI Donor Services until 2002 when he accepted a position as a Traveling Organ Recovery Coordinator with Clinical Consulting Associates (CCA). In 2007, Mr. Bearden became one of the first Virtual Organ Transplant Coordinators in the country for CCA and he continues his work today. He has been certified by the American Board of Transplant Coordination for 34 years. He is a member of the Advisory Board of Organize.org and was a participant in the 2016 White House Summit on Organ Donation and Transplantation. In 2019 he was awarded the Outstanding Civilian Physician Assistant of the Year by the Veterans Caucus of the American Academy of Physician Assistants. "For his concern, caring, and devotion towards patients, profession, and country his commitment is our profession's future."

**Yolanda T. Becker, M.D.** (*until September 2021*), is a professor of surgery and director of kidney and pancreas transplantation at the University of Chicago. She has served in many roles throughout her career as a Transplant Surgeon. Dr. Becker is a Past President of the OPTN/UNOS (Organ Procurement and Transplant Network/United Network for Organ Sharing) board of directors. She has served on the UNOS corporate affairs committee, the nominating committee and the board governance subcommittee. She has chaired the policy oversight committee. Dr. Becker began her involvement with UNOS as a member of the Membership and Professional Standards Committee, and certification maintenance workgroups, co-chairing the latter. Dr. Becker has served as an elected member of the American Society of Transplantation (AST) board of directors, co-chairing its winter symposium, chairing its education committee, and additionally serving on the minority affairs committee. She has served on the American Society of Transplant Surgeons (ASTS) scientific studies committee and on the AST/ASTS American Transplant Congress program planning committee. She also has served on the board of directors of the National Kidney Registry. She earned her medical degree at the Johns Hopkins School of Medicine in Baltimore. Dr. Becker has received additional leadership training, completing the Executive Leaders in Academic Medicine program at Drexel University College of Medicine in Philadelphia.

**Alexander M. Capron, LL.B. (NAM),** is a university professor at the University of Southern California where he teaches public health law and policy, bioethics, and torts, and occupies the Scott H. Bice Chair in Healthcare Law, Policy and Ethics in the Gould School of Law, is professor of medicine and law in the Keck School of Medicine, and is Co-Director of the Pacific Center for Health Policy and Ethics. He previously taught at Georgetown University, the University of Pennsylvania, and Yale University. His ten books and hundreds of articles cover a wide range of topics in law, medicine, and ethics; he has written on human organ transplantation since 1972, including, with Jay Katz, *Catastrophic Diseases: Who Decides What* (1975, paperback 1978). Capron received a B.A. from Swarthmore College and an L.L.B. from Yale University, where he was an officer of the *Yale Law Journal.* He was appointed by Congress as the chair of the Biomedical Ethics Advisory Committee, and by President Bill Clinton as a member of the National Bioethics Advisory Commission. From 1980 to 1983 he was the Executive Director of the President's Commission for the Study of Ethical Problems in Medicine and Biomedical and Behavioral Research, which was established by Congress and appointed by Presidents Carter and Reagan; in one of its numerous reports, *Defining Death: The Medical, Legal and Ethical Issues in the Determination of Death* (1981), the commission set forth the Uniform Determination of Death Act which it had developed with three medical and legal organizations. From 2002 to 2006, he served as director of the Department of Ethics, Trade, Human Rights and Health Law at the World Health Organization, where he co-led its global work on human organ, tissue, and cell transplantation. He is an elected member of the National Academy of Medicine, the American Law Institute, and an elected Fellow of both the American Association for the Advancement of Science and the Hastings Center. He has served as President of the American Society for Law, Medicine and Ethics, and of the International Association of Bioethics. Professor Capron currently serves as a member of an advisory panel on ethics and public policy for a National Science Foundation–funded Engineering Research Center (ERC) at the University of Minnesota on Advanced Technologies for the Preservation of Biological Systems (ATP-Bio). The panel examines the issues that may arise in research on means to preserve and use human and non-human cells, tissues, and organs, publishes the results of its analysis, and provides advice to ATP-Bio investigators about such matters but has no operational authority for the ERC or its investigators.

**Bernice Coleman, Ph.D., ACNP-BC, FAHA, FAAN,** is director of the Nursing Research Department and Performance Improvement Department, assistant professor of medicine and biomedical sciences, and a nurse practitioner for the Heart Transplantation and Mechanical Circulatory Support at the Cedars-Sinai Smidt Heart Institute. She is a member of the American Heart Association Leadership Council on Cardiovascular and Stroke Nursing, past chairperson of the Nursing Health Science and Allied Health Council of the International Society of Heart and Lung Transplantation, and a member of the Nominating Committee for the International Society of Nurses in Genetics. Dr. Coleman was formerly a member of the U.S. Department of Health and Human Services Advisory Committee on Organ Transplantation. She researches health disparities with a focus on exploring the racial outcomes of post–heart transplantation African and Caucasian Americans. Dr. Coleman is a board-certified Acute Care Nurse Practitioner with a master of science in nursing from the Yale School of Nursing and a Ph.D. from the UCLA School of Nursing. She completed her postdoctoral studies in the HLA Laboratory at Cedars-Sinai and the National Institute of Nursing Research Summer Genetics Institute. She is a fellow of the American Academy of Nursing and has presented her work in heart transplantation nationally and internationally.

**Leigh Anne Dageforde, M.D., M.P.H.,** is an abdominal organ transplant (liver, kidney, and pancreas) and hepatobiliary surgeon at Massachusetts General Hospital who specializes in the care of patients with end-stage kidney and liver disease needing organ transplantation, living kidney donors, pancreas transplant patients, and patients with liver and biliary cancer. Dr. Dageforde attended medical school at Vanderbilt University School of Medicine and completed her general surgery residency at Vanderbilt University Medical Center in Nashville, Tennessee. She completed her fellowship in Abdominal Organ Transplantation and HPB surgery at Washington University in St. Louis. In addition to liver, kidney, and pancreas transplantation, her clinical interests also include living kidney donation and treatment of liver and biliary cancer. Dr. Dageforde completed her master of public health degree at Vanderbilt University School of Medicine with a focus on research in improving access to transplantation. She serves on national committees in both the Association of Academic Surgery and the Americas Hepato-Pancreato-Biliary Association. She has recently been appointed co-chair of the American Society of Transplant Surgeons Pipeline Taskforce, focusing on the development of the rising surgical workforce in transplant surgery with an emphasis on mentorship of medical students and residents.

**Sue Dunn, R.N., B.S.N., M.B.A.,** is former chief executive officer of Donor Alliance. She led the Denver-based organ procurement organization (OPO) serving Colorado and Wyoming for more than 15 years, and retired in June 2020. Ms. Dunn joined Donor Alliance in 1989, after 5 years as an organ procurement coordinator in Minnesota. She served as the organization's vice president of Organ Procurement Operations/Compliance and Regulatory Affairs before being named CEO in 2004. She also served as OPTN and UNOS board president from 2018 to 2019, leading semiannual meetings of the board, as well as chairing the Executive Committee and UNOS' Corporate Affairs Committee. She is formerly the president of the Association of Organ Procurement Organizations (AOPO) and has served on numerous industry boards and committees. Until June 2020, Ms. Dunn served in an unpaid capacity on the Board of Directors for AlloSource, a nonprofit tissue processor. Under Ms. Dunn's leadership, Donor Alliance was recognized as a 2018 Malcolm Baldrige National Quality Awardee, the only nonprofit organization of that year, and only the second organ procurement organization to be recognized. She has earned widespread recognition for her leadership at Donor Alliance, and was awarded the 2021 Baldrige Foundation Excellence in Leadership Award in the nonprofit sector. Ms. Dunn received her bachelor of science, nursing in 1978 from Creighton University and her master's in business administration in 2005 from Regis University. She currently mentors OPO leaders through the Gift of Life Transplant Institute's Art and Science of Leadership Program and serves as an unpaid advisor to the UNOS Corporate Affairs Committee.

**Robert D. Gibbons, Ph.D. (NAM),** is the Blum-Riese Professor of Biostatistics and a Pritzker Scholar at the University of Chicago. He has appointments in the Departments of Medicine, Public Health Sciences, and Comparative Human Development. He also directs the Center for Health Statistics. Dr. Gibbons is a Fellow of the American Statistical Association, the

International Statistical Institute, and the Royal Statistical Society, and is a member of the National Academy of Medicine of the National Academy of Sciences. He has authored more than 300 peer-reviewed scientific papers and six books. His statistical work spans the areas of longitudinal data analysis, item response theory, environmental statistics, and drug safety and has led to thousands of applications in the biological and social sciences. Dr. Gibbons has received life-time achievement awards from the American Statistical Association, the American Public Health Association, and Harvard University. He is a founder of the Mental Health Statistics section of the American Statistical Association. Dr. Gibbons has co-authored many publications, including *Full-Information Item Bi-Factor Analysis, Waiting for Organ Transplantation,* and *Weighted Random-Effects Regression Models with Application to Inter-Laboratory Calibration.* He earned his Ph.D. in statistics and psychometrics from the University of Chicago, and his B.A. in chemistry and mathematics from the University of Denver.

**Elisa J. Gordon, Ph.D., M.P.H.,** is professor in the Department of Surgery—Division of Transplantation, Center for Health Services and Outcomes Research, and Center for Bioethics and Medical Humanities at Northwestern University Feinberg School of Medicine. Dr. Gordon completed her doctorate in medical anthropology at Case Western Reserve University. Thereafter, she completed a Fellowship in Clinical Medical Ethics at the University of Chicago. Dr. Gordon obtained her master's degree in public health from the University of Illinois, Chicago, specializing in community health sciences. She is a Fellow of the American Society for Applied Anthropology, and the American Society of Transplantation. Dr. Gordon has received funding from the National Institutes of Health, Health Resources and Services Administration, Department of Defense, and Department of Veterans Affairs as principal investigator for her research on organ transplantation and donation, for reducing health disparities in access to health care and health outcomes, and for developing culturally targeted interventions to enhance patients' informed consent and treatment decision making. She was recognized as an Expertscape world expert in patient education in 2021. Dr. Gordon served as the chair of the UNOS Ethics Committee from 2017 to 2020, and as an appointed member of the American Society of Transplantation's Inclusion, Diversity, Equality, and Access to Life Task Force (2020–2021). She currently serves as co-chair of the American Society of Transplantation's Psychosocial and Ethics Community of Practice, as an Associate Editor of the *American Journal of Transplantation,* as a member of the Data Safety Monitoring Board for the National Institute of Allergy and Infectious Diseases, and as a member of the federal Advisory Committee on Blood and Tissue Safety and Availability.

**Renée Landers, J.D.,** is a professor of law, Faculty Director of the Health and Biomedical Law Concentration, and Faculty Director of the Master of Science in the Law Life Sciences program at Suffolk University Law School in Boston. She was a Distinguished Visiting Fellow at the National Academy of Social Insurance during her fall 2018 sabbatical leave. She was also the President of the Boston Bar Association from 2003 to2004, and was the first woman of color and the first law professor to serve in that position. Professor Landers has worked in private practice and served as Deputy General Counsel for the U.S. Department of Health and Human Services and as Deputy Assistant Attorney General in the Office of Policy Development at the U.S. Department of Justice during the Clinton Administration. Professor Landers served as chair of the Section of Administrative Law and Regulatory Practice of the American Bar Association from 2016 to 2017 and chaired the Section's Nominating Committee from 2018 to 2019. She is a Trustee of the Massachusetts General Hospital and a former Trustee of New England Donor Services and the Massachusetts Eye & Ear Infirmary. In 2019, she rejoined the board of Planned Parenthood League of Massachusetts and became President of the Board beginning in July 2020. Recently, she co-chaired the Boston Bar Association's Task Force on Judicial Independence which issued a report in August 2019. She was a member of the Massachusetts Commission on Judicial Conduct and served as Vice Chair of the Commission from 2009 to 2010. She also served on the task force that drafted the revised Massachusetts Code of Judicial Conduct, effective in 2016, and currently is a member of the Committee on Judicial Ethics, which advises judges on compliance with the Code. Previously, she was a member of the Supreme Judicial Court's committees studying gender, racial, and ethnic bias in the courts.

**Mario Macis, Ph.D.,** is a professor of economics at the Johns Hopkins University Carey Business School. He is also a core faculty member of the Hopkins Business of Health Initiative, affiliate faculty at the Johns Hopkins Berman Institute of Bioethics, and Faculty Research Fellow at the National Bureau of Economic Research. Dr. Macis is an applied economist and his work focuses on how economic incentives interact with psychological factors and social norms to drive individual behavior and policy-relevant outcomes. His main research interests are in prosocial behavior, ethics and economics, and experimental economics. Much of his recent research involved multidisciplinary collaborations with medical and public health scholars and psychologists. He regularly engages with policy makers and practitioners, including national and international agencies as well as associations related to blood, plasma, stem cell, and organ donation. In particular, he conducted studies in partnership with the American Red Cross and the National Marrow Donor Program. His work was published in leading academic journals including the *American Economic Review*, *Management Science*, the *Journal of Health Economics*, the *American Economic Journal: Economic Policy*, and *Science*. Dr. Macis has been a consultant for the World Bank, the International Labor Organization, the National Marrow Donor Program, and the United Nations Development Program.

**Jewel Mullen, M.D., M.P.H., M.P.A.,** is Associate Dean for Health Equity at University of Texas at Austin Dell Medical School, as well as an associate professor in the school's population health and internal medicine departments. She also serves as Director of Health Equity at Ascension Seton to help meet health equity goals across its system. Mullen is an internist, epidemiologist, public health expert, and the former principal Deputy Assistant Secretary for Health in the U.S. Department of Health and Human Services (HHS). While at HHS, she also served as the acting assistant secretary for health and acting director of the National Vaccine Program Office. Prior to HHS, she served as commissioner of the Connecticut Department of Public Health. Her career has spanned clinical, research, teaching, and administrative roles focused on improving the health of all people, especially those who are underserved. She is recognized nationally and internationally as a leader in building effective community-based chronic disease prevention programs and for her commitment to improving individual and population health by strengthening coordination between community, public health and health care systems. A former president of the Association of State and Territorial Health Officials, Dr. Mullen is a current member of the Centers for Disease Control and Prevention's (CDC's) *Morbidity and Mortality Weekly Report* Editorial Board, the ChangeLab Solutions Board of Directors, and the Robert Wood Johnson Foundation's Policies for Action National Advisory Committee which she chairs. She also is a member of the Study Committee on the Equitable Allocation of COVID-19 Vaccine at the National Academies of Science, Engineering, and Medicine, as well as a former member of the Advisory Committee to the CDC Director and its subcommittee on health disparities. Dr. Mullen received her bachelor's and master of public health degrees from Yale University where she also completed a postdoctoral fellowship in psychosocial epidemiology. She graduated from the Mount Sinai School of Medicine, and completed her residency at the Hospital of the University of Pennsylvania. She also holds a master of public administration from Harvard University's John F. Kennedy School of Government and has completed intensive and advanced bioethics courses at the Kennedy Institute of Ethics.

**Neil R. Powe, M.D., M.P.H., M.B.A. (NAM),** serves as leader of the University of California San Francisco Medicine Service at the Priscilla Chan and Mark Zuckerberg San Francisco General Hospital, a leading medicine department in a public hospital with strong basic, clinical, and health services research programs focused on major diseases affecting diverse patients locally, nationally, and globally. His interests are in improving discovery, education, and clinical practice in medicine, making academic organizations function better, enhancing scholarship and multidisciplinary collaboration, and developing future talent and leadership in the health professions. He has a particular interest in cultivating young scientists who are addressing major problems in science, health, and health care delivery. His primary intellectual pursuits involve kidney disease patient-oriented research, epidemiology, disparities, and outcomes and effectiveness research. His research unites medicine and public health with the goals of saving and improving the quality of human lives. It involves the knowledge of fundamental discoveries in biology and clinical medicine to advance the health of patients and populations affected by kidney disease. He has conducted research on disparities in organ donation and interventions to improve access to kidney transplantation. Dr. Powe earned his medical degree at Harvard Medical School and his master's in public health at Harvard School of Public Health. He completed his residency and his master's in business administration, and was a Robert Wood Johnson Clinical Scholar at the University of Pennsylvania.

**Dorry Segev, M.D., Ph.D. (NAM),** as of February 1, 2022, is Professor of Surgery and Population Health and Vice Chair for Research in the Department of Surgery, New York University. Previously, Dr. Segev was the Marjory K. and Thomas Pozefsky Professor of Surgery and Epidemiology and Associate Vice-Chair of Surgery at Johns Hopkins University. He is the founder and director of the Epidemiology Research Group in Organ Transplantation, the largest and most prolific group of its kind in the world. Dr. Segev was the first to demonstrate the survival benefit of incompatible kidney transplantation across the United States, and is responsible for the first HIV-to-HIV transplants in the United States. His National Institutes of Health–funded research includes kidney exchange, desensitization, long-term donor risk, access to transplantation, expanding transplantation including HIV+ donors, geographic disparities, posttransplant outcomes, and the intersection between transplantation and gerontology. With a graduate degree in biostatistics, Dr. Segev focuses on novel statistical and mathematical methods for the simulation of medical data, analysis of large health care datasets, and outcomes research. Dr. Segev is a senior staff member for the Scientific Registry of Transplant Recipients, as well as an advisor to a number of pharmaceutical companies regarding ways to improve solid organ transplantation through machine learning, big data, risk prediction and clinical decision-making tools.

**Dennis Wagner, M.P.A.,** has served as the Principal and Managing Director for Yes and Leadership, LLC since October of 2020. In this capacity he has served as a speaker and session leader at in-person and online events for a wide array of organizations such as the Iowa Healthcare Collaborative, the Gift of Life Institute for Organ Donation and Transplantation, the Association of Organ Procurement Organizations, the National Association of State

Pharmacy Associations, the University of Southern California School of Pharmacy, and others. Dennis and his colleagues also organize and conduct engaging, highly interactive and content-rich board meetings, state and national conferences, and other events aimed principally at supporting leadership development, quality improvement, action learning and results for participating organizations. Dennis currently serves in an uncompensated capacity on the expert advisory panel of the recently formed Kidney Transplant Collaborative and provides expertise in grant applications for new funding opportunities. Dennis is the former director of the iQuality Improvement and Innovation Group in the Centers for Medicare & Medicaid Services (CMS) Center for Clinical Standards and Quality. Dennis and his team support health care providers who are using systematic quality improvement to make care better in tens of thousands of hospitals, nursing homes, clinical practices, and communities across the nation. This team of public and private quality improvers actively work to spread the best practices of the highest performers, so that "best practices become common practice." Prior to his most recent role at CMS, Dennis served as the Associate Director for Campaign Leadership in the Centers for Medicare & Medicaid Innovation, as Deputy Director, and then Acting Director of the CMS Office of Clinical Standards and Quality. Dennis was successful in supporting cross-departmental work to develop and announce a major national Departmental & Presidential Kidney Health Initiative, which included CMS Innovation Center initiatives to support increased kidney procurement and utilization. While at the Health Resources and Services Administration's (HRSA's) Division of Transplantation, Dennis led a series of major national initiatives, including the Organ Donation Breakthrough Collaborative from 2003 to 2007 to increase the donation and transplantation of organs. This work generated unprecedented and lasting national increases in organ donation over this 4-year period. In addition to numerous honors and awards from CMS, the Department of Health and Human Services, HRSA, and the Environmental Protection Agency, Dennis is a recipient of the Samuel J. Heyman Service to America Medal (known as the "Sammies") 2016 Federal Employee of the Year Award. Dennis received his B.A. and M.P.A. degrees from Montana State University.

**James B. Young, M.D.,** is Cleveland Clinic's Executive Director of Academic Affairs and Academic Vice-Dean, Cleveland Clinic Lerner College of Medicine of Case Western Reserve University. He also holds the George and Linda Kaufman Chair in the Heart and Vascular Institute. He was the Medical Director of the Kaufman Center for Heart Failure, which he and a former surgical colleague established in 1998 at Cleveland Clinic. After joining Cleveland Clinic in 1995, Dr. Young was named Head of Heart Failure and Cardiac Transplant Medicine. He is an internationally recognized heart failure and heart transplant cardiologist with an interest in mechanical circulatory support devices. Dr. Young has participated in more than 150 clinical trials as an investigator and has served as the United States' principal or co-principal investigator for many multicenter clinical trials. He has published more than 700 manuscripts and several textbooks. A member of many professional associations, Dr. Young has served as a board member and past president of the International Society of Heart and Lung Transplantation, and as a board member of the Heart Failure Society of America and the American Society of Transplantation. Dr. Young earned a B.A. with honors in biology from the University of Kansas, where he was a resident of Stephenson Scholarship Hall. He matriculated to Baylor College of Medicine in Houston, where he was awarded his medical degree, cum laude, and was elected to the Alpha Omega Alpha medical honor society. He completed his clinical training at Baylor Affiliated Hospitals. Dr. Young is a Fellow of the American College of Cardiology, American College of Physicians, American Heart Association, and the European Society of Cardiology. He is a Diplomat of the American Board of Internal Medicine and the sub-specialty Boards of Cardiovascular Disease and Advanced Heart Failure and Cardiac Transplantation.

## NATIONAL ACADEMIES STAFF

**Rebecca English, M.P.H.** (Study Director), is a Senior Program Officer in the Board on Health Science Policy. She has directed, co-directed, and staffed a number of projects at the National Academies including, most recently, Assessment of Strategies for Managing Cancer Risks Associated with Radiation Exposure During Crewed Space Missions (2021); Necessity, Use, and Care of Laboratory Dogs at the U.S. Department of Veterans Affairs (2020); Temporomandibular Disorders: From Research Discoveries to Clinical Treatment (2020); Physician-Assisted Death: Scanning the Landscape (Proceedings of a Workshop; 2018); and Mitochondrial Replacement Techniques: Ethical, Social, and Policy Considerations (2016). She has also staffed the Forum on Drug Discovery, Development, and Translation in various capacities since 2009 and has worked on wide-ranging projects related to the United States clinical trials enterprise as well as multidrug-resistant tuberculosis throughout the world. Prior to joining the National Academies, she worked on health policy for Congressman Porter J. Goss (FL-14) and for the National Active and Retired Federal Employees Association. Rebecca holds an M.P.H. from the University of Michigan, Ann Arbor, and a B.A. from the University of Notre Dame, majoring in political science.

**Amanda Wagner Gee, M.S.** (*until November 2021*), is a Program Officer in the Board on Health Sciences Policy, with the Forum on Drug Discovery, Development, and Translation. With the Forum, she leads and oversees workshops, including a series on Real-World Evidence in drug development and collaboration on genetics in discovery and development with the Roundtable on Genomics and Precision Health. She also manages Action Collaboratives within the Forum, including a project to map the network of drug development. She worked at the National Institutes of Health before coming to the National Academies. There, she was a research biologist at National Center for Advancing Translational Sciences (NCATS), adapting experiments for automation to identify potential small molecule treatments for a variety of degenerative diseases, such as Huntington's disease and retinal myopathy. Prior to NCATS, she was at the Harvard Stem Cell Institute researching treatments for neuro and muscular degeneration and collaborating regularly with industry, venture capital funders, and patient advocacy groups for her projects. At Harvard, she also oversaw purchasing and regulatory compliance as the laboratory manager. Amanda earned her M.S. degree in cell biology from Duke University and her B.S. degree, summa cum laude, in biology and chemistry from Florida Southern College.

**Siobhan Addie, Ph.D.** (*until August 2021*), is a Program Officer on the Board on Health Sciences Policy. Dr. Addie serves as a staff member on the Roundtable on Genomics and Precision Health and the Forum on Regenerative Medicine, two standing, convening activities at the National Academies. In her role at the Academies, she has developed public workshops and resulting publications on a wide range of topics including bioethics, drug discovery and development, implementation science, health disparities, and health care policy and economics. In addition, she oversaw the Genomics and Population Health action collaborative from 2016 to 2019, an ad hoc activity of the Genomics Roundtable. Prior to joining the staff of the National Academies, Dr. Addie was a Senior Program Manager in Life Sciences at the New York Academy of Sciences (NYAS). Before joining the staff at the NYAS, she was a postdoctoral researcher at Rockefeller University, where she used genetic and biochemical approaches to learn about a rare genetic disorder, Fanconi anemia. Dr. Addie received her Ph.D. from the University of Pittsburgh, where her research explored the role of DNA repair enzyme ERCC1-XPF and how its absence can lead to cancer and aging. She earned her B.S. in cell and molecular biology from the State University of New York at Binghamton in 2006.

**Meredith Hackmann, B.A.,** is an Associate Program Officer on the Board on Health Sciences Policy at the National Academies of Sciences, Engineering, and Medicine. She joined the National Academies in 2014 and has facilitated public workshops, action collaboratives, and working groups with the Roundtable on Genomics and Precision Health and the Forum on Regenerative Medicine. She has also provided background research and writing support for proceedings and consensus studies within the Board on Health Sciences Policy on topics such as bioethics, implementing genomic screening programs, digital health, and consumer genomics. Prior to joining the Academies, she was an intern with the U.S. House of Representatives. She has volunteered with several nonprofit organizations on projects related to community health improvement in Central America, refugee and immigration issues, and hospice care. Meredith earned a bachelor's degree in international studies from the University of Missouri.

**Liz Townsend, M.P.H.** (*until October 2021*), is an Associate Program Officer with the Board on Health Sciences Policy. Liz has worked in studies and workshops on topics in public health, social and behavioral sciences research, adolescent development, and economic policy. Recent projects include The Clinical Utility of Compounded Bioidentical Hormone Therapy (2020); A Roadmap to Reducing Child Poverty (2019); The Promise of Adolescence (2019); and A Decadal Survey of the Social and Behavioral Sciences: A Research Agenda for Advancing Intelligence Analysis (2019). Prior to joining the National Academies, Liz managed a youth suicide prevention program for the State of Maine. She holds a B.S. from Radford University and an M.P.H. from the University of Alabama at Birmingham.

**Emma Fine, B.A.,** is an Associate Program Officer primarily working on the Board on Health Sciences Policy (HSP), and has worked at the National Academies for 4.5 years. Within HSP, she currently supports research on the COVID-19 pandemic, including work on Rapid Expert Consultations that directly inform the White House Office of Science and Technology Policy. Emma also works with DBASSE's Board on Behavioral, Cognitive, and Sensory Sciences on a project that is designing a tool for intelligence analysts to better understand social polling, attitude measurement, and group behavior in non-Western countries, sponsored by the Office of the Director of National Intelligence. Previously, she staffed a project on the Board on Global Health assessing morbidity and mortality from HIV/AIDS in Rwanda. Prior to joining the National Academies, Ms. Fine interned for the U.S. Department of Health and Human Services in the Office of the Assistant Secretary for Preparedness and Response, where she contributed research to the National Health Security Strategy Implementation Plan as well as studying the intersection between terrorism and public health preparedness. In 2016, Ms. Fine graduated from the University of California, Berkeley, where she earned her B.A. in public health and public policy. She is particularly interested in the nexus between public health, intelligence, and national security, and she plans to pursue a degree in national security and enter the field of intelligence.

**Deanna Marie Giraldi, M.P.H.** (*from October 2021*), is an Associate Program Officer on the Board on Health Sciences Policy, with the Forum on Drug Discovery, Development, and Translation. Deanna joined the National Academies in 2021. Prior to joining the Academies, Deanna conducted health care research in Cuba, Scotland, Ireland, England, and Costa Rica, specifically on the intersections of trauma-informed care of refugees and mental health access. She has also worked extensively on gun safety policy, including the crafting of recommendations for prevention and response interventions at the intersections of intimate partner violence and gun violence in the United States. Deanna holds two bachelor's degrees in biology and political science from Vassar College and is an alumna of the Yale School of Public Health where she completed her master of public health in health policy with a concentration in global health.

**Ruth Cooper, B.A.** *(from June 2021)*, is an Associate Program Officer with the Board on Health Care Services at the National Academies of Sciences, Engineering, and Medicine. She has worked on several National Academies projects including studies on space radiation and cancer risk, building data capacity for conducting patient-centered outcomes research, cancer and disability, and evidence-based opioid prescribing, as well as workshops on organ transplant and disability, companion animals as sentinels for environmental exposures, and diagnostic excellence in acute cardiac events, cancers, and COVID-19. She had also assisted with numerous National Cancer Policy Forum workshops ranging from topics like the cancer workforce to health literacy. Prior to joining the National Academies, Ruth spent a year volunteering at Open Arms Home for Children in South Africa. She also has experience in Arctic science policy and has worked at the U.S. Arctic Research Commission and participated in three Arctic field cruises. Ruth holds a B.A. from the University of Notre Dame in neuroscience and behavior with a minor in Mediterranean Middle Eastern studies, and is currently pursuing her M.A. in international science and technology policy at George Washington University.

**Kendall Logan, B.A.** *(until July 2021)*, is a Senior Program Assistant for the Health and Medicine Division's Board on Health Sciences Policy. She joined the National Academies in 2018, and staffed two consensus studies: the Health and Medical cons of Social Isolation and Loneliness in Older Adults, and Temporomandibular Disorders (TMD): From Research Discoveries to Clinical Treatment. She also supports the standing committee on Medical and Epidemiological Aspects of Air Pollution on U.S. Government Employees and their Families. Kendall received her B.A. in anthropology with a public health minor from Haverford College and is currently pursuing a master of public health degree from Columbia University.

**Andrew Pope, Ph.D.,** is Director of the Board on Health Sciences Policy. He has a Ph.D. in physiology and biochemistry from the University of Maryland; he has been a member of the National Academies of Sciences, Engineering, and Medicine staff since 1982, and of the Health and Medicine Division staff since 1989. His primary interests are science policy, biomedical ethics, and environmental and occupational influences on human health. During his tenure at the Academies, Dr. Pope has directed numerous studies on topics that range from injury control, disability prevention, and biologic markers, to the protection of human subjects of research, National Institutes of Health priority-setting processes, organ procurement and transplantation policy, and the role of science and technology in countering terrorism. Since 1998, Dr. Pope has served as Director of the Board on Health Sciences Policy which oversees and guides a program of activities that is intended to encourage and sustain the continuous vigor of the basic biomedical and clinical research enterprises needed to ensure and improve the health and resilience of the public. Ongoing activities include Forums on Neuroscience, Genomics, Drug Discovery and Development, and Medical and Public Health Preparedness for Catastrophic Events. Dr. Pope is the recipient of the Health and Medicine Division's Cecil Award and the National Academy of Sciences President's Special Achievement Award.

**Sharyl Nass, Ph.D.,** serves as Director of the Board on Health Care Services and Director of the National Cancer Policy Forum at the National Academies of Sciences, Engineering, and Medicine. The National Academies provide independent, objective analysis and advice to the nation to solve complex problems and inform public policy decisions related to science, technology, and medicine. To enable the best possible care for all patients, the Board undertakes scholarly analysis of the organization, financing, effectiveness, workforce, and delivery of health care, with emphasis on quality, cost, and accessibility. The Cancer Forum examines policy issues pertaining to the entire continuum of cancer research and care. For more than 2 decades, Dr. Nass has worked on a broad range of health and science policy topics that includes the quality and safety of health care and clinical trials, developing technologies for precision medicine, and strategies for large-scale biomedical science. She has a Ph.D. in cell biology from Georgetown University and undertook postdoctoral training at the Johns Hopkins University School of Medicine, as well as a research fellowship at the Max Planck Institute in Germany. She also holds a B.S. and an M.S. from the University of Wisconsin-Madison. She has been the recipient of the Cecil Medal for Excellence in Health Policy Research, a Distinguished Service Award from the National Academies, and the Institute of Medicine staff team achievement award as team leader.